Amer-Ind Gestural Code
Based on Universal
American Indian Hand Talk

Amer-Ind Gestural Code Based on Universal American Indian Hand Talk

MADGE SKELLY, Ph.D.

St. Louis University

Assisted by Lorraine Schinsky, M.A.
Illustrated by John Dunivent, B.F.A., M.A.

ELSEVIER · NEW YORK
New York · Oxford

Elsevier North Holland, Inc.
52 Vanderbilt Avenue, New York, New York 10017

Distributors outside the United States and Canada:

Thomond Books
(A Division of Elsevier/North-Holland Scientific Publishers, Ltd.)
P.O. Box 85
Limerick, Ireland

Library of Congress Cataloging in Publication Data

Main entry under title:

Skelly, Madge.
  Amer-Ind gestural code based on universal American Indian hand talk.

  Bibliography: p.
  Includes index.
  1. Communicative disorders—Rehabilitation. 2. Sign language.
  3. Indians of North America—Sign language. I. Schinsky, Lorraine, joint
  author. II. Title. [DNLM: 1. Sign language. 2. Speech disorders—
  Rehabilitation. 3. Indians, North American. WM475.3 S627a]
RC423.S537   001.56   79-19202
ISBN 0-444-00333-9
ISBN 0-444-00331-2 pbk.

Desk Editor   Michael Coffey
Design   Edmée Froment
Art Assistant   Virginia Kudlak
Production Manager   Joanne Jay
Compositor   Waldman Graphics
Printer   Halliday Lithograph

Manufactured in the United States of America

to the memory of
John Storer
who with unfailing courage and cheerfulness
made his own deficit serve others

Contents

Acknowledgments

It is with sincere gratitude that the authors acknowledge the encouragement and assistance of a very large number of persons without whom this work would never have been started, continued, or accomplished. If any of these have been inadvertently omitted from our listing, this is regretted and apology is herewith offered.

The Veterans Administration Hospital system has been a gracious sponsor of our initial projects and has provided continuing encouragement in every way. This support was extended by Dr. Bernard Anderman and Dr. Henry Spuehler of the Audiology and Speech Pathology Service in Central Office, Washington, D.C., and was continued at St. Louis by successive hospital directors, David Anton and Joseph Mackney, and by Chiefs of Staff, Dr. Ralph Biddy, Dr. Robert Donati, and Dr. Francis Zacharewicz. Further support for the project was provided by Dr. Francis Carey, Chief of Research, and by the Chiefs of associated clinical services: Dr. William Newton and Dr. Robert Donaldson of Surgery; Dr. Kun Ken Hu of Rehabilitation Medicine; and Dr. Reuben Hackmeyer and Dr. Bernard Goldstein of Out-Patient Service.

At St. Louis University, opportunities for workshops, meetings, and discussions were provided by Dr. George Newberry, Chairman of the Department of Communication Disorders, Dr. Mary Dasovich of the same department's Developmental Disabilities program, and by Dr. Max Pepper, Chairman of the Department of Community Medicine at the School of Medicine.

The senior author was provided opportunity to conduct workshops and present papers at a number of places where subsequent discussions were most valuable to the growth of the project. These included the Karolinska Institute of Rehabilitation in Stockholm, Sweden; the Queen Elizabeth Medical Center in Birmingham, England; the meeting of the International Association of Logopedics and Phoniatrics in Buenos Aires, Argentina; the International Congress of Rehabilitation in Sydney, Australia; the University of Queensland in Brisbane, Australia; and the Ninewells Hospital School of Medicine, University of Dundee, Scotland. Also of value were several papers and exhibits presented at the various annual meetings of the American Speech and Hearing Association, and at those meetings of the state associations of Missouri, Illinois, Kansas, and Wisconsin. A number of invitations for professional presentations were extended from universities, including California State University, the University of Arizona, Southern Illinois University, Vanderbilt University, Southern Methodist University, the University of Wisconsin, and St. Louis University.

Useful also were professional workshops sponsored by the Regional Medical Education Centers of Birmingham, Alabama, and St. Louis, Missouri, and by the Washington (D.C.) Medical Center. Helpful professional seminars were also sponsored by the Harmarville Rehabilitation Center, in Pittsburgh, and by the Veterans Aministration Hospitals in Dallas, Nashville, North Chicago, Little Rock, Long Beach, Hines, and St. Louis. The VA Hospital in St. Louis has conducted professional workshops over three successive years and has also sponsored three annual conferences on the clinical application of Amer-Ind with invited professional speakers and participants from hospitals, clinics, and universities using the system.

The authors extend thanks to Dr. Macalyne Fristoe and Dr. Lyle Lloyd of Purdue University, and to Randall W. Smith of the University of Illinois for their suggestions, which have been most helpful. Kathy Murphy Geronimo of the faculty of Northeastern University deserves special recognition for her participation in the early development of the clinical use of Amer-Ind and for several creative suggestions concerning its use.

We are especially grateful to all those professional speech pathologists who spent much time and effort on reports for our use and who graciously shared their successes and failures with us for the benefit and improvement of Amer-Ind. These include Gunilla Henningsson of Huddinge University Hospital in Sweden; Margaret Hawkins of the Queen Elizabeth Medical Center in England; Dr. Franklin Silverman of Marquette University; Janice L. Duncan of the Special Education Center of Kenosha, Wisconsin; Robert Dodaro of Lake Forest Hospital in Chicago; Nancy Symington Snead of the Kansas Neurological Institute of Topeka; Jan Robinson of Mount Saint Rose Rehabilitation Center, St. Louis; Linda Bleitz, Julie Burns, and Sharon Cleveland of the Visiting Nurses Association; Jane Podleski, Roxanne Cassim, Leonard Sisul, and Regina Brennan, speech pathologists at the Saint Louis State School/Hospital.

Data were received from the following at the indicated VA Medical Centers: Dr. Gwyneth Vaughn at Birmingham; Dr. Shirley Salmon at Kansas City; Dr. Marilyn Corlew at Wood, Wisconsin; Dr. George Horsfall at Tampa; Meredith DeVault at Nashville; Rosemary Sullivan Smiley at Murfreesboro; Mary Weiler, Don Richardson, and John Sunbeck of North Shore Chicago; Sheila Fitzgerald McMahon of Hines; Yolanda Evans of Memphis; Jill Boehler of Albany; Norma Lou Robinson of Asheville; Dr. Zilpha Bosone of Topeka; Paul Rao, A. G. Basili, J. Kotner, and J. Keller at Fort Howard; Muriel Goldojarb at Sepulveda; Rita Fust and Dennis Fuller at St. Louis; Dr. D. J. Hubbard from Kansas City, now Chief of the Audiology and Speech Pathology Service at St. Louis.

The completeness of our out-of-print resources was due to the patient and persistent efforts of St. Louis VA Hospital Medical Library staff—Anne Thorton, Kate Deberry, and especially Helen Henderson—as well as the staff of the Missouri Historical Society and the Smithsonian Institution. We owe them a debt that cannot be paid.

The Amer-Ind videotapes produced by the St. Louis VA Learning Resources Service contributed significantly to the development of the Amer-Ind system. Mark Grey and Ray Iggulden of the television staff were of inestimable service in the preparation of the cassettes, and in their contribution to both the improvement of signal transmission and the conducting of the seminars for professionals. We also want to thank Dr. Ralph Overman who managed the first of the Regional Medical Education workshops, which prepared the way for the early transmission studies.

The *Archives of Physical Medicine and Rehabilitation* granted permission for use of data from its April 1975 issue; *The American Journal of Nursing* permitted reprinting of its article on aphasia of July 1975; and the *Journal of Speech and Hearing Disorders* approved inclusion of the data published in its issue of November 1974. These courtesies are much appreciated.

The cooperation of Fontbonne College and its duplicating department is gratefully recognized for their assistance in the final production of the manuscript. This was arranged through the kindness of Sr. Marie Damien Adams, Dean of the College. Our thanks are due also to Sr. Dorothea Buchanan for her many services to both the authors and the project.

Mary Loafman and Deanna Schinsky shared the lengthy and onerous task of typing the manuscript. They both contributed the careful eye and professional know-how that prevented many errors. We are grateful for the generous allotment of their off-duty hours in order to meet deadlines.

The list of credits would be very incomplete without recognition of the contribution of Mr. Don Garner, Director of the Fontbonne Theatre, who served as advisor and director of the video cassette series on Amer-Ind. His extensive knowledge of television, theater, and script writing added greatly to the total impact of the cassettes on both workshops for professionals and training programs for families of patients. His kindness and patience in the filming were much appreciated.

The senior author wishes to acknowledge with gratitude the tireless work of co-author Lorraine Schinsky on the many details of the final preparation of this manuscript, as well as for her perceptive contributions to the development of the system. John Duvinent's potent illustrations speak for themselves in many ways and add greatly to the usefulness of this text. His artist's eye enabled him to focus our attention on some specifics in signal precision, thereby contributing immeasurably to transmission success.

All the patients who have participated in clinical use of Amer-Ind have made contributions to this work. Without them, the endeavor would have been meaningless.

The American Indians, who in the centuries of their wanderings first invented and then enhanced the system of hand talk, should really be included as co-authors. They created the system and made it available to their present-day descendants; they are the precursors of its clinical use. We cherish their memory and are proud to be the instrument that brings their ancient art to the attention and service of communication professionals and their speechless patients.

**Amer-Ind Gestural Code
Based on Universal
American Indian Hand Talk**

Introduction:
An Alternative Mode

RECOGNIZING THE NEED

The improvement of human communication is certainly a more realistic clinical goal than the achievement of perfection. Historically, however, the opportunity and the means for improvement have been limited, both politically and educationally, to those who already possess average or superior communication skills. Today, fortunately, the needs of the impaired are becoming more frequently recognized. Much-improved and more available means of rehabilitation are being provided to the communicatively handicapped as society grows increasingly aware of the many problems and inequities within itself, and of its own duty to effect solutions. Programs and services are being developed for the deaf, the hard of hearing, the visually impaired, and for the neurologically damaged who cannot read or write. However, while these services, programs, and funding are expanding for the deaf and visually impaired, comparatively little is being done for the speechless.

It is true that modern technology has recently added numerous instruments to assist the communicatively handicapped whose problems are based largely on impairment of motor skills. But almost all of the effective and productive techniques developed for rehabilitation of communication of patients suffering symbolic deficits have had successful application only to the mildly or moderately impaired. There is little or nothing operative for the severely impaired, as is most notable in cases of aphasia and mental retardation.

Furthermore, the need for new techniques in alleviating the communication problems of the brain-damaged increases constantly, for the number of patients is growing. For example, not only is there an increasing proportion of geriatric patients prone to stroke but also, due to the stress factors characteristic of our modern life, the age level of stroke victims has lowered. The soaring incidence of highway accidents resulting in head trauma is also bringing more and younger victims of aphasia to the speech clinic. The escalating damage to the nervous system from the many undesirable components of our environment, including air and noise pollution, combine to rob many Americans of their priceless and uniquely human behavior: speech. Genetic, natal, and developmental problems add their quota to the total speechless population, too, especially in the severely impaired category.

Fortunately, as professional interest in nonverbal communication accelerates, emphasis is being placed on giving the speechless patient *any means available* to assist him in communication. It is currently understood that communication is not limited to speech, or even to language; it can include many nonverbal approaches. Any mode or method that permits a human being to achieve intellectual contact with other humans, for the transmission or exchange of ideas, should be an acceptable mode of communication. Given the many modes available with which to accomplish this objective, wider choice is provided to meet the specific needs of the individual human being's type and degree of impairment.

Any mode that alleviates (even slightly) one patient's lack of communication—has value. There should be no denigration or derogation of its origin or manner, and it should always be remembered that what is useful for one in communication, is potentially useful for many. Some profitable approaches may have already been abandoned because of inconsistent results, when the failure was really due, not to flaws in the technique, but to unwise selection of candidates or to lack of skill in the clinical application. Furthermore, there is no need to view differing techniques as necessarily in competition with each other. Any method is productive only when a skilled clinician applies it to appropriate populations.

The severely rated aphasic and the severely impaired mentally retarded still remain as the greatest challenges to communication rehabilitation. Customary approaches, on the whole, have yielded little progress, while gestural methods have met with success in an increasing number of cases and syndromes.

To choose an appropriate gestural system for the brain-damaged, however, it is necessary to define our terms and determine our basic criteria.

TERMINOLOGY

APHASIA, APRAXIA, AND DYSARTHRIA

Historically, the modality-bound impairment of the motor expression of language has been included under or known by many names, including motor aphasia, Broca's aphasia, expressive aphasia, subcortical motor aphasia, aphemia, Marie's anarthria, verbal aphasia, cortical dysarthria, and apraxic dysarthria. Brown (1968) describes the central language process as consisting of four components: a vocabulary of symbols, a grammar of linguistic rules for assembling the symbols, a memory storage system adequate for processing them, and an ability to use the linguistic rules for decoding and encoding them. **Aphasia** is defined as an impairment of any combination of these components. It follows, then, that when the central processes are intact and the impairment is restricted to motoric execution, apraxia is indicated, not aphasia.

Brain (1964) defines **apraxia** as the "inability to carry out purposive movement, the nature of which the patient understands, in the absence of severe motor paralysis, sensory loss and ataxia" (p. 104). Goodglass and Kaplan (1972) write: "apraxia refers to the loss of the capacity to carry out purposeful movement, when motor strength and coordination are adequate" (pp. 51–52). Wechsler (1958) expands these definitions of apraxia as the "inability to carry out purposive movements in the absence of paralysis or other motor impairment, sensory impairment or mental defect" (p. 323).

Profitable discussion of diagnosis and treatment also requires differentiation of **dysarthria** from apraxia. Perkins (1971) provides a concise summary: "Speech effects of disability of the output transmission system take two major forms: apraxia, difficulty in motor formulation of articulated languages, and dysarthria, incoordination in execution of the speech act" (p. 134). He expands the description of dysarthria by stating that it is "characterized by weakness and incoordination of the speech apparatus itself" (p. 135). Wechsler (1958) writes, "Apraxia is used to designate that loss or impairment of skilled movement in which only the conceptual motion formula is lost, while the motor apparatus for performing the act is intact" (p. 13). He adds that when the peripheral speech musculature or its innervation are impaired, the defect is known as dysarthria. Nielson (1962) describes the apraxic patient as "unable to connect his ideation and motion, although both are intact" (p. 29). DeReuck and O'Connor (1964) classify dysarthria as a "a motor disorder independent of language" (p. 329).

When apraxia affects the voluntary initiation and sequencing of the movements necessary to phonation and articulation, it is frequently labeled **apraxia of speech**. It is also referred to, in the literature of several disciplines, as **verbal apraxia**. Some authors include graphic language output under *verbal*. In some presented papers and publications, the term *speech* is apparently considered synonymous with expressive language. It is important to include the concept of "purposive" in the definition of apraxia. Differential diagnosis centers on this voluntary control. The apraxic patient exhibits many motor sequences at the involuntary level that he is unable to replicate voluntarily. Adequate jaw and tongue action for chewing is an example. Since he cannot repeat this sequence on demand or for speech production, his behavior may be characterized as inconsistent. The dysarthric patient, however, *is* consistent, having the identical movement problems in eating that he experiences in speaking. In this text, the term **oral apraxia** refers to problems in any voluntary sequencing of movement of the oral structures. The term **oral–verbal apraxia** is used to indicate such problems with production of spoken language. Although aphasia, apraxia, and dysarthria, are thus distinguished as discrete syndromes, the diagnostic problem may be compounded; a patient may exhibit symptoms of more than one or even of all three.

AMERICAN INDIAN HAND TALK AND AMER-IND CODE

American Indian Hand Talk (or **American Indian Code**) in this text refers to the original manual system used by the American Indians. **Amer-Ind Code** (or simply **Amer-Ind**) is based on American Indian Hand Talk but has been adapted slightly for modern clinical use.

CRITERIA FOR A USEFUL GESTURAL SYSTEM

Six areas appear critical in judging any gestural system for the speechless:

1. Since so many brain-injured patients are candidates for gestural communication, the first criterion should be a **low level of symbolism**, plus a concomitant **concrete reference base** for the gestures.
2. **Ease of acquisition** of the system by the speechless patient is desirable since it both facilitates a speedier implementation of the system and tends to alleviate the patient's anxiety about learning performance.
3. A third criterion is **ease of interpretation** by viewers attempting to communicate with the speechless patient. (If interpretation is achieved at a widespread level with the general public rather than confined to the patient's personal milieu, the integration of the communicatively handicapped person into society can be greatly facilitated.)
4. As a fourth criterion, it is desirable to have a system that provides the greatest possible **flexibility in the encoding of concepts**, rather than of words, of a lanaguage. The code will be most useful to the greatest number of speechless patients if it is independent of the restraints inherent in syntactic structure and grammatical rules. Brain-damaged patients in particular usually have great difficulty when they are limited to specific forms for the expression of meaning.
5. The fifth criterion requires a system with a high degree of **adaptability to existing gestures**, human gestures that can be easily recognized and shaped into a single uncomplicated code, preferably already field-tested for its usefulness under even the most challenging situations and conditions.
6. A sixth criterion should be added especially for those speechless patients who retain or acquire language and are able to write: its **potential speed of execution** must exceed that of written communication in the conversational setting.

These criteria describe a necessarily simple, even primitive code, which can provide for both the immediate requirements of the moderately impaired during the early post-trauma period preceding a recovery of speech and/or language, and for the more demanding life-long needs of those very severely impaired persons who may be unable to master any other mode of human communication.

MANUAL SIGN SYSTEMS CREATED FOR THE DEAF

Various manual sign systems for the deaf have been developed throughout the world with considerable degrees of success. They were designed primarily to accommodate to or substitute for a specific sensory reception loss. They have provided an adequate mode for many users and have assisted a fairly large proportion of the users in learning the printed and written language of their environment.

These various manual sign systems satisfy the fifth and sixth criteria listed above for a useful gestural format to serve the speechless. All gestural systems are usually speedier than writing and therefore satisfy the sixth criterion. Also, these systems are usually well-structured internally for effective transmission of meaning and thus satisfy the fifth criterion. Some appear to differ with the others in structure and rules, with the divergences aimed at specific educational objectives. However, there is some question of satisfaction of the fourth criterion: flexibility. In each of these manual systems there is structure as well as rules which must be formally learned both by the impaired person and by those wishing or needing to communicate with him. These rules are somewhat comparable to the grammatical restraints of any linguistic system. Persons with intact cognition who also have language comprehension experience little difficulty with this condition, but it presents extensive problems for the brain-damaged person operating on a low concept level or on a restricted retrieval base. The majority of speechless patients are in these latter two categories.

When measured by the first three criteria, these systems appear less useful. All the manual systems for the deaf employ signs that are predominantly (90 percent) highly symbolic, either arbitrary or conventional in design. These arbitrary signs comprise 70 percent of the total; 20 percent are conventional. Whether arbitrary or conventional, these signs represent a high level of symbolism, comparable to that of the language, spoken and written, of the country in which the particular system is used.

Because specific meaning is not obvious in either the arbitrary or conventional signs, these gestures are seldom spontaneous; they must be learned. This presents as difficult an undertaking as the acquisition of any new, strange language. For brain-damaged patients, the high symbolic level alone renders this task almost impossible. In some cases, such patients master only the concretely based signs, which constitute approximately 10 percent of the total system.

Even with excellent public relations efforts, extensive public education programs, and in some cases, the intervention of the law, the deaf still need to use interpreters of sign for much of their communication beyond their immediate circle of family, friends, or other deaf signers. The numerous and varied efforts to induce the general public to learn these systems have not been very productive to date, since only those with personal need or desire to communicate with the deaf signer have been willing to make the effort to acquire expertise in the very complex sign language of the deaf. Even for these interested persons, the meaning of signs can be deduced only for the concretely based 10 percent. The other 90 percent of the signs must be learned, just as the words of any foreign language are acquired, with considerable effort rather than ease. For the brain-damaged patient, interpretation presents the identical difficulties inherent in acquisition.

For those wishing to explore further the various sign languages developed for use of the deaf, several useful works are cited in the reference list.

The results measuring the available manual languages used by the deaf against these criteria led to consideration of a very old hand signal system developed by the American Indians.

AMERICAN INDIAN HAND TALK

DEVELOPMENT

In *Man's Rise to Civilization as Shown by the Indians of North America*, Peter Farb (1968) says that at the time of the discovery of the new world, there were in all the Americas about 2200 different spoken languages. In North America alone there existed more than 550 distinct languages, as dissimilar from each other as Swahili from English. These languages were no more primitive nor limited in vocabulary than any of the European languages.

To accommodate to the wide variance of spoken languages and the absence of any common tongue, a variety of Indian tribes used a gesture system they called "Hand Talk" which developed at the time of the great migration from Asia. During the nomadic phase of migration and vast geographical dispersion people of varying origins and with widely different spoken languages encountered each other in a manner that did not foster bilingualism. The basic hand signal code that developed was based on easily understood pantomime, with meaning demonstrable in action rather than in words. The untutored viewer must comprehend easily since there was no common language in which to explain.

Those gestures that were successfully transmitted perpetuated themselves by their very utility. They were exchanged and adopted. Any mild variants must have remained close to the original concrete referents. Unsuccessfully transmitted gestures were dropped. A concrete base, rather than a language or word base, controlled this development. Action became the prime component because it was so easily demonstrated. Names evolved, when necessary, in relation to action, paralleling most of the American Indian spoken languages. The gesture system was shaped (a) by its origin in the need for a basic communicative method, and (b) by its primary purpose of transcending numerous and different spoken languages.

CHARACTERISTICS

Despite variations, the system became informally codified, which kept it coherent and serviceable, and was continually extended to meet the needs of cross-language communication. Any new idea could be expressed by the agglutination of priorly used gestures and strings of descriptive gestures.

According to the Bureau of American Ethnology of the Smithsonian Institution, the system became so highly developed that "for all practical purposes, [it] hardly fell short of a spoken language" (Hodge, 1960).

But no matter how developed it became, the American Indian Code never lost its intrinsic clarity. Even as imaginative new descriptive gestures were added, all gestures had to be so clear that the majority of viewers could easily guess their meaning. This need for clarity tended to preserve a simplicity of structure in the system and at the same time limit the levels of abstraction and symbolism. Also, the system's telegraphic style, using the fewest possible gestures to convey a meaning, engendered no need for rules or grammar.

The American Indian manual system was well developed and widely disseminated by the time Columbus arrived. Early sixteenth-century European historians, reporting on the voyages of Columbus as well as of Spanish, French, Italian, and English explorers, agree that the natives communicated well with their hand signals and that the foreign visitors had no difficulty understanding them. The basic differences between the languages of the European visitors and the languages of the American Indians appeared to have little adverse effect on mutual gesture exchange. Most European languages are nominally oriented, while American Indian languages are action oriented. In the latter, naming derives from the doing. This makes the American Indian kinetic transmission system easy both to interpret and to acquire.

CODE, NOT LANGUAGE

At its inception and during its long development and use, American Indian Hand Talk had as its sole purpose communication across language barriers. No matter how well it serves this purpose, however, the system should not be labeled a language, but rather regarded as a signal system or preferably a code. It may, for contemporary clarification, be compared to the recently adopted international highway directives. These, too, are a code that can be understood easily, regardless of the viewer's language.

A similar misunderstanding, possibly due to the use of the word 'sign' for the gestures involved, is the assumption that the ancient hand talk of the American Indians had the same basis and shares the same characteristics as the manual communication systems developed for the use of the deaf. This assumption is erroneous for, while the deaf signers and their viewers share a common national language, American Indian Hand Talk was founded on the absence of a shared linguistic background.

MODERN APPLICATION

The American Indian Code's low symbolic level, ease of acquisition, flexibility, speed, lack of grammatical structure and rules, and use of concrete, demonstrable referents, which enable the viewer to interpret without formal instruction, make it adaptable to the use of many patients who are unable to speak. It can also be of special value to those speechless patients who, through brain damage, are unable to use other gestural systems.

American Indian Hand Talk (especially in its modern form, Amer-Ind, which has been modified for the speechless) thus appears to satisfy all six criteria for a useful gestural system for speechless persons, and particularly for those with symbolic deficits.

REVIEW OF THE LITERATURE ON
AMERICAN INDIAN HAND TALK

The customary literature search presents unique problems here, since the American Indian tradition was largely oral. Even those documentations that may have been included in circular pictographs on skins, or in the formal designs of bead or shell records, or in the tales preserved in wood carvings are no longer available. These tenuous threads of Indian history were lost or destroyed in the many migrations. American Indian Hand Talk has, in a sense, undergone similar obliteration. Those who knew it well and used it routinely have today been reduced to a very small number of aged and widely scattered Indian persons. Only an isolated few are left to monitor a modern revival for accuracy. The only surviving written records from the nineteenth century based on direct contact with the system in actual use are by three white men: Colonel Garrick Mallery, Captain William Philo Clark, and Reverend Lewis F. Hadley. In the early twentieth century, the noted naturalist, Ernest Thompson Seton, added another volume.

MALLERY

Colonel Garrick Mallery was a man of scholarly approach. He attempted a thorough search for the factors common to all human gestural communication. In 1879 he presented to the Smithsonian Institution a progress report titled "Sign Language Among the North American Indians Compared with that Among Other Peoples and Deaf-Mutes." His point of view was linguistic and his purpose anthropological.

Mallery says his researches in sign were inspired by "the high development of communication by gesture among the tribes of North America and its continued extensive use by many of them." (p. 269)

A number of the observations made by Mallery are highly relevant to our purpose of communication rehabilitation today:

> The insane understand and obey gestures when they have no knowledge whatever of words. It is also found that semi-idiotic children who cannot be taught more than the merest rudiments of speech can receive a considerable amount of information through signs, and can express themselves by them. (p. 276) "Sufferers from aphasia continue to use appropriate gestures after their words have become uncontrollable. (p. 276)

Mallery also mentions the ease of interpretation of American Indian Hand Talk:

> Without having ever before seen or made one of their signs, he [the non-Indian] will soon not only catch the meaning of theirs, but produce his own, which they will likewise comprehend, the power remaining latent in him until called forth by necessity. (p. 280)

> Nearly all that is absolutely necessary for our physical needs can be expressed in pantomime. Far beyond the mere signs for eating, drinking, sleeping, and the like, anyone will understand . . . washing, dressing, shaving, walking, driving, writing, reading, churning, milking, boiling, or frying, shooting, fishing . . . and, in short, an endless list. (p. 281)

Modern communication rehabilitation can usefully apply Mallery's recognition of the significance of *action* in this context. He says:

> there is little distinction between pantomime and a developed sign language, in which thought is transmitted rapidly and certainly from hand to eye. Pantomime acts movements, reproduces forms and positions, presents pictures, and manifests emotions with greater realization than any other mode of utterance. (p. 281)

Despite his scholarly approach and his recognition of action as element primary to the expression of basic human needs, Colonel Mallery in his descriptions of Hand Talk does not credit its American Indian developers with the imagination and intelligence obvious in its invention as a *codified* pantomime system of great flexibility. He presents accurate observation of the hand positions and movements of hand talkers he observed, but fails to note the basic *concepts* which are so kinetically pictured by the hands. Only when a concept is envisioned are both the signaler and viewer able to communicate without an interpreter; only then is effective communication by the manual mode possible.

Colonel Mallery is handicapped by his linguistic point of view. **Code** is different from **language**. The latter has extension by synonym; the former by flexibility. For example, to the American Indian signaler, *man* can be expressed in an almost endless variety of ways: the animal walking upright, the two-leg walking animal, the strong one, the protector of the infant, the provider of meat and fish, the orator, etc. Similarly, *woman* is signaled as the provider of babies, the gardener, the herbalist, the milk-giving breast, the double-curved one, etc. Almost any single idea can be expressed in the code in a variety of ways. Concomitantly, almost every signal can, by agglutination or modification, express a variety of concepts quite distinctively. Apparently, Mallery not only failed to observe the conceptual rather than linguistic base of American Indian hand talk, he also did not realize its codification. He saw its flexibility as the liberty of the individual to invent personal signals. This viewpoint, unfortunately, has been adopted by a number of speech pathologists who are aware of and interested in the code as a useful communication tool. Whatever value the code may have can be destroyed by proliferation of *personal* dialects. The freedom that code offers in expressing a particular idea in a number of different ways may be compared to the modern use of a thesaurus for vocabulary variety rather than constant invention of new personal words. The acceptance by modern users of the system's codification is necessary if it is to continue to serve its ancient use for modern people.

CLARK

Captain W.P. Clark's book, *Indian Sign Language*, published in 1885, also describes American Indian Hand Talk as a pantomimic language. He states that he was "strongly impressed with its value and beauty." (p. 5)

> I observed that these Indians, having different vocal languages, had no difficulty communicating with each other, and held constant intercourse by means of gestures ... The gesture speech was easy to acquire and remember ...

> Although individuals may obscure these gestures through carelessness and awkwardness, or efforts to secure a super abundance of graceful execution, yet one skilled in the sign language will instantly recognize them, provided that they possess the radical or essential part. (p. 5)

Captain Clark points out developmental characteristics of the American Indian system that have considerable significance in its clinical adaptation to the rehabilitation of communication: "Even in my comparatively short experience with the Indian, I have observed the birth, growth and death of many gestures. Before the introduction of the coffee-mill, coffee was represented as a *grain*." (p. 15) The introduction of the coffee-mill killed off these gestures at once. He reports that the gesture of cranking the mill then becomes the significant signal. Today, of course, it is usually designated as MORNING DRINK HOT.

One of Clark's other examples illustrates a common misinterpretation of American Indian thought as evidenced in a particular signal: "I have heard Indians declare that they had always located the Great Spirit in the heavens, and yet in gesture they would indicate that this was the location of the white man's God and for their Great Mystery would point to the North, South, or East for its location." (p. 16) He failed to see that the Indians were indicating that God is everywhere, not just in the sky overhead. The same writer, however, displayed great sensitivity in perceiving something of value in the difference between the races.

> To become, in short, accomplished (in hand talk) one must train the mind to *think*, like the Indians, *in action*. Vividness of description is secured by exactness, earnestness, and vigor of gesture; a graceful execution can only result from long practice. . . . It must be borne in mind that this is in a great measure a pantomimic language, and the air-pictures must at least be a fair imitation to be worthy of recognition. (p. 17)

Clark also points out that the system is not grammatically structured. "Articles, conjunctions and prepositions are omitted. . . . Verbs are used in the present tense, nouns and verbs in the singular number, the idea of plurality being expressed in some other way". (p. 17). Past and future, as well as gender, are also expressed differently than in English. Mark L. Knapp in *Non Verbal Communication in Human Interaction* (1972) endorses this when he points out that current evidence suggests that kinesics is not a communication system with the same structure as spoken language. "We must view any nonverbal behavior in context—the meaning ultimately depends on the context. We must see these separated parts of nonverbal study as an integrated whole in any given situation—a reminder to avoid oversimplification in analyzing nonverbal behavior." (p. 112)

HADLEY

In 1893, Reverend Lewis Hadley published a very limited edition of *Indian Hand Talk*. His intention was to teach English to hand-talking American Indians through "their almost universal gesture system" (Title page). He also proposed to develop a schema to represent signals pictographically, with the intention of using it to print the Bible in American Indian Hand Talk. He made a notable attempt to draw the gestures, but his lack of artistic ability destined the endeavour to failure. His drawings, because of their flaws in perspective and emphasis, create some very false impressions concerning the manual execution of the signals.

SETON

Ernest Thompson Seton (1918) was interested in the universality of sign communication. "Many thoughtful men have been trying for a century, at least, to give mankind a world speech which would overstep all linguistic barriers, and one cannot help wondering why they have overlooked the Sign Language, the one mode common to all mankind, already established and as old as Babel. . . ." (p. xv)

As far back as the records go, we find human gesture in use, Seton reports, citing nineteen examples in Homer. Egyptologists remind us, he says, that the oldest records show a manual code in use very similar to current gesture systems. He cites the concept of *hunger* as an example of the arbitrariness of words as opposed to the concreteness and logic of gesture, which at once indicates the pain, the place, and then shows cause and remedy.

"Nor can sign talk have changed radically," he states, "for it is founded on the basic elements of human make-up [and] is so perfectly ideographic that no amount of bad presentation can completely divert attention from the essential thought." (p. xvi)

"Being so fundamental, ancient and persistent, Sign Language is, perforce, universal. In some measure it is used by every race on earth today, Eskimo and Zulu, Japanese and Frenchmen, Turk and Aztec, Greek and Patagonian. And whenever two men of hopelessly diverse speech have met, they have found a medium of thought exchange in the old Sign Language—the pantomimic suggestion of ideas." (p. xvii)

The American Indian, asserts Seton, is undoubtedly the best hand talker the world has known. Their simple and convenient manual system was used in early western trade and diplomacy as far back as records go. Every traveler needed to study and practice the gestures and all attest to the system's simplicity, picturesqueness, grace, and practical utility.

Seton defines a true manual system as *an established code of logical gestures to convey ideas without reference to words or letters of a language*. He points out that the distinctive difference between American Indian Code and the sign systems of the deaf lies in this linguistic facet. He notes that the deaf sign systems assume a knowledge by signer and viewer of a common language, while the American Indian Code conversely assumes the absence of a shared spoken or written language. He adds that the majority of signs in the deaf system are arbitrary or conventional, while in American Indian System, the gestures are never arbitrary, but rather the product of the slow evolution of ages of use, with roots deep in human behavior and therefore so logical and reasonable that they are easily and quickly understood, learned, and used.

Two principal attitudes toward the study of manual systems are presented briefly by Seton:

1. The scholarly view, which Seton characterizes as academic, is described as being devoted to preservation of faithful, unchanged versions of the oldest gestures. This view precludes modifying or changing the recorded forms. Its followers devote themselves to analysis of structure, comparison of similarities, and determination of differences among various users, as well as speculation on origins and development. Its practitioners usually are linguistically oriented and look upon the system as a relic from the past, studying it principally from a historical point of view.

2. According to Seton, the second group of American Indian Hand Talk proponents realize that this ancient system is not a dead communication mode, but rather a system approaching its renaissance, and which therefore needs to be brought up to date in its repertoire to become useful today. This view accepts the idea that the ancient signals, like any current additions, *were invented by people who had need of them*. It matters little, avers Seton, whence come new elements of the code, so long as they be needed, serviceable, and constructed on the original premises of human communicability where no other mode exists. In this event, he prophesies, hand talk, fully developed, will find much good work to do.

The authors of this book believe that American Indian Hand Talk, "fully developed" and modernized into Amer-Ind, has indeed found much good work to do in serving the rehabilitation needs of the speechless. It is very intriguing, in view of the favorable results of recent pilot studies of application with those speechless persons diagnosed as mentally retarded, to find this early twentieth-century naturalist stating that the American Indian system has "a sweet reasonableness, a mathematical accuracy" that has "an insistent and reactionary effect on the mental processes and [mental] pictures of those who use it. Therefore, it is valuable for the kind of mind it makes." (p. xxxiv)

Although not a linguist, Seton points out with accuracy and perception the significant factors of the system's structural simplicity, which serves the proposed clinical purpose. The relation of one idea to another within the system is indicated chiefly by proximity and sequence, rather than by elaborate rules of grammar and syntax. A signal may be interpreted as an action (verb), object (noun), or descriptor (adjective or adverb). Case is determined by context, sequence, and logic. Possession and gender may be readily identified by appropriate additive signals. The present tense is always understood in the action signal unless additive past or future signals are employed. Number is shown by context. Voice is always active, never passive, since the American Indian mode of thought always sees the *human being* as in charge and as *acting* rather than being acted upon. The imperative is indicated by the additive signal for COMMAND and the subjunctive by that for PERHAPS.

Possibly because Seton is the only artist among the four mentioned chroniclers of American Indian Hand Talk, it is natural that he saw more clearly the innate conceptual basis of the system. He realized that it was important to observe the hand movements as pictures of meaning. He regrets the conventionalization of signals which did occur and which destroyed, in many instances, the great virtue of the system—ease of comprehension by the untutored viewer. He advocates that "it is well worthwhile in each case to note the original concept as fully as possible; first, as a help to the memory (and understanding) and second, as a guard against slovenly gesture." He contends that this produces signals of "point, power, and accuracy." (p. xliii)

Seton states, "the fact that most signs are capable of logical explanation does not mean that they are self-explanatory. Indeed, nearly all have become conventional, and each must be learned separately before it can be rightly used." (p. xliii) It is an exaggeration to say "nearly all" have become conventionalized. Recent transmission tests show the more accurate figure to be 10 percent. The *memorization* of *undesirable* conventionalizations will never serve modern clinical use. *Rather, the conventionalized signals should be restored to their original logic* and, therefore, to their original forms. Mere memorization, however, has never yet made anyone a competent user of any communication system. One must grasp the system's underlying logic, and the logic and propriety of individual expressions, for human communication to assume its full stature.

Regrettably, from the American Indian point of view, Seton perpetuates two errors that are firmly embedded in much other reporting of Hand Talk. First, while he states correctly that abstract ideas are not copiously rendered in code, he adds that "it often happens that a gesture with the index [finger] alone is specific, [but] the same gesture with the flat hand becomes abstract." (p. xli) While the first half of this statement is true, the American Indian sees a gesture with the flat hand not as an abstraction of the finger signal but as an extension of the concept to more people and more occasions, all of which are concrete. (Incidentally, the flat hand must be palm down for this application, which is the signal for ALL. The flat hand, palm up, is the additive signal for *object* or *thing*, when the situation requires distinguishing object from action. The logic is that we can hold an object in the hand but we cannot hold an action. Action is seen or experienced kinetically, not tactually.)

The major misinterpretation concerns the often repeated statement that American Indians believed intelligence to be located in the heart. Seton says, "Signs which make the heart the seat of the mind are, I think, older than those which give the place of honor to the brain" (p. xliii). American Indians never saw the heart as the locus of thought! Like whites, the American Indians characterize the heart as the seat of emotion. They may occasionally misuse code in this context as many erudite speakers misuse English when they say, "I feel that . . ." when they really mean, "I think that. . . ." The signal for "feel" is HEART, that for "think" is BRAIN.

OTHER LITERATURE

More recent publications do not contribute appreciably to the present-day clinical use of Amer-Ind. *American Indian Sign Language,* published in 1926 by its author, William Tompkins, focused on American Indian culture of the past, with its vocabulary emphasis in that direction. Mr. Tompkins was a scout and learned the art of hand talk from Indian friends. While many of his descriptions are accurate, an almost equal number are distorted. His reference is only to the signal use of a limited tribal area.

Indian Sign Language by Robert Hofsinde, published in 1956, shifted from the original concrete basis of signals to a stylized and therefore much more arbitrary and symbolic level. Hofsinde's work reports on usage of only one tribe. Apparently, as an artist he was most attracted to the more graceful (but also more formal or ceremonial rather than the coloquial) versions of many of the gestures. In ritual usage, because viewers generally have knowledge of content, transmission of meaning is sacrificed in the interests of beauty of execution and the pictorial effect of large and dance-like gestures.

Neither of these texts indicate any possibility of modern use of the American Indian Code, although Tompkins does suggest that the Boy Scouts could use it for secret language and for nature study.

In 1908, Aline Amon's *Talking Hands* portrayed American Indian woods life. As in Tompkins' book, the vocabulary centers on the past with no mention or implication of any other possible use, other than for the entertainment of children. Though charmingly written, the illustrations are naive and idealistic, portraying both an unrealistic version of the past and an inaccurate account of Hand Talk and its use.

None of these three books is directed toward a specific adaptation for the use of speechless patients in daily modern communication. In the majority of instances, the conventional and even arbitrary modifications of the original concrete signals make them useless for inclusion in a clinical version where the goals are quick, easy acquisition and execution by the speech-impaired person, and effective interpretation by the untrained viewer.

IN CONCLUSION

These reports were written by whites in limited contact with American Indian cultures. Even the most accurate and scholarly of these, Mallery, misunderstood the code's basis. Consequently, when they attempted to describe the signals in words, they focused on exact hand positions or movements, failing to realize that the signals were *manual kinetic pictographs of ideas*. Because of this basic misunderstanding, they were unaware of the flexibility of American Indian Code, in which the same idea may be expressed in several different ways; and also, conversely, in which the same signal can express a variety of different ideas. Even the most meticulous white writers made these mistakes in their reports because of their linguistic bias. When they encountered unexpected variants, they assumed that different tribes had different signals. Since those whose records have survived were associated only with plains tribes, the writers quite naturally assumed that this system was peculiar to the plains inhabitants. So the erroneous idea that only American Indians of the plains used the code was perpetuated, despite numerous historical references (including the works of other white writers) to coastal Indians and their use of the code with new settlers.

As the American Indians of the East rapidly learned the languages of the European settlers, the colloquial use of the manual code did deteriorate among the various eastern tribes, since the basic need for it had disappeared. Yet, almost all of them preserved it in their ceremonials. Here, beauty of execution took precedence over preservation of meaning, so that today the ceremonial signals are no longer easy to read. (Human beings appear to share this tendency across many cultures; ceremony almost always tends to become ritualistic and therefore mysterious, hence uncommunicative, except to the initiates. Usually, considerable misunderstanding ensues. Many incorrect ideas about American Indians have been sustained and disseminated in this fashion.)

To restore the original high level of transmission of ancient American Indian Code is a primary intention of this project. Only with an understanding of the basic characteristics of restored American Indian gesture can the Code become adapted as a rehabilitation tool to serve the needs of the speechless. To this end then, it was proposed to delete from the repertoire of Amer-Ind those signals that were corrupted into arbitrary or conventional form as well as those no longer relevant to today's needs. This same viewpoint dictated expansion of the Amer-Ind repertoire by the addition of signals for the modern, industralized society of today, just as they might have developed had American Indian Hand Talk continued until the present as an active, colloquial, communication mode. To these purposes, then, were directed the clinical investigations reported in the following section.

CLINICAL INVESTIGATION

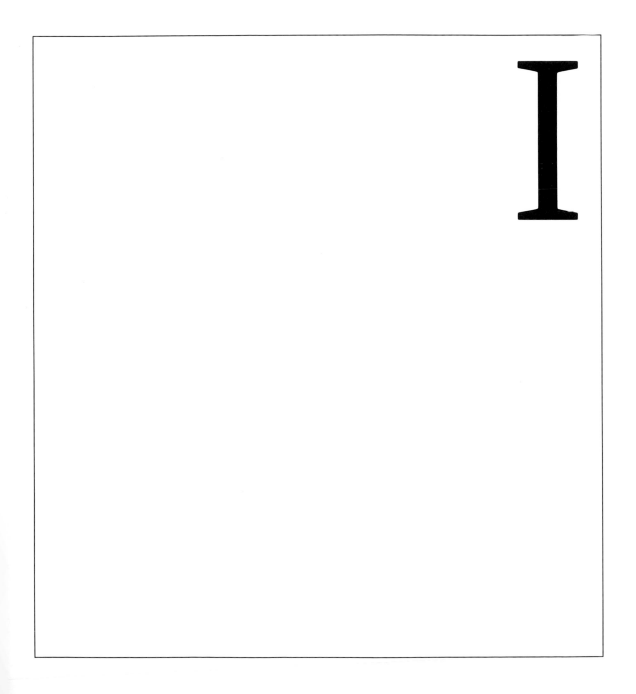

I

Preclinical Questions
and Preparations

1

QUESTIONS

As for most innovative rehabilitation approaches in the early stages of their clinical application (the first five years), many pertinent questions remain unanswered for a considerable time. Meanwhile, exploratory projects continue to add gradually to the general base of knowledge. To date, a number of queries concerning the clinical use of Amer-Ind Code for speechless patients have been proposed and some helpful answers have been obtained. Though these answers are as yet not definitive, they nonetheless serve to improve current usage and to locate crucial areas for further investigation.

Initial relevant questions may be grouped under four general concerns: (1) *authentication* and *modernization* of the ancient hand talk of the American Indian tribes for current clinical use with speechless patients; (2) *acquisition* of the signals by speechless patients of varying syndromes; (3) *transmission* of the signals to viewers in the patient's life; and (4) *conclusions* concerning professional approaches to secure for each patient acquisition and transmission levels that produce some improvement in the patient's communication in daily-life situations.

Each of these areas generates a variety of queries. Who today knows the American Indian Code of the past? How well have its basic virtues been preserved since need for them ceased? What records exist and how reliable are they? What adaptations may be needed for current communication in a quite different societal frame? What modernization might have occurred had the hand talk continued as a living communication mode? What modernizations of this ancient art can best serve the proposed clinical purpose? Who is best qualified to make the necessary adaptations? What tests can we use for prognostic selection of patient candidates? What kind of speechless person can learn and use the system for daily communication? At what levels can it be so utilized? In what span of time can it be acquired? Can it help the more severely impaired for whom so little is available? Can oral–verbal apraxic patients profit from it? Can aphasics? Can the brain-damaged and mentally retarded? Can the motorically handicapped? Can the surgically impaired? Also, what methods can best inculcate code usage with these patients?

For those acquiring Amer-Ind, how well will it transmit? To whom and under what circumstances? What effect will motoric problems have on transmission? Are there specific signals which are difficult to acquire and/ or transmit? Is a one-hand version possible for the hemiplegic patient?

What instructional methods best prepare the speech pathologist to induct patients into clinical use of the code? How should such methods prepare hospital and educational personnel as well as families, friends, and even the general public to accept, recognize, interpret, and utilize the signaling of the speechless patient?

And finally, will development of manual code communication in any way affect the speechless signaling patient's potential for oral verbalization in his own language?

Accounts of some of the initial preparatory undertakings and early pilot studies, as well as the clinical exploratory procedures and their accompanying experimental treatment projects follow. They are reported in varying degrees of detail and with expanding awareness of the magnitude of as yet unexplored realms. Brief descriptions of field results from a number of contributors are also included. The cumulative clinical knowledge gained is summarized in the recommendations in Part II as a base for clinical application in treatment.

AUTHENTICATION

Unfortunately, no organization within or among tribes has been established for the preservation of the ancient art of American Indian Hand Talk. Some western tribes, however, have made efforts to preserve and teach hand code, and interest appears to be growing in all American Indian arts.

The best preservation of hand code has been for ritual purposes. But while the code used in rituals is beautiful in its execution, its formalization does not provide a base for clinical daily life use. Also, there is some variance in how the signals are remembered, if remembered at all, among many tribes.

American Indians of advanced age, who were taught code in their youth when active daily use of the code was common and there were many accomplished signalers to teach it, are now the principal resource. A number of these people have been consulted at varying steps of the clinical program. Among these advisors have been signal practitioners from tribes of the eastern woodlands, the Great Lakes, the plains, the Northwest, and the Southwest.

The repertoire currently represented in the clinical program has accrued from the memory of a member of the Iroquois Confederacy and has been measured by the memories of still-living practitioners from around the country. Each signal admitted to the clinical repertoire has been checked with the records of both Clark and Mallery, which are the best available written records.

MODERNIZATION

The clinical team has eliminated signals considered applicable only to human needs and activities of the past, except in the case where these signals are so universal across time as to be modifiable for current use. Each signal admitted to the clinical repertoire has been checked for current usefulness, ease of execution, and transmission success.

A small percentage of new signals, not found in either the literature or among the Indian elders, has been developed to accommodate the technical needs of twentieth-century communication. They have accrued from experimental pantomime, based on the principles of the ancient art: *concrete reference* in action or object and *ease of interpretation* by the uninstructed viewer. They have also been submitted to one or more tribal elders for approval. (As in other human communication modes, some such signals would have been added had hand talk continued as a living communication code.) Their transmission has been tested to meet the standard set by the ancient signals in the repertoire.

The senior author has had experience in using the clinical repertoire for communication across language barriers during the past six years on four continents. The language populations involved, in addition to English, were Spanish, French, Portuguese, Italian, German, Japanese, Hawaiian, Swedish, Danish, Dutch, and the languages of the aboriginal peoples of Australia. These, of course, were informal, social situations where the hand talk served very well for communication.

In one instance, however, the group consisted of persons of varying language backgrounds. The occasion was professional, requiring communication of paramedical content. An examination on the material was administered in the language of each viewer after the lecture in code. All participants passed at a level equal to that achieved in a normal lecture situation. This was a single instance, of course, and with a highly intelligent, highly motivated group of people.

Only time and extended clinical application by many expert speech pathologists in varying locations with numerous, appropriately chosen patients can convincingly validate the code for clinical use.

Acquisition: Projects 1–10

2

PROJECT 1: A CANCER SURGERY PATIENT

In the clinical projects in speech rehabilitation for the total glossectomee at the St. Louis VA Hospital, some patients exhibited surgical residual deficits of such magnitude as to preclude oral speech rehabilitation by the compensatory methods previously developed (Donaldson, Skelly, and Paletta, 1968; Skelly et al., 1971; Skelly et al., 1972; Skelly and Donaldson, 1972; Skelly, Donaldson, and Schinsky, 1972; Skelly and Donaldson, 1973; and Skelly, Donaldson, and Fust, 1973). One such speechless-voiceless case was transferred for plastic reconstruction after prior extensive cancer surgery in several stages. This 44-yr-old man had first reported to a physician in March 1969, with a two month history of a lesion of the anterior floor of the mouth. The biopsy revealed a well-differentiated infiltrating squamous cell carcinoma. During the following year, the patient was treated at several locations by a variety of approaches including direct cryosurgery. In April 1970, a total mandibulectomy, total glossectomy, total laryngectomy, and a bilateral upper neck dissection was carried out. When the patient was referred for reconstructive surgery, he exhibited a defect of the entire lower face and oropharynx. The only articulator preserved was the upper lip, which was almost immobile.

Eight months after completion of the reconstructive surgery, the patient had an intact lower face and mouth, resulting in a socially acceptable appearance. He also had a water-tight, funnel-shaped oropharynx which permitted self-feeding with a rubber catheter. There was adequate camouflage of the anterior neck by a bearded visor flap (Griffin, Donaldson, and Skelly, 1973). At this point, the patient presented a considerable challenge to the speech pathologist.

The patient's communication problem was acute. His only method was graphic. Since he was an intelligent, imaginative man, with a better than average command of language, he naturally tended in his writing toward complete and rather lengthy comments and replies. The delays inherent in this method deterred continued conversation of any duration. Normal speakers in his environment displayed impatience with this labored mode of communication and avoided the occasions for such conversations. Consequently, there was a lack of any real social satisfaction for the patient.

In the speech clinic he used a few spontaneous gestures to supplement his written communication. While these gestures were basically meaningful, they were very limited. They were randomly variable and inconsistent, unreliable in relation to specific referents, and confusingly indefinite in execution.

An exploratory project was undertaken to formalize and refine these gestures. The patient rejected a proposal to utilize a sign language of the deaf on the rationale that he did not know many persons with whom he could use it. When American Indian Hand Talk was suggested to him as an alternative, and its origin and history explained, he decided that it might prove useful.

Since motivation for persistence is usually directly related to satisfaction of needs, the initial signal repertoire was designed for the immediate personal use of this patient. He was asked to accumulate in a pocket notebook dated entries of all his written communications. This material was analyzed for word use, frequency of word repetition, use of synonyms, and range of subject matter. An individual repertoire based on daily-life need evolved from this.

The patient was then instructed by an American Indian member of the staff in the specific signals that would serve his daily conversational needs. As soon as he developed adequate precision of execution, he was asked to signal rather than write, and to resort to writing only when the code communication failed. His notebook yielded the number, occasion, and specific transmissions involved in his failures. Success and failure percentages from these data were used to refine, improve, and score the patient's reliability of transmission and his progress. Communicability was checked daily in hospital situations outside the speech clinic with the widest possible variety of viewers. The patient's transmission failures were also used to assess the communicative potential of each signal involved. Alternative signals were compared for transmission success.

In the course of the instruction, both the mirror and videotape were used to allow the patient to view his own signaling. The videotapes yielded faster, more permanent, and more discrete results in effecting precision and consistency. While drill before the mirror yielded visual reinforcement for the kinetic, the viewing of the videotapes appeared to provide the patient with a more objective view of his own performance, and contributed greatly to the patient's understanding of the dynamics between signaler and viewer.

This patient received two individual one-hour sessions in Amer-Ind Code daily, five days a week, for a period of three months. By that time, he had acquired a signal repertoire of approximately 200. With this repertoire he achieved the normal, swift, casual interactions of daily life in his hospital environment. He communicated successfully with doctors, nurses, other hospital personnel, volunteers, patients, and visitors, none of whom had received any instruction in interpreting the code.

The patient assessed the code as more useful to him than writing since it was swifter, maintained eye contact, and tended to limit his own units of transmission so the other person could participate more completely and satisfactorily. The learning and use of this limited but specific repertoire had both psychologically and socially desirable results. The patient joined several organizations, used the code for shopping, banking, traveling, and his other daily needs. He reported that he had little or no difficulty in communicating with the majority of the people he encountered, and that he very seldom needed to resort to writing.

On his checkup a year later, he revealed a few undesirable code habits. Since he was very much at ease with signaling, he executed signal sequences with such rapidity that some viewers could not easily follow him. His speed tended to cause some elisions in the complete signal so that many were elliptically shortened. This speed also encouraged lack of precision. He concurred with the comments on his signaling and agreed to monitor it with the goal of improvement.

The patient was invited to attend group sessions with other patients and to assist by demonstrating precise, consistent signals, executed at a speed appropriate to the particular viewer. In these sessions, he has been of great service to others in the program and has profited himself from his participation.

It was concluded from this study that the motivated speechless patient with a surgical deficit could learn easily and use profitably Amer-Ind Code as an alternative communication mode to writing.

PROJECT 2: A RIGHT HEMIPLEGIC ORAL–VERBAL APRAXIC PATIENT

Of all the syndromes represented among the speechless patient population, that of severe oral–verbal apraxia appears most resistent to therapeutic intervention. Therefore, the second exploratory project attempted to assess the feasibility of Amer-Ind Code for a 50-yr-old, severely impaired, oral–verbal apraxic patient with complicating mild aphasia and right hemiplegia. This patient was unable to walk and was confined to a wheelchair. He was unable to write or to speak. He produced some phonation and some meaningless gestures. He had received six months of twice-a-week out-patient treatment for speech with no observable results. He also demonstrated a mild to moderate receptive difficulty through the auditory channel, which was later diagnosed as hearing loss.

The patient was asked to match objects with pictures of those objects, and he succeeded. Action shots depicting the use of the objects were then presented. As a matching activity, the patient was asked to correlate with the object and the action picture of the object. These objects included a wheelchair, water, food, a bed, a blanket, a fan, and a wrist watch.

Following the successful matching drills, the signals BATHROOM, THIRSTY, HUNGRY, HOT, COLD, TIRED, and TIME were demonstrated one by one, associated with the relevant pictures. When the patient reproduced a signal, he was immediately reinforced with the appropriate result; he was wheeled to the bathroom, he was presented with a glass of water, he was offered toast and jelly, he was fanned, he was given a blanket around him or over his knees, he was wheeled to the sofa, and a pillow was brought out. The signal TIME was associated with the arrival of his transportation: "time to go home."

At the session following the one in which the patient had learned a signal, he was offered an alternative choice between the thing it represented and something else. Each was signaled to him, and he was expected to make a choice using a signal. After DRINK and HUNGRY, for instance, he was offered choices of water, milk, and cola, or toast, cookie, doughnut. If he signaled THIRSTY he was presented with a tray with the three drinks. If he signaled HUNGRY he was offered a selection of the three foods. From this point on, the patient progressed rapidly in acquisition of signals. At the beginning of the project he was simply randomly pointing, but he gradually acquired selective skills as well as constantly improving command of his hand movements. Many of the two-hand signals were successfully adapted to a one hand version for his left hand. He rapidly added PAIN, YES, NO, MAYBE, REJECT, OK, HELLO, GOODBYE, WALK or GO, HOME, DOCTOR, YOU, ALL, and QUESTION.

At the end of the six-month period of twice-a-week, hour-long sessions, he had accumulated a total repertoire of sixty signals, and was using them to serve his needs and satisfy many of his wishes. He not only answered questions in signal, but he both asked questions and volunteered spontaneous comments. His family and friends reported very satisfactory use of signals for general communication at home. He continued in group sessions for an additional six months, where he grew more adept at using combinations of signals to express additional meanings. To date, his hand control and his signal precision have improved, and he is now walking with a cane. The auditory deficit noted on admission appears to have undergone considerable amelioration, since he responds appropriately in signal to all spoken cues. His current repertoire of about seventy signals appears adequate for his daily-life needs.

It was concluded from this study that the oral–verbal apraxic patient might learn and use the Amer-Ind Code, and that a one-hand version of the two-hand signals could be developed for the left hand, to accommodate the right hemiplegic patient. Further exploration of application appeared justified.

PROJECT 3: A TWELVE-PATIENT GROUP OF VARYING SYNDROMES

A group approach was explored next in a pilot study involving twelve patients with varying etiologies of speechlessness: two glossectomees, one laryngectomee, two dysphonic patients, one dysarthric patient, and six apraxic patients. The two glossectomees in the group were simultaneously attending the rehabilitation program for compensatory oral speech. One, however, had an unfavorable prognosis because of the extensive surgery and adjunctive problems in dysphagia. The other had a very favorable prognosis for the compensatory method but wished to develop an alternative mode in code, as during damp weather he had problems in controlling oral mucous and consequently experienced difficulty in producing intelligible compensatory speech. One laryngectomee in the group had a poor prognosis for esophageal voice; although he produced esophageal sound, it was highly unreliable. His problem was compounded by the fact that the electrolarynx failed to provide suitable vibration through his scarred tissue.

One of the two dysphonic patients had a history of recurrent voice loss and desired to develop an alternative mode. The second dysphonic had a good prognosis for voice rehabilitation and did, in fact, make a complete recovery, but meanwhile wished to learn the code as a means of alleviating the silence of voice rest.

A severely dysarthric patient whose speech was highly unintelligible was asked to experiment with the code. Six oral–verbal apraxic patients, all of whom had prior sessions with other approaches (with no improvement in speech), were added to the group. None of these was diagnosed as aphasic. All were right hemiplegics.

The project began with a presentation to the group of a wide variety of uses of gesture in American life by persons who have command of language. Because people relegate gesture to an inferior status in communication, it is important that the patient attempting to learn and use it realize that it has many respected uses already in American life. It is used regularly by construction workers, sports referees, policemen, sailors, television and radio directors, to mention a few. The patients were then encouraged to demonstrate any of these gestures with which they were familiar. Following this, ten simple basic gestures of Amer-Ind Code were introduced by clinician demonstration. Videotapes were consistently used to film each participant's signaling for the patient's own criticism and for group reaction; each tape was viewed for the purpose of refining the precision, consistency, and transmission of the signals. These gestures were then utilized as replies to questions structured to elicit them. Finally, the signals were assigned for use in daily life. At each session the repertoire was extended by several signals. These were organized in order of need for the individuals in the group. The repertoire was next increased to serve satisfaction of wishes, as well as need. Weekly signal lists centered about a stated topic to stimulate spontaneous comment. Preplanning of hospital mock situations provided opportunities for patient success in use of code and for reinforcement of interest and persistence. The mock-situations also provided opportunity for rehearsal of signals needed in specific daily-life situations. The process of **agglutination** (the linking of two or more signals to express a new and different concept) was explained, demonstrated and incorporated in the sessions. Home and hospital assignments provided opportunity for the participants to use and test the success of their signaling.

Throughout the program, as each signal was introduced its single-hand adaptation was emphasized for the right hemiplegic participants. Demonstrating clinicians alternated two-hand and one-hand versions. They also used the *left* hand for single hand signaling to encourage the hemiplegic signalers.

Informal reports were received from hospital personnel on successful (or unsuccessful) use of code by patients in daily-life situations. The reporting viewers included physicians, nurses, social workers, physical and occupational therapists, aides, technicians, secretaries, canteen employees, other patients, volunteers, and visitors. While formal testing or score rendering was not feasible or even desirable at this stage of the program, the feedback from these informal reports was highly favorable.

Each member of the group had some success in using this gestural system in life situations with viewers uninstructed in the code. Among these viewers were many who were also unfamiliar with the patient. In each case, the degree of success varied in accordance with the individual's handicap and abilities.

The program was scheduled over a six-month period, with two sessions each week (each session lasting two hours with a ten-minute break). One hundred signals were presented during the first three months, and an additional hundred, including agglutinates, during the second three-month period. One glossectomee achieved 100 percent mastery of the signals presented, the other 92 percent. One dysphonic learned 100 percent the other 87 percent. The laryngectomee developed 67 percent of the signals usefully, the dysarthric 60 percent. The apraxic scores were 72, 67, 67, 55, 50, and 17 percent on the left-hand variant signals.

During the first quarter, the apraxic patients were all below the median and the other patients all above. It is notable, however, that during the second quarter, five of the six apraxics matched or exceeded scores of the patients with other syndromes. This higher improvement differential between the first and second quarters has important therapeutic implications for patients with this disability. Among other factors, adaptation to the single-hand, left-hand variant signals may account for some of the early delay. (Lengthier treatment of patients with certain impairments may be indicated. In many cases, termination of treatment may occur too soon.)

One of the important differences between research and clinical interpretation of data is exemplified in the percentage scores reported in this project. While the patient with 17 percent may be considered a failure on paper, in the clinical interpretation he is not. The patient's family is delighted that the patient has thirty-five signals that can be reliably used to communicate concepts. All of these signals concern his immediate needs and desires. In context and combination, the signals provide him the equivalent of about a two-hundred-word spoken vocabulary. When the family learns to use the appropriate questions and make the relevant extrapolation, the communication level becomes significantly higher than it was before the patient acquired the signal repertoire.

It was concluded from this study that Amer-Ind Code might well provide a usable supplementary communication system, on either a temporary or permanent basis, for patients with speech deficits consequent to cancer surgery. It also appears to warrant further exploration of Code use for the oral–verbal apraxic. The following table summarizes the group's progress.

PROJECT 3: SIGNAL ACQUISITION BY SYNDROME PILOT GROUP

Patient Syndrome	Quarter 1 100 signals presented, no. acquired	Quarter 2 100 signals & agglutinates presented, no. acquired	Of 200 presented, no. acquired	% acquired
1. glossectomy	100	100	200	100
2. dysphonia	100	100	200	100
3. glossectomy	90	95	185	92.5
4. dysphonia	85	90	175	87.5
5. laryngectomy	65	70	135	67.5
6. dysarthria	60	60	120	60
7. apraxia	55	90	145	72.5
8. apraxia	55	80	135	67.5
9. apraxia	50	85	135	67.5
10. apraxia	40	70	110	55
11. apraxia	35	65	100	50
12. apraxia	15	20	35	17.5

PROJECT 4: NINE DUALLY IMPAIRED CANCER SURGERY PATIENTS

Cancer patients who have had complete excision of the larynx as well as complete excision of the tongue, with accompanying total or partial mandibulectomy and possibly bilateral neck dissection, have severe problems in voice and speech rehabilitation. Although there are now techniques that can provide intelligible speech for them, the process is a slow and lengthy one. There are also times, even after development of very adequate voice and speech, when either or both voice and speech fail them due to various factors related to the degree of their surgery. This project was inititated to investigate the usefulness of Amer-Ind Code as a supplementary (or even alternative) mode of communication for such impaired persons. Nine dually impaired patients were instructed in the use of code by the methods previously described. These patients attended code group sessions twice a week for one hour each session. They also received two or more hour-long treatment sessions per day on the techniques of glossectomy compensation for oral speech. During these latter sessions, ten minutes on Amer-Ind Code were interpolated in each half hour. This provided approximately eighty minutes a day on compensation and forty minutes a day on code (in addition to the code group participation) over a twelve-week period. The rationale for this division was that code would provide faster communication than writing, would preserve eye contact (as writing fails to do), might motivate persistence on the compensations for speech. It would also provide a success cushion against the early failures in the compensatory techniques. (The oral surgery patients had difficulty enduring more than 20 minutes on the compensatory motor sequence without rest. The Amer-Ind Code profitably filled the ten-minute oral rest period.)

Four of the nine patients mastered and used approximately 100 signals.

They reported that they found them useful while learning the compensatory speech, and that they anticipated that the signals would be valuable in certain future situations should their compensatory speech for any reason fail. (These four patients also achieved the highest intelligibility scores for their compensatory speech.)

Three patients developed and used about eighty of the basic signals. They reported them as being useful in the early stages of their treatment, when they had no intelligible compensatory speech. As their intelligibility scores increased in the compensatory oral speech, they still found the signals valuable in improving communication with people who did not always understand their early oral efforts. They predicted that the code would continue to help them in this way.

The eighth patient learned about forty signals, but did not make much use of them outside the demanded use in the clinic. He was indifferent in his attitude toward code, and doubtful of its use to him at home. Unfortunately for his life communication, his intelligibility score in compensatory speech was among the lowest.

The ninth patient was making excellent progress in both code and compensatory speech, and attempting to use both in life communication situations, when he decided that he must go home. He lived at such a distance that out-patient treatment was not possible. He reports that his combined use of the signals and the compensatory speech that he mastered afford him adequate communication in his life situation. His decision to terminate was regrettable clinically as his prognosis in both compensatory speech and signal transmission was highly favorable.

It appears that Amer-Ind Code may be a valuable adjunctive communication mode for cancer surgery patients. The project results also indicate that motivation, patience, and persistence on the patient's part are essential to success. Acceptance of manual communication may be a highly important factor in success. The motivational aspect of treatment should probably receive more structured planning and occur very early in the treatment sequence. This aspect of treatment is not limited to surgery patients but applies also to the oral–verbal apraxic patients.

PROJECT 5: SIX ORAL–VERBAL APRAXIC PATIENTS

During the past decade, approximately four hundred veterans were diagnosed as oral apraxics or oral–verbal apraxics or as both. Sixty-five percent were classified as severely apraxic. The oral–verbal output of these patients, even after extensive treatment, has frequently been minimal with consequent discouragement to the patients, their families, and their clinicians. Since 75 percent of these severely impaired patients were also agraphic, they were able to achieve only limited, highly unsatisfactory communication.

THE PROJECT

To find some way to improve communication for such dually impaired apraxics, a clinical pilot study was begun to explore the expanded use of

Amer-Ind Code. This system had already demonstrated, in four previous projects, a strong usefulness in serving the communication needs of speechless patients with problems of varying etiologies (Skelly et al., 1972).

A project devoted to development of a one-hand code for hemiplegics (Skelly et al., 1973) revealed varying types and degrees of oral movement accompanying the manual gestures of some of the patients. Occasionally these gestures were associated with unintelligible spontaneous vocalization. It was hypothesized that these spontaneous articulatory movements and vocalizations might be employed clinically to facilitate speech production. Since successful use of Amer-Ind Code necessitates adequate voluntary control of hand movement, we assumed that patients whose gestural scores exceeded their verbal scores on the Porch Index of Communicative Ability (PICA) (Porch, 1971) would be most likely to benefit from the proj-project. The six patients whose gestural and verbal scores showed the widest differences were chosen from the current register. In each case there was more than a four-point gap between gestural and verbal scores on the PICA (Table 1). These patients had all been diagnosed previously as having severe oral and oral–verbal apraxia on the Goodglass and Kaplan test, the Assessment of Aphasia and Related Disorders (1972), which contains a segment on apraxia.

THE PATIENTS

Patient A was a 36-yr-old male veteran who had suffered a ruptured cerebral aneurysm, treated with surgical intervention within two years prior to the project. Evaluation of his communication on admission to the clinic (not the project) showed intact auditory and visual comprehension but severe oral and oral–verbal apraxia. His oral and graphic functions were much inferior to his performance on the PICA tests. In six months of individual group treatment, he made a slight gain in oral scores and a limited but slightly better gain in graphic scores. These were not sufficient, however, to serve his daily communication needs. On his admission to the project his scores on the PICA were gestural 13.20, verbal 8.70, and graphic 9.55. His gestures with objects were accurate but delayed. He was able to speak some words in imitation but not able to replicate them reliably. The stimulus for imitation was effective only after three repetitions of the pattern. His writing was distorted and was produced only after repetition of the pattern.

Patient B was a 41-yr-old male right hemiplegic who three years previously had suffered a thrombotic cerebrovascular accident, with consequent severe dysarthria as well as oral and oral–verbal apraxia. He had received nineteen months of speech treatment elsewhere with no oral speech ensuing. His attempts at writing were highly inaccurate, though recognizably related in simple tasks (such as copying one-syllable words). In the test on his admission to the project his attempts at speech produced sounds that were comprehensible but not related to the task. Control of oral movement was highly unreliable and frustrating to the patient. His gestures on testing were accurate but incomplete, and these gestures were elicited only with objects. He essayed a few social gestures, without such stimulation, but did

TABLE 1. PROJECT 5: SIX ORAL VERBAL APRAXICS

Data	Patient A	Patient B	Patient C	Patient D	Patient E	Patient F
PICA Rank on admission	1	2	3	4	5	6
Age	36	41	52	48	52	48
Prior trauma	——	——	——	3 CVA	CVA	
Time lapse				3 yr	5 yr	
Admission trauma	Ruptured cerebral aneurism, surgery,	CVA	CVA	CVA	CVA	Car accident, 4-mo coma
Time lapse	2 yr	3 yr	3yr	3 yr	1 mo	3yr
Prior therapy	6 mo	19 mo	20 mo	12 mo	none	6 mo
Gestural-verbal differential	4.50	6.55	6.29	8.36	10.80	9.53
PICA scores on admission:						
Gestural	13.20	11.93	12.52	12.01	14.22	12.78
Verbal	8.70	5.38	5.23	3.65	3.42	3.25
Graphic	9.55	6.90	3.25	4.26	10.31	7.63
Diagnosis	Oral and oral–verbal apraxia	Dysarthric, oral, and oral–verbal apraxia	Oral and oral–verbal apraxia and aphasia	Oral and oral–verbal apraxia	Oral and oral–verbal apraxia	Oral and oral–verbal apraxia and aphasia

not succeed in transmitting meaning; nor did he replicate any of these attempts so far as clinical observation could determine. His PICA scores on admission to the project were gestural 11.93, verbal 5.38, and graphic 6.90.

Patient C was a 52-yr-old Air Force veteran who three years before had experienced a sudden cerebrovascular accident, with consequent right hemiplegia. He had been diagnosed as having severe aphasia, with moderate-to-severe oral and oral–verbal apraxia. For over two years he was a wheelchair patient, and for the past eight months he had been on braced ambulation with a cane. Despite almost two years of speech treatment elsewhere, he had no usable speech on admission to the clinic. Suitable behavioral responses indicated adequate auditory reception, but testing revealed limitations of auditory memory span. The patient used his glasses to examine the newspaper, with apparent enjoyment. He was unable to write anything but an illegible version of his name. On testing, his attempts at speech were partially comprehensible but not related to the task. His PICA scores on his admission to the project were gestural 12.52, verbal 5.23, and graphic 3.25.

Patient D was a 48-yr-old veteran who had experienced three cerebrovascular accidents: one hemorrhagic and two thrombotic. Three years pre-

TABLE 1. PROJECT 5: SIX ORAL VERBAL APRAXICS (continued)

Data	Patient A	Patient B	Patient C	Patient D	Patient E	Patient F
Presenting speech	Speech: one-word imitation; writing, one word, all distorted	No speech; low-level; graphic	No speech; signature only—illegible	No speech; low-level; graphic	No speech; no writing	No speech; no writing
PICA scores on termination:						
Gestural	13.52	13.09	12.75	13.63	14.25	14.15
Verbal	11.85	12.15	11.52	10.72	8.30	4.85
Graphic	9.55	9.63	9.81	10.23	11.15	9.35
Gestural-verbal differential	3.15	6.77	6.29	7.07	4.98	1.60
Speech on project termination	3-word sentences; over 200 words	3-word phrases; over 200 words	3-word sentences; over 200 words	2-word phrases; approx. 175 words	Single word use; approx. 50 words	No use; occasional word, not always intelligible.
Contributing data	——	——	Hearing notch at 4000 Hz; R 40 dB, L 50 dB.	——	——	Hearing notch at 4000 Hz; R 45 dB, L 75 dB; left visual field defect; impaired auditory memory span.

vious to the project, he had suffered another thrombotic attack resulting in right hemiplegia with oral and oral–verbal apraxia. After that, he received twelve months of individual and group treatment in the speech clinic. On his admission to the project his attempts at speech were minimal. His gestures on testing were accurate and responsive but not organized; they were elicited only by presentation of a concrete object as stimulus. His writing was incomprehensible but differentiated (although not at a useful level). His scores on admission to the project were gestural 12.01, verbal 3.65, and graphic 4.26.

Patient E was a 52-yr-old veteran. Five years before, he had experienced a cerebrovascular accident, after which he had completely recovered his speech and language. One month after his second attack he was admitted to the project. Evaluation showed complete loss of spoken language, including phonation. He was able to copy one-word graphic tasks, but these showed spelling confusions such as letter substitutions, omissions, and order inversions. His gestural responses when concrete objects were presented as stimuli were accurate although limited and delayed. To simple auditory commands he responded with appropriate but limited manual behavior. His

PICA scores at the time of his admission to the project were gestural 14.22, verbal 3.42, and graphic 10.31.

Patient F was a 48-yr-old Air Force veteran who had an accident three years prior to the project. He was comatose for seven months. After his recovery from the coma he was diagnosed as severely aphasic. At that time he was transferred to a second hospital, where the diagnostic report recorded "no clots, no neurological evidence of lesion producing aphasia." He received six months of speech treatment, after which he was transferred to the reporting clinic. Before participation in the project, he had right hemiplegia and was wheelchair-bound, but he was eventually moved to energetic braced ambulation with a cane. On his admission to our clinic, evaluation revealed moderate impairment of auditory comprehension and limited auditory memory span. His visual recognition appeared impaired, and right visual-field defect was present. Severe impairment of oral expression included lack of ability to imitate the simplest orofacial movements. The patient was totally agraphic. He received ten months of speech treatment at the clinic, including individual and group sessions. During the first half of this period he appeared to be unmotivated and uncooperative. His behavior slowly changed to a high level of motivation and cooperation. On admission to the project, he made the following PICA scores: gestural 12.78, verbal 3.25, and graphic 7.63.

All six patients were ambulatory at the time of their admission to the experimental code project. Their hearing was determined to be within useful normal limits, but both Air Force men revealed a 4000-Hz drop: Patient F at 40 dB on the right and 50 dB on the left, and Patient C showing a 45-dB level on the right and 75 dB on the left. All six patients were cooperative and enthusiastic about the project. (The six patients had some preliminary exposure in the use of Amer-Ind Code prior to this project.)

INSTRUCTION

The patients' instruction in code began with a description and demonstration of signals in daily use by many people, such as a head shake (yes, no), a shoulder shrug (maybe, perhaps), finger pointing (that person, that thing), an extended hand, palm up (give me), an extended hand, palm out, wrist flexed (stop), finger crooking (Come here), and a finger over the lips (quiet, hush). Imitation and use of these gestures by the group were explored. Members were encouraged to suggest additional gestures. By demonstration, the need to develop precision and consistency was explained and emphasized.

The beginning signaler must realize several characteristics of gestural communication: (1) Code is not a language; signals do not represent discrete words. (2) Signals are interpreted in whatever language the viewer uses. (3) Since Code is not a language, it has no grammatical structure but uses a logical associative order to the same purpose. Consequently, it has a telegraphic style. (4) There is no one *correct* signal for an idea. Any signal or group of signals from the repertoire that conveys an idea adequately to a number of viewers reliably on different occasions is acceptable. (In a prior project, each patient able to write had kept a daily notebook log of the communicative writing used daily for analysis of vocabulary needs. The most useful signals list that evolved was used with the apraxic patients in this project.)

The initial goal was to have the patients use, as frequently as appropriate and with precision and consistency, all the natural gestures already mentioned as they are signaled in Amer-Ind Code. The procedure was to integrate them in every patient–clinician contact, to stimulate them in all patient–patient contacts, and on ward visits to introduce them in patient–personnel contact. The patients' families were also apprised of the program.

The next goal was to develop a group of topic-related signals. This was achieved in three steps: (1) use of these signals in a question/answer drill; (2) practice in a structured conversation; (3) eliciting the signals in a spontaneous conversation. Frequent conferences of the clinician with family members and hospital personnel yielded information about the patients' use of the signals.

The clinician introduced a topic and demonstrated the appropriate gesture. The patients imitated the gesture in concert, then individually. A series of gestures was so presented, followed by retrieval probes, where each patient was asked to recall and demonstrate one of the gestures. The clinician asked appropriate questions to elicit use of the gestures in the patient's response. Patients then were asked to volunteer to use the gestures to ask questions. The clinician finally led the session into a conversational pattern about the topic. Similar progressions were used to lead the patients to combine signals to increase the code repertoire. A videotape of each session was reviewed at the close of the session with constructive comment by the clinician. Patients were also encouraged to comment in code. At the beginning of the next session, parts of the prior tape were reviewed by the group as a base for correct retrieval preceding the presentation of new material.

METHODS OF FACILITATION

At the beginning of this attempt to use the Amer-Ind Code as a possible facilitator of oral verbalization, previously acquired signal repertoires were swiftly reviewed. Then the purpose of the project was explained. The following methods were applied to a limited number of signals at each session. Appropriate drills, reviews, and integration into daily use were included.

The clinician demonstrated a signal; then the patients replicated it. The clinician presented the signal, speaking a one-word meaning. This was repeated, with the patients performing the signal simultaneously with the clinician but focusing their attention on the clinician's articulatory movements. The patients then repeated the manual signal in unison, attempting to replicate the clinician's oral movements. Next, the patients were encouraged to attempt vocal synchronization with the manual signal and the oral movement. Within the first month, with two group sessions of two hours a week, some speech was elicited from all six patients.

Immediate repetition of any success was requested. Self-observation by mirror was explored as a facilitator, with negative results. Self-observation by videotape appeared to assist progress. Self- and peer judgment of success contributed positive reinforcement. Recitation in unison accelerated progress. When the group speech efforts were followed at once by individual trials seriatim, the successful patients were usually able to retain and later to reproduce the successful effort. Clinician and peer approval were given generously for any spontaneous oral attempts accompanying presentation of a signal.

All six patients mastered fifty signals within the first two months. Additional useful, modernized signals were added, ranging from seventy to one hundred in the group. All six group members easily interpret over two hundred signals used by the surgical patient with highly developed gestural skill. All six apraxic patients developed some spontaneous oral–verbal production synchronous with their signaling. At the end of a six-month period, the gestural and verbal achievement was again assessed by the PICA.

All six patients made progress in using speech accompanying signaling. Two of them (Patients A and C) are currently attempting three-word sentences of propositional speech related to daily needs and activities without signals. Patients B and D are now using approximately two hundred individual words and placing some of them in phrases; Patient E uses approximately fifty words. They revert to Amer-Ind when words fail but persist in attempts to substitute the oral–verbal for the gestural. Patient F currently approximates production of ten words. While he has made this limited progress in oral production, his communication has profited from the use of Amer-Ind and the accompanying reduction of frustration. PICA scores at the initiation of the pilot project are compared with scores at the termination of the project in Table 2. All six patients are continuing on the clinical schedule.

DISCUSSION

It was expected that the project would increase the gestural scores. While the group's verbal scores increased by a range of low 1.60 to high 7.07, the increase in gestural scores ranged from only 0.03 to 1.62. Although it may be valid, then, to use the gestural–verbal gap on the PICA as a criterion for choosing an apraxic patient for a code group, this group's mastery of ideational signals appears to have had little effect on their scores in manually demonstrating the use of objects in the test.

If the patients' progress is compared by their relative ranks on admission and termination, there is consistency in the verbal score application. Only Patients A and B exchanged ranks. The special deficits of Patient F in vision and audition, plus possible residual effects of his car accident injury, may account for his slower rate of progress. The group's graphic scores increased by a range from zero to 6.56. No pattern of relationship was observed. Except for Patient C, the graphic scores on admission exceeded the verbal scores. On termination, the verbal scores exceeded the graphic scores except for Patients E and F. Patients A and B remain static in graphic score; the others improved.

Five of the six patients made progress, as measured by the verbal scores

TABLE 2. PROJECT FIVE: Differences in patients' scores on admission to the project and on termination.

Patient	Gestural Rank			Verbal Rank			Graphic Rank		
	A	T	D	A	T	D	A	T	D
A	2	4	0.32	1	2	3.15	2	5 (3b)	0
B	6	5	1.16	2	1	6.77	4	4 (3a)	−0.27
C	4	6	0.23	3	3	6.29	6	3	6.56
D	5	3	1.62	4	4	7.07	5	2	5.95
E	1	1	0.03	5	5	4.98	1	1	0.84
F	3	2	1.37	6	6	1.60	3	6 (3c)	1.72

A = admission score, T = termination score, and D = differential. The termination scores of 4, 5 and 6 were all very close.

on the PICA. Comparable improvement in practical daily use was also noted by hospital personnel, family members, and friends. The results of this study warrant further exploration of Amer-Ind as a facilitator of oral verbalization for apraxic patients. Application of similar approaches may be useful for the aphasic.

PROJECT 6: TWENTY APHASIC PATIENTS

The twenty patients listed in this report were all diagnosed as primarily aphasic. Although some patients had additional complications, these were generally characterized as mild. Each patient had undergone previous traditional language rehabilitation programs, ranging in duration from six to twelve months. On the date of admission to the Amer-Ind project, none had any usable verbalization or effective gestures, except in a few cases where a wife or daughter apparently understood some of the patient's self-generative gestures.

All the patients, except patients 19 and 20, were exposed to presentation of a minimum of fifty signals throughout a series of approximately fifty sessions. Patients 19 and 20 received presentation of only forty and thirty signals, respectively, at a similar number of sessions. Additional signals were available through social use, special topic sessions, and video presentation, although not all patients attended the latter.

Results, in summary, show that one patient developed high competence in code and achieved accompanying verbalization on more than 50 percent of his communication attempts. He was considered to have advanced beyond the need of code except for facilitation when in difficulty.

Nine additional patients achieved facilitation of verbal output somewhat consistent with the code level at which they expressed their needs.

Of the twenty patients listed, twelve achieved propositional use of code.

TWENTY APHASIC PATIENTS

Patient No.	Signals Presented to Patient	Imitation (I)	Replication (R)	Social Signal (S)	Answers to Questions (Q)	Need Level (N)	Wish Level (W)	Propositional Equivalent Level (P)	Facilitation (F)	Verbalization (V)
1	200	200	200	200	200	200	200	200	F	
2	200	200	200	200	200	200	200	200	F	V30%
3	200	200	145	145	80	40	40	——	——	——
4	200	185	150	125	140	150	150	150	F	V50%
5	95	95	95	30	60	90	90	80	F	
6	95	95	95	85	65	45	65	15	——	——
7	85	85	40	12	40	48	30	14	F	V40%
8	75	75	75	30	50	60	40	25	——	——
9	65	65	63	30	50	55	55	55	F	V30%
10	65	65	50	3	40	30	30	25	F	V25%
11	65	65	65	30	50	50	50	——	——	——
12	65	64	64	30	50	45	50	——	——	——
13	65	64	64	30	50	60	60	20	F	——
14	60	60	45	30	15	10	10	——	F	——
15	50	50	50	30	30	30	30	——	——	——
16	50	50	50	15	50	50	50	50	——	——
17	50	50	50	20	25	50	50	——	——	——
18	50	50	50	30	35	15	10	——	F	——
19	40	40	40	30	38	40	40	40	——	——
20	30	30	30	30	30	30	30	——	——	——
Mean	——	——	76	57	67	65	64	72	——	——

Of these twelve, eight were among the facilitated verbalizers; the other four have not produced any verbalization as yet. Among the twelve patients signaling at the propositional level, the highest number of signals involved was two hundred, the lowest was twenty (of the sixty-four this patient replicated). It is expected that this score will eventually elevate, as he used sixty of his sixty-four-signal repertoire to express needs.

The relationship among signals presented, replicated successfully, and used propositionally, appeared to be a highly individual one, with no reliable trends apparent in the current data. There appeared to be a high relationship between the number of signals successfully replicated in clinical sessions and the actual use of signals to express needs and wishes: seventeen of the twenty patients used more than half their code repertoire for the latter purposes.

Nineteen of the patients used more than half of their acquired repertoire to respond to questions. Fifteen used social signals at 50 percent of their repertoire. One patient used only three social signals (of his fifty signals acquired) but he had progressed to verbalization at the social level.

All patients involved achieved, to varying degrees, a repertoire of signals and practical use of it. The number of patients achieving each level, and the high, low, and mean (where appropriate) on each use level was:

Level	No. Patients	No. Signals		Level Mean
		High	Low	
Replication	20	200	30	76
Social use	20	200	3	57
Question reply	20	200	15	67
Needs	20	200	10	65
Wishes	20	200	10	64
Propositional	12	200	20	72
Facilitation	10	Not quantified by signal		
Verbalization	5	Not quantified by signal		

Note: A treatment strategy that emphasizes life use of the signals a patient is able to replicate rather than quantitative extension of signals in mere replication may be more profitable to the patient. Certainly mere replication of signals is not very satisfying and contributes nothing to life communication.

PROJECT 7: FIELD REPORTS ON APHASIA

Section A. Forty Patients   Section D: Ten Patients
Section B. Sixty-seven Patients   Section E: Seven Patients
Section C. Twenty Patients   Section F: Seventeen Patients

SECTION A

Eight clinicians contributed data on the forty patients summarized in Section A. All these patients were exposed to instruction on approximately one hundred signals. The time spans varied from three to six months, the sessions from two to four times per week. Usually, sessions were approximately an hour in length, although in some instances they were as brief as a half hour. In general, individual sessions outnumbered group sessions. Most patients were exposed to both individual and group sessions.

No facilitation of verbalization was reported for any of the forty patients. Twenty-five used code at a communication level equivalent to propositional speech, ranging from 112 to 9 signals, with a mean of 28. Fifteen used more than half of their acquired code repertoire in this fashion. Thirty-seven of the forty used signals to satisfy their needs, with twenty-two of them applying more than half their repertoire for this purpose. They ranged from 112 to 4 signals, with a mean of 30. To obtain their wishes, twenty-seven patients ranged from 112 to 4 signals with a mean of 25. Fifteen of them used more than half of their code repertoire at this level. Twenty-nine used social signals with eighteen employing more than half of their repertoire. The range extended from a high of 112 to a low of 10, with the mean at 41.

SECTION B

Reports on a total of another sixty-seven aphasia patients were received from ten additional clinicians in the field. They are reported separately from those in Section A, as their data varied in format. All were highly inform-

FIELD REPORTS ON FORTY APHASIC PATIENTS
INVOLVING EIGHT CLINICIANS—continued

Patient No.	Signals Presented	Imitation (I)	Replication (R)	Social Signals (S)	Answers to Questions (Q)	Need Level (N)	Wish Level (W)	Propositional Level (P)	Facilitated (F)	Verbalization (V)
1	100	——	112	112	112	112	112	112	——	——
2	100	——	100	——	100	100	——	——	——	——
3	100	——	80	30	50	80	75	71	——	——
4	100	——	80	30	40	75	75	71	——	——
5	100	——	72	——	72	72	——	——	——	——
6	100	——	63	——	63	63	——	——	——	——
7	100	——	52	——	52	52	——	——	——	——
8	100	——	50	40	20	33	33	23	——	——
9	100	——	50	35	——	15	15	25	——	——
10	100	——	50	25	——	10	10	20	——	——
11	100	——	50	20	——	10	10	15	——	——
12	100	——	50	20	——	10	10	15	——	——
13	100	——	50	17	15	32	26	26	——	——
14	100	——	48	30	20	10	10	20	——	——
15	100	——	46	10	20	30	24	24	——	——
16	100	——	44	30	——	15	15	30	——	——
17	100	——	44	10	23	25	23	23	——	——
18	100	——	43	15	——	10	10	8	——	——
19	100	——	42	25	——	10	9	15	——	——
20	100	——	41	41	41	41	41	41	——	——
21	100	——	40	40	40	40	40	40	——	——
22	100	——	40	20	——	20	20	20	——	——
23	100	——	38	20	——	8	8	10	——	——
24	100	——	38	38	38	38	——	——	——	——
25	100	——	30	5	10	20	18	22	——	——

ative on an individual basis but not easily transposed for comparison. Some were subjective and descriptive, contributing greatly to estimation of code impact on aphasic patients, but not serving a specified quantification.

From a summation of the clinical information, it appears that results approximated those reported in Project Six and in Section A of this project in terms of patient acquisition of signals and ability to retrieve and replicate them on cue.

In most instances, a very large number of signals was presented to the patients—in a great many instances the entire 193 signals in the video repertoire. The clinicians expressed satisfaction with the number of signals acquired, imitated, and replicated. They reported a lower level, in general, of use of social signals.

There was almost universal dissatisfaction expressed concerning transfer from the cued retrieval/replicative stage to self-initiated use. It is clear that these patients, although able to replicate numerous signals, either could not or would not use signals without the cues associated with acquisition

FIELD REPORTS ON FORTY APHASIC PATIENTS
INVOLVING EIGHT CLINICIANS—continued

Patient No.	Signals Presented	Imitation (I)	Replication (R)	Social Signals (S)	Answers to Questions (Q)	Need Level (N)	Wish Level (W)	Propositional Level (P)	Facilitated (F)	Verbalization (V)
26	100	—	30	15	—	7	8	15	—	—
27	100	—	20	20	—	6	5	10	—	—
28	100	—	20	—	10	17	17	17	—	—
29	100	—	20	5	—	12	—	9	—	—
30	100	—	20	18	2	—	—	—	—	—
31	100	—	20	17	—	—	—	—	—	—
32	100	—	20	15	—	—	—	—	—	—
33	100	—	20	12	2	4	4	—	—	—
34	100	—	20	—	—	2	20	20	—	—
35	100	—	20	20	20	20	20	—	—	—
36	100	—	20	—	—	20	20	—	—	—
37	100	—	20	—	—	20	—	—	—	—
38	100	—	20	—	—	20	—	—	—	—
39	100	—	10	—	10	10	—	—	—	—
40	100	—	10	—	10	10	—	—	—	—
# pts on the level			40	29	22	37	27	25	—	—
$\bar{M}$ for = on level			41	25	32	30	25	28	—	—
$\bar{M}$ for total 40			41	18	19	27	17	18	—	—
Range - High			112	112	112	112	112	112	—	—
- Low			10	5	2	4	4	9	—	—
- Zeros	- none			11	16	3	13	15		

and replication. Usually, they did not respond even to the cueing outside the speech clinic.

Except for their acquisition of a much larger number of signals, results with these patients seem to equate them with the lowest quartile of the forty patients in Section A. As yet, however, no common background factors have been identified for future prognostic use. Search continues for such significant indicators. Further analyses of clinical methods are also indicated. These will be discussed in Part II of this text.

SECTION C

Six clinicians agreed to pool clinical data on aphasic patients in code treatment over a twelve-month period, with initiation of a code program for appropriate patients on admission to the speech clinic. At the end of the twelve months, status data on patients were reported (listed here as termination of project).

The twenty patients in this section were all diagnosed as aphasic. Two were accident victims with head injuries. One had a myocardial infarction, one a subcortical hematoma with craniotomy. The other sixteen had cerebrovascular incidents. Three patients were diagnosed as having accompanying mild oral apraxia, and another was diagnosed as suffering from severe dysarthria. Age levels were widely distributed from 27 to 66, with the two accident victims at 27 and 41. The 33-year-old was a CVA.

Lapse of time between onset and initiation of treatment varied from one to thirty-two months. Treatment schedules varied from one to twelve months, with sessions varying from eight months up to eighty-three, with no consistent relation between time span and number of sessions.

Criteria for admission was speechlessness and diagnosis of aphasia. Patients 11 and 12 had received six months of language rehabilitation prior to the project, with no results. The other patients had no prior speech treatment.

Seven of the twenty patients were untestable on the PICA on admission. Five of these continued as untestable after treatment, although all of them achieved progress in code communication. In two instances, patient's pre- and post-scores remained unchanged, despite progress in code. In one other case, there was no change in verbal score, but a slight increase in gestural score. In three instances, with an untestable report at admission, both verbal and gestural scores were obtained on the project terminal reporting date, with the gestural scores higher than the verbal scores. In all cases where PICA scores were obtained, the gestural scores improved and, except in one case, were higher than the verbal scores. This differs from the report in Project 5 on oral–verbal apraxic patients, where signaling *improvement* did not appear to affect the gestural scores.

Of the twenty patients in the project, nine achieved use of code at the level regarded as equivalent to propositional speech. Five of these used two hundred signals, two used one hundred and one used sixty. Five also were verbalizing. Five other patients were also verbalizing with the signals, although they had a lower level of use: that is, initiating signals in the social context to satisfy needs and wishes, but not otherwise, either conversationally or propositionally. An additional three patients achieved social, need, and wish use of signals and the remaining four used signals to serve their needs. The following table 7C lists the data.

Note: Restoration of normal speech is, of course, the desirable goal in all cases of speechlessness. The Amer-Ind program was developed, however, because realistically many speechless patients do not re-acquire oral speech. For them, the use of Amer-Ind Code at a level of propositional equivalence is the top goal. Therefore, the data table lists the patients in this project in order of success with Amer-Ind. The highest level is the (P) propositional equivalent. The next is use of signals to satisfy wishes (W), lower is its use to satisfy needs (N), lowest is its use socially (S), where possibly the signals are merely conditioned.

Where patients are at the same signal level, they are listed in descending order in terms of number of signals so used. Where more than one patient had the same level and number of signals, these are listed in descending order of time (months/sessions) required to achieve this.

TWENTY PATIENT/SIX CLINICIANS—PICA SCORES

| | | | | | | | | | PICA Scores | | | |
| | | | | | RX | | Results | | Verbal | | Gestural | |
Patient No.	Etiology	Diagnosis	Patient Age	Months Onset–RX	Rx Sessions	Months	Level of Signal Use	No. Signals In Use	Admission	Termination	Admission	Termination
1			49	1	20	3	P F	200	3.87	9.62	7.40	7.92
2		X	46	8	56	7	P F	200	5.57	11.60	13.67	13.80
3			54	5	70	3	P F	200	3.65	11.90	12.01	12.88
4			54	5	60	5	P F	200	9.50	13.75	12.05	14.03
5	TR		41	8	60	4	P F	200	Fluctuating Results			
6			60	13	56	6	P F	100	9.77	SAME	11.95	SAME
7			33	8	28	4	P	100	FLUCTUATING			
8	HC	X	51	4	48	10	P	100	4.95	No Change	12.66	13.25
9			60	8	40	5	P	60	U	Signaled Fluctuating		
10			53	8	64	8	SNWF	120	U	4.32	U	11.82
11			61	24	50	6	SNWF	50	3.20	11.60	10.80	12.78
12			56	32	56	12	SNWF	50	6.70	12.35	10.75	12.97
13			48	2	26	2	N F	50	4.70	10.37	3.53	7.08
14		X	66	7	19	3	SNW	50	U	3.34	U	10.25
15			54	1	96	11	SNW	50	U	11.20	U	10.25
16	M		60	3	83	6	SNW	40	2.60	3.00	10.92	13.90
17			61	1	70	11	N	75	3.12	3.37	9.00	12.36
18		D	56	8	1	1	N	40	U	U	U	U
19			56	12	26	6	N	30	8.64	10.47	12.52	13.56
20			27	2	26	12	N	30	5.58	10.12	10.86	12.58

Etiology: TR = head injury from accident; HC = hematoma (subcortical)/craniotomy; M = myocardial infarction; all others are CVA.
Diagnosis: X = apraxia;
D = dysarthria; all others are Aphasia.
PICA scores: U = untestable.
Results: F = Verbal Facilitation; P = Propositional level; S = Social Signal; N = Needs; W = Wishes.

SECTION D: FIELD REPORTS—FORT HOWARD VA HOSPITAL PROJECT WITH APHASICS*

Introduction

The Audiology and Speech Pathology service (A&SP) of the Fort Howard Veterans Administration Hospital has offered a program in Amer-Ind code since February 1976. The goal of treatment was to teach nonverbal, gestural signals as an alternative means of communication. Facilitation of

*Reported by P.R. Rao, A.G. Basili, J. Horner, and J. Koller, Amer-Ind Conference, St. Louis, October 1977.

oral–verbal expression was a complementary treatment goal. The population was comprised of severe, chronic aphasic individuals. Progress in traditional therapy had plateaued and patients were nonfunctional in the oral–verbal modality at the time of admission to the project.

Description of Patients

Ten male veteran patients were enrolled. They ranged in age from 38 to 65, with a mean age of 54 years. Nine of the ten patients had suffered a single cerebrovascular accident to the left hemisphere, while one patient suffered left hemisphere traumatic insult. All ten patients presented aphasia as measured by the Aphasia Language Performance Scales (ALPS) (Keenan and Brassell, 1975) and as diagnosed by a certified speech–language pathologist. As indicated in Table 1 three patients were classified as presenting profound language involvement, six were classified severe, and one was moderate-to-severe. Each patient exhibited limb apraxia and/or apraxia of speech. With respect to limb apraxia, two patients were classified as profound, four as severe, one as moderate-to-severe, and one as mild. With respect to apraxia of speech, four patients were classified as profound, five as severe, and one as moderate-to-severe. Thus, each of the ten patients exhibited some degree of limb apraxia. Table 1 also includes the ALPS overall score received when the test was administered to each patient at the time of initial evaluation.

Amer-Ind Program

Performance criteria for admission were: (1) failure to achieve anticipated gains from traditional therapy, and; (2) presence of one or more positive prognostic indicators warranting continued inclusion in a speech pathology rehabilitation program, e.g., short time post-onset, moderate age, and/or stimulability. All patients in the program participated in group treatment for at least two half-hour sessions per week, involving direct training of a core Amer-Ind repertoire (approximately 150 signals), comprised of single

TABLE 1. PATIENT PROFILE UPON ADMISSION TO A&SP

Patients	Age	Etiology	Aphasia Classification	Apraxia Limb	Classification: Speech	Admission Overall ALPS
1	59	L CVA	Severe	Severe	Profound	2.25
2	55	L CVA	Severe	Moderate-/Severe	Moderate-/Severe	2.75
3	59	L CVA	Severe	Profound	Profound	3.25
4	59	L CVA	Profound	Mild	Severe	1.5
5	53	L CVA	Moderate-/Severe	None	Severe	4.38
6	57	L CVA	Severe	Severe	Severe	1.63
7	65	L CVA	Severe	Profound	Severe	2.25
8	46	L CVA	Profound	Severe	Profound	1.0
9	51	TRAUMA	Profound	Severe	Profound	1.15
10	38	L CVA	Severe	None	Severe	2.38

object, action and descriptive signals and basic agglutinations. Initial treatment involved eliciting imitative gestures and progressed to spontaneous signaling through the use of real object, picture, and printed word cues. Verbalization was reinforced only in a gestural context and only when the verbal response was appropriate and intelligible. Verbalization was neither discouraged, nor actively encouraged. This complement to gesture was accepted as an attempt at total communication and was measured independently of gestural communication.

Results

Background. As Table 3 (p. 47) shows, eight patients had previously received less than six months of traditional therapy and one patient received more than one year. All ten patients failed to achieve functional communication with traditional therapy alone. Table 3 also reports the length of Amer-Ind treatment and indicates which patients achieved anticipated gains. Of the ten subjects, three were terminated because of apparent failure to benefit. The remaining seven patients showed continuous positive changes in language abilities.

Severity. Table 2 presents ALPS performance data chronologically from project admission to the most recent ALPS. Prior to the project, each patient's overall ALPS score was stable (+ or −.05 out of 10 overall) for at least two consecutive months. A comparison of each patient's preproject overall ALPS score with the most recent overall ALPS score is seen in Table 3. These data show that seven of the ten patients improved beyond the plateau observed during a unitary, traditional therapy regime. Therefore, these data offer support for the view that participation by these select patients in Amer-Ind facilitated continued language recovery.

The greatest improvement in overall performance was 2.0 (on a scale of 10), with five patients achieving an overall improvement of 0.5 or greater. A comparison of pre- and postproject performances shows a marked reduction in severity in aphasic involvement, as well as reduced severity of both apraxia of speech and limb apraxia. The most positive changes were noted in patients at the lower end of the severity scale. Preproject ratings found four out of the ten patients exhibited a severe limb apraxia, while postproject ratings found only one patient in the severe range; three patients improved to a moderate-severe level. Similarly, nine out of the ten patients presented profound severe apraxia of speech prior to the project, while postproject assessment found only seven of the ten patients in this range. Thus patients who had failed to achieve anticipated gains from a regime that excluded gestural expressive stimulation exhibited positive changes once enrolled in group gestural therapy. Amelioration of oral apraxia was also noted clinically a posteriori.

In addition to the ALPS, nine of the ten patients were administered two other independent measures: the *Peabody Picture Vocabulary Test* (PPVT) (Dunn, 1959), a test of receptive vocabulary, and the *Raven's Coloured Progressive Matrices* (RCPM) (Raven, 1956), a test of visual abstract reasoning (see Table 4, p. 47). Of the nine patients who were administered the

TABLE 2. SUMMARY OF LANGUAGE TEST RESULTS

Patients	Scale	Original ALPS	Change	Before Amer-Ind	Change	During/After Amer-Ind
1	L	3.0	+	5.0	-0-	5.0
	T	0	-0-	0	-0-	0
	R	3.0	+	5.0	-0-	5.0
	W	3.0	+	3.5	+	5.0
	O	2.5	+	3.38	+	3.75
2	L	3.0	+	5.0	+	5.5
	T	1.0	-0-	1.0	+	4.5
	R	3.0	-0-	3.0	+	5.5
	W	4.0	-0-	4.0	+	4.5
	O	2.75	+	3.0	+	5.0
*3	L	2.0	+	6.0	+	7.5
	T	1.0	-0-	1.0	+	3.0
	R	5.5	—	4.0	+	6.5
	W	4.5	+	5.5	+	6.5
	O	3.25	+	4.13	+	6.0
*4	L	2.0	+	6.5	+	7.5
	T	2.0	+	3.0	+	4.0
	R	0	+	4.5	+	6.0
	W	2.0	+	4.0	+	6.0
	O	1.5	+	4.5	+	5.88
*5	L	5.0	-0-	5.0	+	8.5
	T	4.5	-0-	4.5	—	3.0
	R	2.5	+	3.0	+	4.0
	W	2.5	+	4.5	+	5.0
	O	3.63	+	4.25	+	5.12
*6	L	1.0	+	2.0	-0-	2.0
	T	1.5	+	2.0	—	1.5
	R	2.0	-0-	2.0	—	1.5
	W	2.0	-0-	2.0	+	2.5
	O	1.63	+	2.0	—	1.88
7	L	2.0	-0-	2.0	—	1.5
	T	3.0	—	1.5	+	2.5
	R	2.0	+	3.0	—	2.0
	W	2.0	+	2.5	-0-	2.5
	O	2.25	-0-	2.25	—	2.13
8	L	2.0	—	1.5	-0-	1.5
	T	0	+	1.5	—	1.0
	R	1.0	+	2.0	-0-	2.0
	W	1.0	+	3.0	+	4.0
	O	1.0	+	1.88	+	2.12
9	L	2.0	-0-	2.0	-0-	2.0
	T	0	+	1.0	-0-	1.0
	R	1.5	+	2.0	-0-	2.0
	W	1.13	+	1.5	-0-	1.5
	O	1.15	+	1.63	-0-	1.63
*10	L	2.0	-0-	2.0	+	3.0
	T	3.5	—	2.5	+	3.5
	R	1.0	-0-	1.0	+	2.0
	W	3.0	—	2.5	-0-	2.5
	O	2.38	—	2.0	+	2.75
Range	L	1.0 5.0		1.5 6.5		1.5 8.5
	T	0 4.5		0 4.5		0 4.5
	R	0 5.5		1.0 5.0		1.5 6.5
	W	1.0 4.5		1.5 5.5		1.5 7.0
	O	1.0 4.38		1.63 4.5		1.63 6.0

*Received both traditional therapy *and* Amer-Ind. L=Listening; T=Talking; R=Reading; W=Writing; O=Overall.

TABLE 3. FAILURE TO ACHIEVE ANTICIPATED GAINS FROM THERAPY (TRADITIONAL VS AMER-IND)

Patient	Months of Traditional Rx	Failure To Achieve Anticipated Gains From Traditional Rx	Months of Amer-Ind Rx	Failure To Achieve Anticipated Gains From Amer-Ind Rx
1	1	Yes	10	No
2	1	Yes	15	No
3	3	Yes	12	No
4	2	Yes	12	No
5	2	Yes	3	No
6	5	Yes	3	Yes
7	2	Yes	5	Yes
8	12	Yes	20	No
9	16	Yes	12	Yes
10	1	Yes	4	No

Patient	Received Traditional & Amer-Ind Rx Concurrently	Improvement Following Cessation of Traditional Rx Only	Gains As Measured by Overall Most Recent ALPS
1	No	Yes	+ .37
2	No	Yes	+2.0
3	Yes	Yes	+1.77
4	Yes	Yes	+1.38
5	Yes	Yes	+ .87
6	Yes	No	− .12
7	No	No	− .12
8	No	Yes	+ .24
9	No	No Change	-0-
10	Yes	Yes	+ .75

TABLE 4. RESULTS OF OTHER MEASURES

Patient	First PPVT (Raw Score)	First RCPM (Raw Score)	Last PPVT (Raw Score)	Last RCPM (Raw Score)
1	32	28	59	29
2	75	19	87	23
3	83	30	123	34
4	37	32	93	36
5	74	18	78	25
6	63	20	56	26
7	3	20	7	*
8	0	12	20	22
9	*	*	*	*
10	4	26	75	27

*Test was not administered.

PPVT on admission and post Amer-Ind, eight exhibited positive changes, with raw score changes from 4 to 71 (out of 150). Only one patient exhibited regression on the PPVT, with a decrease in raw score of 7. Notable increments in receptive vocabulary were noted in three patients: patient 3's raw score improved 30 points; patient 4, 56 points; and patient 10, 71 points. The RCPM also showed positive changes. Admission and post-project RCPM scores were obtained on eight patients (one patient was administered the RCPM on admission only, and one patient was not tested using the RCPM). For the eight patients reported, initial RCPM raw scores ranged from 12 to a maximum of 36 with a mean score of 23.12. Final RCPM scores ranged from 22 to 36, with a mean score of 27.75. Each of the eight patients for whom RCPM performance is reported exhibited progress in visual abstract reasoning ability as measured by the RCPM, while two of these patients showed notable improvement: patient 4 received a final score of 36, and patient 8 nearly doubled his original score (12 to 22).

Summary

Data on ten patients who were enrolled in an Amer-Ind group program over a two-year period have been summarized. These patients had failed to achieve anticipated gains from traditional treatment alone, and were subsequently enrolled in an Amer-Ind program.

Available standardized and clinical data obtained before, during, and after participation were reported on overall language abilities as measured by the ALPS, apraxia of speech, limb apraxia, receptive vocabulary, and visual abstract reasoning ability. Improvements were noted in one or more areas in most patients. This favorable clinical impression was corroborated by over half of the spouses or significant others who communicated with these individuals on a daily basis. The complaint, "I don't know what he's trying to tell me, it's so frustrating," was alleviated following the patients' participation in AAP. Thus, the project appears to have enhanced the receptive and expressive abilities of these patients to some degree.

Several factors may limit conclusions: the heterogeneity of subjects; the various lengths of treatment; the failure, in some cases, to administer supplementary language tests immediately prior to enrollment; and the lack of standardized evaluation of limb and oral apraxia. However, the strong trend toward significant continued gains in language in this group of severe chronic aphasics suggests the need for continued investigation.

SECTION E: FIELD REPORTS—ALBANY VA HOSPITAL*

Patients and Treatment

Seven aphasic patients received treatment with Amer-Ind code from October 1976 to August 1977. Six of these patients had cerebrovascular accidents, the other suffered from post-infectious leuko-encephalopathy. The

---

*Reported by Jill Boehler, Amer-Ind Conference, St. Louis, October 1977.

latter was 31 years old. The others were 67, 50, 73, 49, 59, and 74 years old. Patients had individual sessions, which varied according to their needs and tolerances. All were involved in weekly group meetings, primarily structured to encourage and elicit use of signals previously acquired. The group session included a brief review of previously acquired signals and the introduction of some new signals, according to group needs. Where appropriate, signals in the same category were also included on an association basis. The major portion of the group meeting was devoted to a club-like schedule with activities encouraging the appropriate use of code in the particular situations arranged by the clinician.

Results

Five of the patients, including the 31-year-old, achieved use of self-initiated code to serve their daily communication needs. Signals were acquired easily, retained, and used effectively. In uncontrolled situations, these patients tended to attempt verbal communication initially, but finding this unproductive, substituted code immediately and successfully. The other two patients had no difficulty imitating the signals, but were unable to retain them from session to session. They did not produce any self-initiated signals.

Patient 6 had little contact with people other than ward personnel. He was a long-term nursing home care patient who appeared to have little desire to communicate. He had had prior extensive speech treatment for many months without effect.

Patient 7 functioned at a very low receptive level. Although unable to repeat any verbal patterns, respond verbally to cues, or retain signals, he did produce some appropriate verbalizations when attempting to imitate signals.

The major factors in a patient's success in this project appeared to be the patient's need or desire to communicate, the number and frequency of communicative situations in which he was placed, and the reception his efforts received from the people in his environment, especially their acceptance of the gestural mode. Successful signaling appears to be highly related to reinforcement of the patient's signaling. The patient retains those signals that afford him rewarding communication. His progress appeared highly related to the amount of time he was placed in situations requiring communication or response from him. It may be very important to orient both family and ward personnel to afford the patient this type of opportunity for communication and reward.

SECTION F: FIELD REPORTS—TOPEKA VA HOSPITAL*

Patient population. Primarily moderate to severe dysphasia, with accompanying dyspraxia (oral and frequently manual) and occasionally, significant dysarthria, were the diagnosed impairments of the patients.

---

*Reported by Zilpha T. Bosone, Amer-Ind Conference, St. Louis, October 1977.

Goals

1. To develop the *concept* of using gestures for communication:
   a. to initiate meaningful, intelligible signals as a means of self-expression;
   b. to initiate meaningful, intelligible signals that are adjunctive to spoken language.
2. To enhance language training in auditory/visual comprehension by using a multimodal approach.

Methods. A multimodal approach was used for most patients, emphaing those concepts that are most useful in the patient's milieu. The patient was encouraged to use gesture, speech, writing, and drawing as a means of self-expression. If one of these modalities emerged as the most successful means of communication, that modality received additional, or even exclusive, attention.

The group setting was found to be especially helpful for inculcating gestural communication. All meaningful, appropriate signals were accepted. Specific techniques that were used to elicit gestures include:

1. Videotapes with clinicians demonstrating specific concepts. The patients described and discussed what they had seen.
2. Patients were encouraged to use gestures to describe their activities for a particular time period (a weekend, a home visit, morning, etc.).
3. Group activity sequences were used for gestural comprehension and expression. For example:
   a. One patient described a picture using gestures; another patient selected the picture he believed had been described.
   b. Patients used gestures to ask for a specific object from another patient.
   c. Items were removed from a tray of common, useful objects, and each patient guessed, using gestures, which objects had been removed.
4. Objects were manipulated or actions were taken by the clinician according to the directions given in gesture by the patient(s).
5. Expansion of gestural communication was encouraged by having the patient provide more detail by gesturing quantity, color, and object label.
6. Generalization of responses were attempted through in-service training of hospital staff and the patients' families. Follow-up reports of patients' communication skills were obtained periodically.

Problems:	Solutions:
1. Manual dyspraxia	Direct patient to look at his hand(s) as he executes the gestures. Manipulation of the patient's hand(s) is also used.
2. Incomplete agglutinated signs	Simplify signals to only one movement, when possible.
3. Poor motivation to learn or use gestures	(a) Group the sessions so that patient can see and be inspired by the attempts of others.
(a) due to primary desire to speak, even though speech may be completely unintelligible;	(b) Provide opportunity for success in using gestures to manipulate his environment.

(b) due to the idea that hand signaling is silly, childish, or a mark of failure to regain speech.

4. Lack of opportunity to communicate.

(c) Explain that the use of gestures may aid in developing more meaningful speech.

(d) Explain or show many occasions in sports, etc. where hand signals are customary.

In-service training for hospital staff; training for family members.

Results: Levels of Use. Seventeen patients were involved in the program. Four patients had such severe problems, including manual apraxia, that gesture was unsuccessful at any level. Six of the patients used some gestures in the clinic situation with success in expressing the concepts under consideration that day. However, these patients did not gesture outside the clinic. Three patients used self-initiated gestures for communication outside the clinic for expression of basic, immediate needs. One patient used gestures successfully as his sole means of communication at a level approaching propositional speech. Three patients achieved some improvement in spoken language, both in quantity and appropriateness.

PROJECT 8: THREE SECTIONS

SECTIONS A & B*

The Patients

Ten speechless persons diagnosed as mentally retarded were chosen for a pilot program in Amer-Ind as an alternative mode of communication. Three of the subjects were classified as profoundly retarded, the others as very severely retarded. Intelligence quotients were not obtainable. The project was planned for ten weeks, with four sessions per week of at least twenty minutes each. Two of the profoundly retarded patients were dropped from the program in its early stages, one because of psychotic attacks, the other for additional eye contact and attention training, which is a preliminary requirement. There were some unavoidable interruptions of the planned schedule, resulting in a reduction of the total treatment sessions to thirty rather than the planned forty.

All sessions were individual, as initially there were behavior control problems not consonant with group treatment. Procedures were all based on concrete referents. Usually the signals for EAT and DRINK were demonstrated first, with various types of food and liquids, which were also used for rewards. Other early signals included STOP/WAIT, SIT/STAND, COME/GO, TIRED/REST, WASH, and TOILET. As quickly as possible with each patient, attempts were made to demonstrate that the patient's signaling could control the conduct of those around him. SIT/STAND appears the best initial signal for this purpose. It provided a variation on the typical food reward; also, there was a built-in reinforcement when the clinician obeyed the patient's signaling. Social signals were introduced in appropriate situations, and imitation was elicited when possible. Tactile or kinetic assistance was provided where needed.

*Reported by J. Podleski, of the staff of the St. Louis State School/Hospital, on "Amer-Ind with the Mentally Retarded," Amer-Ind Conference, St. Louis, October 1977.

At the end of the initial pilot of ten weeks, there was enough progress to warrant continuance. The patients were scored and summated, and then continued for an additional ten-week period. Each ten-week project was scored individually, and the two compared.

Results

All eight patients elevated their level of signal use in the second project, although in three cases there was no increase in the number of signals used. The level of use is regarded as the more important of the two scorings. (See pp. 97–107 for detailed explanation of levels on the Amer-Ind Scale.) The mean for the group was nineteen signals and the range 29–5 for the thirty signals attempted. Level use ranged from level I to level V. Seven of the eight patients exhibited desirable behavior changes during both projects. Even with those who had signal use at a low level, there was apparently greatly improved signal comprehension. Directives that previously had been ignored when spoken were now obeyed when signaled. Seven of the patients demonstrated this increased understanding of signals. Three attempted verbalization when signaling and had stabilized three words orally in this fashion. Two others had produced phonation when attempting to signal. Five increased their use of signals. While three patients showed no increase in number of signals, two of these (patients 6 and 7) were among the verbalizers, and they, too, modified their behavior. Incidentally, patient 6 was the patient rated as profoundly impaired. Progress with this type of patient has been slow and the increments small. With improved methods it is hoped that progress can be accelerated in both directions. Patient data and scores are summarized in the following table.

SECTIONS A AND B

Project No.	Age	Desirable Behavior Change	Signal Levels	Verbalization	Phonation	Self-gesture	Physical facilitation	Comprehension of Signals	Execution of Signals
1	21	Yes	(I–V)			Yes	/k,	(25–29)	(25–29)
2	18	Yes	(I–IV)	Yes, 3	Yes	Yes		(16–27)	(16–27)
3	24	Yes	(I–IV)		Yes			(14–40)	(14–40)
4	22	Yes	(I–IV)			Yes	/k	(17–19)	(17–19)
5	24	Yes	(I–III)				/k	(10–12)	(10–12)
6	24	Yes	(I–III)	Yes 3			/k	(11–11)	(11–11)
7	20	Yes	(I–III)	Yes				(6–6)	(6–6)
8	20	No	(I–III)					(5–5)	(0–0)

In all bracketed scores (Project A) the first figure is the number at the end of the first ten weeks, second is the number at the end of the second ten weeks (Project B).
Level V is transition to self-initiated signal use. Level IV indicates signal retrieval from memory for use. Level III indicates ability to execute signals with cues. /k indicates need for kinetic assistance.

SECTION C*

The same clinician who conducted Sections A & B of this project, also conducted Section C simultaneously with B. In Section C, an additional six patients were chosen; five were diagnosed as very severely retarded, one as profoundly so. The same methods and procedures were used as in Section A.

Results

Three of these patients made suitable changes in behaviors, where needed. The other three were cooperative and did not require change. One patient produced some verbalization with two of his thirty-nine signals. Two others acquired some social signal use. Two required kinetic assistance to execute the signals. Three reached level III in execution and three achieved level V with some of the signals (transition to self-initiated use). The mean for the group was twenty signals with a range of 39 to 10.

PROJECT 8

	Age	Sign level	Phon. Verb	Compre-hension	Execution
1	22	III & V		39	39
2	22	III & V		33	33/k
3	22	III & V		16	13
4	23	III		14	9
5	22	III		11	5/k
6	21	III		10	8

PROJECT 9: AMER-IND IN MENTAL RETARDATION**

This project in the use of Amer-Ind with mentally retarded subjects involved a population of twenty severely and profoundly mentally retarded physically handicapped children and adults, hereafter referred to as "residents." The age range was from 8 to 47 years with one eight-year-old, ten teenagers, five in their 20s, two in their 30s, and two in their 40s.

The project was divided into two ten-week segments. Sessions were scheduled daily, five days per week, for a projected total of forty sessions. Because of many interfering factors, this was reduced so that the mean number of sessions was twenty-four.

METHODS

Methods followed the levels and steps proposed in the Amer-Ind Scale (see pp. 97–107). Emphasis was placed on signaling meaningful to the residents

---

*Reported by J. Podleski on "Amer-Ind with Mentally Retarded—the Severe to Profound Range, Amer-Ind Conference, St. Louis, October 1977.
**Reported by Janet Freese and Victoria Frerker of the St. Louis Developmental Disabilities Center, with the assistance of Jo Ann Johnson and Dennis Caldwell.

within their environment and experience. This included skills (washing hands, brushing hair, etc.), enjoyment (music, toys, activities, etc.), and individual needs and wishes. Emphasis was also placed on dealing with interfering behaviors. Since the residents enjoyed the individual attention received in the signaling sessions, whenever deviant behavior was exhibited, the resident was removed from the session for the remainder of that day. Emphasis was placed on physically manipulating the resident. Physical assistance, both tactile and kinetic, was given in shaping the signals. Sustained eye contact was required before initiating signaling. Extraneous stimuli of all kinds were eliminated from the clinical setting.

RESULTS

Failures

Selection of inappropriate candidates for signaling occurred in some instances. Physical imitation, pointing and shaping skills probably should be developed prior to sessions in code.

Resident use of signals with other staff did not occur, due to lack of reinforcement by staff. Future in-service emphasis will be placed on rapport with ward staff and other professionals to secure their cooperation.

Problems

1. The proposed procedure for concept generalization through presentation of three items related to a signal may have been overstimulating to the residents in this specific project. The residents appeared more interested in appropriating the items than in attending to the signal representing them. We are now presenting only one item at a time, but changing the item in each category daily. In this fashion, the residents are presented with various items for generalization, but confined to the one on each occasion which will secure the related reward.
2. Residents do not understand the basic principle of communication. They have no need to communicate, as everything is done for them routinely. In-service staff education may assist in changing this, so some pressures will be exerted socially for signal communication of which each resident is capable. The residents have never been able to manipulate other people. Signal sessions may be structured to help residents learn this cause and effect relationship of communication.
3. Initially, it was difficult to distinguish some of the residents' self-stimulatory behavior from some of the signals. More observation of residents outside the clinical setting is planned for future programs.
4. Deviant behaviors were a problem. Eliminating such behaviors prior to signal sessions may improve the signal acquisition.
5. Some residents had developed self-created gestures for *bathroom*, *eat*, and *drink*, so there was confusion in acquisition of the coded signals. We plan to accept such gestures and gradually shape them to the code.

Successes

1. The residents involved in the program have become more attentive and are extending the attention span.
2. More imitative skills have been acquired.
3. Residents are exhibiting less self-stimulatory behavior.
4. Residents have developed more awareness and use of their hands in many ways.
5. There has been a noticeable decrease in deviant behaviors in signal sessions and also in many instances on the wards. Some of the residents at first exhibited such undesirable behavior (as temper tantrums), but now check themselves and resume control.

The residents have acquired an average of twenty-five signals during the two ten-week projects. The individuals range from 47 to 9 signals. Their levels range from level I to level IX. One resident uses signals at level IX, facilitating oral speech. One uses it at level VIII which is the equivalent of propositional speech. Thirteen use their signals at level VI, which expresses their needs and wishes and assists them in answering questions. One resident is at level IV, which is transitional to use. Two are at level III, imitation of the clinician's signals, and one is at level I, which is presignal stimulation for attention and eye contact.

PROJECT 10: IMPACTS OF LEARNING AMER-IND ON MENTALLY RETARDED CHILDREN*

Many mentally retarded children, particularly those with IQ's below 50, fail to acquire enough speech for even their basic communication needs. There has been considerable interest during the past few years in the use of total communication approach (i.e., simultaneous speech and manual signing) with such children. The manual system used by almost all investigators with these children is American Sign Language (AMESLAN), the system of finger spelling and manual signing used by the deaf. While this system is extremely flexible, the gestures are not highly intelligible to untrained interpreters. Recently, an alternative manual system has been introduced by Skelly (1975) known as American Indian Code (Amer-Ind) that is reported to be more concrete than AMESLAN and *over 80 percent* intelligible to untrained observers. This report summarizes the impacts of a ten-week total communication program using Amer-Ind on thirty-two moderately retarded children.

Ss ranged in age from 3 to 19 years with a mean age of 10.5 years. Their *MA*s ranged from 2 to 5 years. The judged intelligibility levels of their speech at the beginning of the program ranged from 0 percent to 25 percent.

Ss participated in four to five thirty-minute individual and group sessions

*Reported by Janice L. Duncan of the Columbus Special Education Center, Kenosha, Wisconsin, and Franklin L. Silverman, Marquette University, Milwaukee.

per week. Emphasis was on teaching Amer-Ind signals they could use in their school or home environments. The *Ss* classroom teachers reinforced their use of total communication throughout the day. Both the speech clinician and the classroom teacher charted each child's verbal and gestural communication daily.

The therapy outcome criteria suggested by Silverman (1977, pp. 250–251) were used to assess the impacts of the Program on *Ss*. Of the thirty-two *Ss*, twenty-seven were observed by the clinician and/or teacher using Amer-Ind spontaneously for communicative purposes. The number of signals learned by *Ss* during the ten-week period ranged from 15 to 200 with a mean of 48. Fifteen *Ss* were reported by their teacher, clinician, and/or parents to have increased their attempts to communicate by speech; none were reported to have reduced their attempts to communicate in this manner. Thirteen *Ss* were reported to have made noticeable changes in overall behavior, including (1) reduced frustration behavior, such as temper tantrums, and (2) increased willingness to participate in language activities. All of the children seemed to accept the use of Amer-Ind and all of the families appeared to be supportive of their children's participation in the program.

The results were considered encouraging enough by staff and parents to warrant continuing the children in the Program. The results to date suggest that Amer-Ind may be preferable to AMESLAN for mentally retarded children because of its concreteness and, more importantly, because of its high intelligibility to untrained observers.

Transmission: Projects 11–19

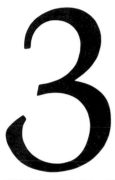

PROJECT 11: SIGNAL TRANSMISSION TO 110 UNINSTRUCTED VIEWERS

Both American Indian tradition and European historians supported the high level of viewer understanding of American Indian Hand Talk without specific instruction in it. Early projects with speechless patients gave evidence of such ease of acquisition. For implementation of the program in general clinical use, however, it appeared desirable to test transmission success in a more structured and measurable situation.

The first project was concerned with a general population of 110 persons. This group was formed by requesting cooperation from persons encountered during one week of hospital duty. Lack of any formal connection with speech pathology or medicine, lack of any knowledge of any manual system, and willingness to cooperate were the only criteria. The group included seventy females and forty males. They ranged from 14 to 70 years in age, with a median in the 40s. The educational mean was high school graduation.

Each viewer was given an answer sheet on which numbers represented the signals. Category cues were provided. The stimulus was a pre-prepared video cassette, presenting a competent patient signaler demonstrating fifty signals, which were randomly chosen from two hundred used with patients to date. Each signal was presented twice, with its accompanying identifying number. Each viewer was instructed to write the English word that best represented the meaning of the signal. It was stated emphatically that there was no one correct answer, but a wide conceptual range from which to choose a particular word. The examiner demonstrated three samples.

Only two of the participants scored less than 75 percent correct interpretation of the signal concept. Sixty-three of the participants scored above 80 percent, eleven scored above 90 percent. There was no correlation between test scores and age, educational level, or sex. Viewer success is summarized in the accompanying table.

SIGNAL TRANSMISSION TO 110 UNINSTRUCTED
VIEWERS BY ONE COMPETENT PATIENT-SIGNALER

| Viewers | | Score range |
%	#	in %
	4 · · ·	95–100
11.8	9 · · ·	90–94
	14 · · ·	85–89
50.9	42 · · ·	80–84
	39 · · ·	75–79
36.36	1 · · ·	70
0.91	1 · · ·	66

PROJECT 12: TRANSMISSION TO SPEECH PATHOLOGISTS BY PATIENT-SIGNALER

At the introductory session of a professional workshop, sixteen speech clinicians who were assembled for the workshop, witnessed a pretest of a videotape of fifty randomly selected signals, presented by a patient-signaler. No cues were given. The viewers were informed that the signals were intended to convey concepts, not particular words. Three example signals with lists of associated English words were provided. Each viewer was to write an identifying word for each signal presented, attempting to choose the label that embraced the widest range of the associated concept.

Seven of the professional viewers had no prior experience with any manual system. Five had minimal exposure to a brief video demonstration of Amer-Ind a year previously. Four persons had moderate exposure, having witnessed the video presentation of Amer-Ind at the ASHA convention two years previously.

The seven with no prior experience averaged ten errors (range 3–14) with an 80 percent success score. Those with the minimal exposure averaged 9.6 errors (range 5–13) with success score of 81 percent. Those with moderate exposure averaged six errors (range 5–7) with success score of 88 percent. The total group averaged 8.5 errors (range 3–14), average of 83 percent success (range 94 to 72 percent).

While these viewers may be considered better prepared than the general public, the scores are encouraging for comparatively uninstructed viewers.

TRANSMISSION TO 16 SPEECH PATHOLOGISTS
OF VARYING FAMILIARITY WITH SIGNALING

No exposure	Range	Errors	Success %
7	3–14	10	80
Minimal Exposure			
5	5–13	9.6	81
Moderate exposure			
4	5–7	6	88

PROJECT 13: TRANSMISSION AT PROFESSIONAL WORKSHOPS

A more formal testing of transmission with a larger population was undertaken in connection with five scheduled workshops for professional speech pathologists at various locations in the United States. Twenty participants with no training or experience in manual systems were chosen to attend each workshop for instruction in Amer-Ind and its clinical use. At the first session a preworkshop transmission test was administered. A video of a competent patient-signaler was presented, demonstrating fifty randomly chosen signals, each of which was listed by number only. Signals were grouped in broadly related categories, and a category cue was indicated on the test sheet. Participants were instructed to write the first English word that came to mind when the signal was completed. Each signal was presented twice.

Following completion of the test, the video was repeated, accompanied by a variety of English words related to the concept demonstrated. Time was alloted for discussion of any English words listed that differed from the established concept labels in clinical use. Participants scored their own tests, with the workshop director reviewing all.

In workshop A the highest score was 90 percent, the lowest 70 percent, in each case representing one person. Two participants scored 76 percent; the other sixteen were all in the 80–88 percent bracket.

In workshop B, the high score was 98 percent, the low 64 percent, with one person high and two low. Two participants scored 90 percent, one 78 percent, the other fourteen were all in the 80–88 percent group.

In workshop C, the high score was 92 percent, the low score 80 percent. Four persons scored 90 percent, the other nine were distributed throughout the 80–88 percent bracket.

In workshop D, the high score was 98 percent, the low score 60 percent, in each case representing one person. This group had the most widely distributed scores, with one at 96 percent, one at 90 percent, one at 62 percent, one at 70 percent, three at 78 percent, and eight in the 80–88 percent bracket.

In workshop E, the high score was 100 percent, the low 78 percent, with one in the high, and two in the low. Six additional participants scored in the 90–94 percent bracket, with the remaining eleven in the 80–88 percent group.

When the scores are summated for the five groups, the high score is, of course, 100 percent, and the low 60 percent. Since 100 participants are involved, each represents 1 percent of the summated figures. Nineteen percent of the participants scored in the 9th decile (90–100), 64 percent scored in the 8th decile (80–88), 13 percent scored in the 7th decile, and 4 percent

TRANSMISSION OF SIGNALS—100 VIEWERS
(50 SIGNALS, RANDOM, COMPETENT PATIENT-SIGNALER)

		Number of Viewers	Viewers' Score	Professional Viewer Groups				
				A	B	C	D	E
83%	19%	1	100					1
		2	98		1		1	
		1	96				1	
		1	94					1
		2	92			1		1
		12	90	1	2	4	1	4
	64%	8	88	1	2	2		3
		9	86	4		2	2	1
		11	84	4	2	2	1	2
		14	82	3	4	3	4	
		22	80	4	6	6	1	5
13%		6	78		1		3	2
		2	76	2				
			74					
			72				4	
		5	70	1				
4%			68					
			66					
		2	64			2		
		1	62				1	
		1	60				1	

in the 6th decile. Additional summation shows that 83 percent of the participants scored at or above 80 percent success in interpreting the signals. Conversely, we can state that only 4 percent scored below 70 percent success, while 96 percent scored above 70 percent.

It appears from this study that speech pathologists, uninstructed in this code, can and do interpret it at a highly successful level. Many acoustic studies performed by the Bell Telephone Laboratory indicate that 50 percent reception of the acoustic signal can carry a meaningful message. Various studies in reading indicate that the meaningful message may be grasped by scanning, which covers approximately 60 percent of the visual stimuli. We may hope that the higher level achieved here will carry the visual message of Amer-Ind.

In applying the results of this assessment of transmission success, it is well to remember that it has been presented in the most difficult frame of reference: individual signals out of context. This probably accounts for the rather constant clinical statements that the patient is understood better in the clinic and at home than the patient's test scores would indicate.

PROJECT 14: COMPARISON OF PRE- AND POSTWORKSHOP SCORES—EFFECTS OF TRAINING

It appeared desirable at the five workshops reported in Project 13 to have the participants' success in interpreting signals assessed at the termination of the seminar. Again, fifty signals were randomly chosen. They were not cued categorically, or otherwise, but presented in a random order by a competent patient-signaler.

The scores could not be exactly compared with those of the pre-test, because the first had cue assistance. However, it seemed logical that at the termination of the workshop the participants should not require cue assistance. Due to the inherent understandability of Amer-Ind, it was predicted that, on the whole, score increase would not be large.

In general, the hypothesis was supported; the average over-all gain being 7.5 percent. In Group A, the low score moved from 70 to 86 percent, for Group B from 64 to 70 percent, for Group C from 80 to 82 percent, for Group D from 60 to 86 percent, and for Group E from 78 to 80 percent. Overall, gains appeared to be in general proportion to the pretest score. However, there was some very interesting variations from this.

In two instances, the participant appeared to regress instead of gain, moving in one case from 88 percent to 84 percent, and in the other from 88 to 80 percent (the small regression may be due to any one or more of several factors. The most probable factor appeared to be differences in transmission of *specific* signals. This hypothesis was later explored). Both of the participants that regressed were in Group E.

In two other cases, the pretest score exactly equaled the posttest score; in Group A this occurred at 86 percent and in Group B at 82 percent. The most dramatic gains appeared of course, in cases of low pretest scores. In Group D, the three participants making the three lowest pretest scores of 62, 60, and 60 gained in each case thirty points for final scores, respectively, of 92, 90, and 90. Another with a pretest score of 70 gained twenty-eight for a posttest score of 98. Another in this group gained twenty points from 78 to 98.

The average gain by groups were 9.3 for A, 6.4 for B, 4.3 for C, 10.7 for D, and 7.1 for E. The average gain across the five groups was 7.5.

In terms of individuals, five persons (or 5 percent of the participants) made gains of 30 percent. Thirty persons gained from 10 to 20 percent, sixty persons gained from 2 to 8 percent. Two persons regressed one by 4 percent, the other by 8 percent. Three remained unchanged, one at 86 percent, one at 82 percent, and, of course, the person who scored 100 percent on the pretest.

PROJECT 14: TRANSMISSION SCORES

Pre- and Post Test Scores
50 Signals, Same Patient-Signaler

A		B		C		D		E	
Pre	Post	Pre	Post	Pre	Post	Pre	Post	Pre	Post
90	96	90	96	92	94	98	100	100	100
88	100	88	98	90	96	96	100	94	96
86	96	88	92	90	96	96	98	92	98
86	94	88	90	90	94	86	96	90	96
86	92	84	90	90	92	86	94	90	94
86	86	84	86	88	94	84	92	90	94
84	98	82	90	88	92	82	98	90	92
84	92	82	84	86	92	82	98	88	90
84	92	82	82	86	90	82	96	88	84
84	90	80	92	84	88	82	96	88	80
82	98	80	92	84	88	78	98	86	96
82	88	80	90	82	88	78	94	84	94
82	88	80	88	82	88	78	94	84	92
82	88	80	86	82	86	70	98	80	96
80	98	80	84	80	88	70	98	80	94
80	88	80	84	80	88	70	96	80	94
80	88	80	82	80	86	70	86	80	94
76	88	78	84	80	84	62	92	80	94
76	86	64	72	80	82	60	90	78	92
70	88	64	70	80	82	60	90	78	92

We conclude from this comparison that there are as yet some factors concerning signal transmission and improvement in signal recognition that are unknown to us, and which require further investigation. It is apparent that the signals are, on the whole, easily interpreted without instruction. Instruction appears, for the most part, to add only a slight percentage increment. However, there are some who profit greatly from it. To date, the latter are all persons who made lower scores on the pretest.

If we are to apply this to the training of hospital personnel in contact with speechless patients, and to family members who must cope with patient speechlessness, it appears that some instruction in code will improve viewer ability to interpret the speechless patient's signaling.

The workshops for the professional speech pathologist were, of course, devoted to many other aspects of code as a clinical tool, and such investigation should be continued. The workshops were involved in having the speech pathologists learn to signal but also emphasized methods of inducting the speechless patient into the code as a communication mode.

PROJECT 15: EFFECT OF BRIEF TRAINING BY VIDEO ONLY

In the interests of patients introduced to Amer-Ind as a communication mode, it appeared advisable to learn the level at which uninstructed persons in their daily-life environment interpreted signals. It also seemed appropriate to inquire concerning improvement in understanding code.

A project involving twenty persons, including wives, relatives, and friends of patients was undertaken. This population was asked to view a video cassette showing the same fifty signals used in workshop pretesting, and to write one English word that each signal suggested to them. The score sheets were category cued, and the signals were presented in category groups. They were clearly and precisely demonstrated by an accomplished clinician signaler.

As a second step, the participants were asked to view four half-hour video cassettes that had been filmed to explain and demonstrate the code. In the course of the viewing, the participants were exposed to approximately 150 signals, and were briefed on both the origins of American Indian Hand Talk and its present-day clinical application in Amer-Ind.

As the concluding step, the participants were asked to complete a posttest following the video instruction. This test consisted of the same fifty signals as the pretest, but it was presented with the signals in random order, without cues, and executed by a patient-signaler. The rationale here was that during the pretest and instruction, it was desirable for the participants have the signal executed as precisely and clearly as possible. Since the intent in the posttest was to assess not only improvement in interpretation but also competence in interpreting signals executed by an impaired relative or friend, the use of patient-signaler appeared useful. Although the patient executed the signals correctly, they were not as precise as in the pretest film in which a clinician was the signaler.

On the pretest, 17 of the 20 participants scored at or above 70 percent. Eleven scored in the 70s, five in the 80s, one in the 90s. Only three were

PROJECT 15: TRANSMISSION EFFECT OF BRIEF TRAINING BY VIDEO
ONLY: PATIENT RELATED POPULATION (WIVES, RELATIVES, FRIENDS)

Pretest		Posttest		% Gain
5%	94	100	5%	6
	86	94		8
	82	98		6
25%	82	98		16
	82	96		14
	82	96		14
85%	78	94		16
	78	94		16
	76	98		22
55%	76	96	90%	20
	76	94		18
	74	94		18
	72	92		20
	72	90		18
	70	96		26
	70	94		24
	70	94		24
10%	64	96		32
	62	92		30
5%	50	88	5%	38

below 70 percent success. On the posttest, one scored 100 percent, one scored 88 percent, and the other eighteen all scored in the 90s. It is interesting to note the extensive gain of the pretest low scorers: the 64 percent became 96 percent, the 62 percent moved to 92 percent, and the 50 percent rose to 88 percent.

In contrasting the pre- and posttest scores, it is evident that on the pretest only one person scored above 88 percent, while on the posttest 88 percent was the lowest score. This impressive gain accrued from one viewing session. It should be noted that this patient related population had high motivation for improvement.

It appears that while family and friends of the impaired signaler, when uninstructed, read the signal at or above the 70 percent level in general, very brief professional video orientation moved 19 of the 20 project participants to the 90 to 100 percent decile. It is projected that the occasional attendance of family or friends at a group session may also contribute to their interpretation skills, especially in interpreting the left-hand signals of the right hemiplegic patient, as well as the less precise execution of the motorically handicapped signaler.

PROJECT 16: PATIENT-SIGNALER WITH 25 PHYSICIAN VIEWERS UNINSTRUCTED IN AMER-IND

During the course of the preliminary clinical testing of Amer-Ind for patient communication use, informal reports had been solicited and received from physicians, nurses, and other hospital personnel. These reported in general that the patients' signals were fairly easy to understand.

At another hospital where code had not yet been introduced, as part of a physician staff meeting the speech pathologist presented a brief description of the system in preparation for its inclusion in the clinic's treatment repertoire. To demonstrate patient use, permission had been given for use of the pretest video cassette. When it was described, the physicians suggested that while viewing it, they respond as testees.

The results show that only one error was made in the entire group. It was on a signal that appeared to be difficult for a number of viewers in the prior transmission studies. A high score was expected from the physician group since, as professionals, they are highly trained to observe and deduce. However, the almost perfect score for a sizeable group was still a pleasant surprise.

PROJECT 17: SIGNALS AS A FACTOR IN TRANSMISSION

In prior studies of signal transmission, emphasis has been placed chiefly on the receiving population. On the hypothesis that some individual signals may be more or less difficult to interpret than others, an analysis of the errors in transmission was made in terms, not of the viewer, but of the individual signals involved.

Data for this was obtained from the score sheets involving five groups of twenty viewers, each exposed to a fifty-signal test. The 193 signals demonstrated in the *Video Dictionary of Amer-Ind,* * prepared by the Learning Resources Service of the VA Hospital, were used as the base. Seven more recently developed signals were chosen from the repertoire for a total of two hundred signals. One competent signaler presented the signals.

The signals were divided into four groups of fifty by random distribution. A fifth group of fifty signals was chosen randomly from the total two hundred. Each group of fifty signals was presented to a group of twenty viewers with no previous exposure to the system. The results were scored according to the concept label lists of English words accepted as appropriate interpretation of the concept denoted by the signal. This scoring produced a method of assessing each signal in terms of its success or error potential as well as the success or error potential in the group of fifty signals.

RESULTS

In the first group of fifty signals, on twenty-four of the signals no interpretation error was recorded. On an additional twenty-two signals, less than five errors were noted. Four signals were associated with higher error scores: 7, 9, 11, and one of 20. By multiplying the number of errors by the number of signals involved in that error, a total error score of 106 evolved for the first group of signals. This occurred in the responses of twenty persons to fifty signals, which produces a potential error score of 1000. Of the actual error score (106) four signals were associated with 47 points of this score.

Similar analysis of the other four groups of signals produced error scores for the groups ranging from 99 to 113. The same twenty-six signals associated with error scores in the first group were also associated with errors

---

*This *Video Dictionary* has been up-dated in 1979, with the new version titled *Amer-Ind Gestural Repertoire.*

in the other groups, although with some slight shifts in the exact number of errors, accounting for the slight variation in range of group error.

Of the two hundred signals examined, only seven appeared to be associated with more than five errors. The most difficult signal, both in terms of this analysis and also in the opinion of clinicians involved in field studies, is that for HARD, which can be interpreted as *stone, wood, metal,* etc. WORK, NAPKIN, and TIME, SECOND/TWO, EASY/FAST, and EAST/WEST, complete the list of seven most likely to be misinterpreted, under certain conditions.

Further clinical explorations of variances in execution have greatly improved the transmission of these signals, as well as the others on the total list of 26: TOP/ON/ABOVE/OVER; BOTTOM/UNDER/BELOW; SNOW/RAIN; OPEN/SHUT; DOWN/HERE; SPREAD/PAINT; PUSH/STOP; BOX; and SMART/BRAIN.

Descriptions of the improvements in execution of these signals for higher levels of transmission, as well as clarification techniques to be used when signals are misunderstood, are explained at length in Part II of this text.

PROJECT SEVENTEEN

# Errors	Signals at this error level	Error Product
zero	24	zero
1	8	8
2	4	8
3	1	3
4	5	20
5	4	20
7	1	7
9	1	9
11	1	11
20	1	20
Total	26	106

PROJECT 18: THE SIGNALER AS A FACTOR IN TRANSMISSION

In addition to the viewing population and the structure of the signals themselves, another factor affecting transmission success is of course the signaler. A comparison of transmissions by competent signalers to those of impaired signalers was obtained from workshop scores where both types of signalers were involved in videotape transmission.

The same randomly chosen fifty signals were videotape recorded by a competent signaler and were distributed among eight highly impaired patient-signalers. Each tape was interpreted by twenty matched viewers untrained in code, who were instructed to write the English word they best associated with the meaning of the signal. It was explained that the signals represented concepts, not specific words. The responses were scored according to the list of English words most frequently associated with the concept. Both series of responses were scored by the same judge. For each type there was a potential error score of 1000. On each signal there was a potential error score of 20.

RESULTS

Responses for the competent signaler paralleled those in Project 16. Transmission error score for the fifty signals for the competent signaler was 113/1000, and for the impaired group it was 243/1000. In the impaired group, thirteen signals were transmitted without error; twenty-three were conveyed with no more than five errors each; five had no more than ten errors each; eight had no more than fifteen errors; and only one exceeded this with sixteen errors. The individual patient error and transmission scores are listed in the following table.

PROJECT 18: TRANSMISSION BY HIGHLY IMPAIRED PATIENTS

Impaired patient-signaler	# Signals	# Observers	Possible error	Actual errors	Error %	Transmission success (%)
1	7	20	140	22	15.7	84.3
2	7	20	140	25	17.8	82.2
3	6	20	120	24	20.0	80.0
4	7	20	140	29	20.7	79.3
5	6	20	120	25	20.8	79.2
6	7	20	140	36	25.7	74.3
7	5	20	100	29	29.0	71.0
8	5	20	100	37	37.0	63.0

PROJECT 19: SIGNAL ILLUSTRATIONS AS A MEDIUM OF TRANSMISSION OF MEANING

Since the illustrations of the signals are included in Part III of this text for learning purposes, they were evaluated for their transmission success (see pp. 199–438 for concept illustrations and labels.) Can uninstructed persons interpret the meaning of the illustrations? Can uninstructed persons execute the signals from the illustrations, and if so, does this have any effect on their ability to interpret the meaning? Are there consistent patterns of success or failure? If failures are observed, can changes in the illustrations involved shift the success/failure ratio? Project 19 was planned in three segments to answer these questions.

SECTION A

Slides of illustrations of Amer-Ind signals were projected onto a viewing screen with no identification, except numbers relating them to concept labels in the text. These slides were viewed by a population of fifty persons who had prior training on the fifty basic signals of the total 250 signal repertoire. These fifty signals were discounted and scoring was based only on the remaining uninstructed two hundred illustrations.

Viewers were asked to interpret each signal illustration by writing a single word representing the concept involved in the signal.

Forty-four illustrations were identified as presenting problems in swift interpretation. All fifty viewers had some difficulty with some of the illustrations in a range extending from forty-four illustrations (22 percent) to thirty-four illustrations (17 percent), with a mean of forty-one illustrations (20.5 percent).

SECTION B

A second, similar population of fifty persons was also presented the slide projections of the illustrations of the 250 signals. They were directed to use the illustration first solely for execution of the signal manually, regardless of meaning. Then they were asked to write the meaning.

Fourteen signals presented problems in execution and in interpretation. They were all included in the forty-four reported in Section A. Twenty-five of the fifty subjects were involved in the difficulties presented by these fourteen illustrations of signals. The other twenty-five (of the fifty subjects) all executed the total two hundred signals and interpreted them correctly.

SECTION C

The fourteen illustrations that had continued to present difficulty in Section B were reexamined by the authors and illustrator. Modifications were made of each illustration, and introduced into the repertoire. The total repertoire was then again tested in the same manner with another viewing audience of fifty persons.

Twelve subjects failed on execution and interpretation of two signal illustrations, but in each case the two signals were different. Twenty-four signals were each involved once. Only one of the fourteen listed in Section B was among them. It appeared that errors were all randomly unique to the viewer, and not attributable to the illustrations.

SUMMARY

It would appear that the illustrations as presented in Section A had an interpretation score of 80 percent success. Section B appears to demonstrate that kinetic execution of the signal may contribute greatly to its interpretation. Section C appears to indicate that the changes in the illustrations have produced improvement in both execution and interpretation. (The modified illustrations rather than the original versions are used in Part III of this book.) These all have clinical implications for treatment. The speechless patient may learn signal meaning more effectively by kinesis than by auditory instruction or pictorial presentation. These same observations may apply to speaking persons who wish to improve their ability to interpret signals. This has important connotations for families and friends of the speechless patients, as well as for clinicians. It also emphasizes the introductory theme of the text: action.

Investigation Conclusions

4

GENERAL CONCLUSIONS

Clinical investigations were directed toward acquisition and transmission of Amer-Ind signals by various patient populations, as well as transmission reception by various viewing populations. In the clinical investigations reported, **acquisition** is defined as successful use by the patient-signalers in conveying a message. **Transmission** means successful reception of the message by the viewing populations.

It appears that some results of these investigations may be used as a base for treatment planning for certain speechless patients. It is advisable also that it be used for further studies to eliminate or reduce the problems still inherent in the change to a markedly different communication system for those patients who have lost (or never acquired) the linguistic mode that is considered normal.

The principle syndromes covered were surgical excision (cancer), oral–verbal apraxia, aphasia, and mental retardation. It appears that three quite different rehabilitation patterns are needed among these groups.

Certainly the surgical cases, with adequate hearing and intact intelligence, may be approached on the auditory instruction level, and inducted at once into signal use. Their progress appears to depend entirely on their motivation to learn and use. Those who wish to do so quite quickly master the code both quantitatively and qualitatively.

The oral–verbal apraxics who have no complicating aphasic involvement (or a very mild one) may be treated by the same methods. While their progress is much slower than that of the surgical cases, they can and have equalled the use levels with the auditory approach.

Where there appears to be any reduction in the symbolic competence of the patient as in aphasia, the treatment approaches must center initially on signal association with reality, rather than with any language. Oral apraxics who are also aphasic would, of course, be included here, as well as patients who are classified as speechless and mentally retarded. Concrete approaches centering on conceptualization and concept–signal relationship are indicated. Hence, it appears that similar concept–signal methods are appropriate at least initially for the severe aphasics who are unable to relate their conceptualization to the high symbolic level of language.

SPECIFIC CONCLUSIONS

Interpretation by the viewer will be improved if the signaler indicates the general topic to be discussed. It may improve transmission considerably if a place and time reference are included. If a viewer has difficulty interpreting, the signal should be repeated with greater precision and perhaps a slightly slower pace. Additional signals may help to clarify. Occasionally, it is necessary to approach the presentation from another point of view, using an entirely different signal.

For a viewer attempting to interpret Amer-Ind for the first time, the signaler will find it helpful to indicate the number of signals that will be used, along with the signal ADD for compound or agglutinative use. For example, the signal for SHELTER (or *house*)* added to READ means *library*. The patient extends the index fingers, the other fingers curled (palms down), crosses index fingers to signal the concept ADD and demonstrates the signal for SHELTER and signal for READ. The hemiplegic patient indicates agglutination by first indicating with fingers the number of signals to be joined, then bringing fingers together and demonstrating the signal to be so joined for the new concept.

In the clinical projects, the following approaches appeared to faciliate development and use of Amer-Ind:

1. Videotape recording is excellent for the patient's criticism of his or her execution of the signals. This technique facilitates self-monitoring better than a mirror, since the video image may be repeated. This allows the

---

*In this text, and with all speech pathologists presently using Amer-Ind, concept labels are rendered in capital letters. Each label has a series of synonyms, which are rendered in lower-case, italic letters. The signal for SHELTER, for example, executed by the hands simulating a gable roof line, has the synonyms *build, building, dwell, home, house, residence, roof*. Part III of this text (pp. 197–483) presents and describes the major concept labels and their synonyms. The labels are arranged alphabetically and are numbered consecutively. The signal index (pp. 469–483) can be used to find the proper signal for conveyance of a specific synonym. For more complicated concepts, a series of agglutinations (combinations of signals) are recommended (pp. 467–468).

patient to concentrate on production while executing the signals and on criticism when reviewing the tape.

2. Group work, when possible, provides motivation, greater willingness to experiment, as well as practice in performing the signals in a consistent and precise manner. More suggestions for modifying gestures to meet the motor limitations and problems of individual patients accrue in the group setting. The group approach provides its own social setting for spontaneous communication.

3. Structuring treatment sessions around a particular topic enables the clinician to introduce signals related to the chosen topic, to elicit associations tending to reinforce memory storage and retrieval, and to stimulate participation in conversation structured for use of these signals. The structure provides a meaningful context for the patient, and signals gain intelligibility as they are related to a pattern. This procedure is more effective than gestures presented at random with little or no way to provide reinforcement and daily-life use.

4. Daily practice assignments should relate closely to that day's treatment session as well as to the patient's needs. Assignments should also give the patient an opportunity to test new signals on people outside the clinic, challenging him to attempt difficult transmission. The patient needs to test newly developed signals on willing observers and to note any problems arising from the manner of execution or difficulties in interpretation. The patient will profit from practice in transmitting a specific idea to someone outside the clinic using the methods for increasing clarity discussed in the treatment sessions.

Part II, which follows, attempts to provide information applicable to various types of patient population, and to assist professionals in development of both (1) conceptualization in relation to code and (2) code use itself as a useful alternate to verbal communication. Further studies may improve the suggested methods or replace them with superior techniques.

CLINICAL APPLICATION

II

Clinical Testing

5

INTRODUCTION

A disproportionate amount of the clinician's time, and the patient's, may be spent in testing as opposed to treatment. Sometimes patients are subjected to needless repetition with tests having the same informational objective. Adequate testing is certainly highly desirable, but excessive testing is unwarranted. Any activity in which the patient is asked to spend his time and energy should be directly profitable to the individual's disability and treatment.

Adequate testing is, of course, proper for establishment of diagnosis and base lines. It is possible to incorporate test segments in treatment sequences both legitimately and profitably. Research also can be so included. Every therapeutic plan designed by an expert clinician may be regarded as a clinical investigation based on the hypothesis that if such and such a procedure is carried out in such and such a way, under such and such conditions with this patient, specific results will occur. This is the basis of all effective therapeutic planning by objectives designed to accomplish the desired goal.

The adequacy of the clinician's mastery of the particular technique at issue has seldom been listed among the factors to be considered in evaluating either test or research results. The assumption that every qualified clinician is expert in any and every technique is not necessarily well founded. The most eminent members of clinical professions are among the first to disqualify themselves for certain cases under certain conditions.

A plethora of tests is available in speech pathology for clinical use principally for evaluating patients for admission to a rehabilitation program in the speech clinic. Many of them may be superfluous with certain cases, particularly when the patient is speechless. Tests designed for specific research studies are not necessarily appropriate in some clinical instances.

True criteria for clinical test choice are (1) adequacy in assessing the patient's abilities and deficits, and (2) appropriateness to the patient's needs for rehabilitation. Adequacy implies choice of those tests that will either simultaneously or sequentially provide enough information with which to plan the patient's initial sessions. Extensive testing may frequently be profitably delayed until there has been some clinical assessment of the patient. Overwhelming the patient with numerous tests may result only in frustration and fatigue, which may produce a false picture of the patient's problems. Standard tests are not always appropriate for the speechless patient, as most of these tests assume some verbal level of response. Valid and reliable responses from the patient can be obtained only in the mode or modes available to the patient. They will accrue only if administration is in a mode within the patient's comprehension.

There are a number of reasons, other than mental or physical incapacity, why patients might fail to perform test tasks:

1. The most frequent failures occur because the patient does not know what is expected. In some instances, spoken directives are given to individuals who in screening have displayed some auditory reception impairment. It may be necessary to make some adaptation of the test presentation to compensate for this deficit.

    As an example, consider a test task that requires the patient to demonstrate the use of some common objects. A number of tests have such tasks among their items. Presumably, the tester wishes to know whether or not the patient (1) realizes the use of the object, (2) can express this in behavior, (3) uses the object in expressing the function, (4) pantomimes the function without use of the object. The patient may actually be *able* to perform at all four levels, but may fail to do so if he or she thinks the tester wishes the objects to be named (which the patient cannot do). If directions are given through the auditory channel and the patient is not able to receive, the patient may misinterpret what is required. In administering this type of task to aphasic and other brain-damaged patients, significantly different score results have accrued in the Amer-Ind program when the clinician demonstrated the expected type of reponse with three non-test common objects as a pre-test illustration of expected response.

2. Sometimes test results are aborted because the patient has been provided with the wrong tool. An example is available in graphic tests. A number of aphasic patients on admission testing for Amer-Ind were unable to perform graphic tests with either pen or pencil. Several, however, produced quite adequate results on an electric typewriter. It is, of course, quite accurate to say that this changes the task. But does it, basically? Are we concerned with the mode or the message? What is wrong with using the typewriter, if the patient can communicate on it? It is a quite respectable modern mode of writing. It is true also that the typewriter

gives the patient assistance which the pen or pencil cannot. The machine retains, retrieves and prints the letters. The patient need only *recognize* the letters. In producing letters with pen or pencil, the patient must not only retain, retrieve and produce the letters from visual image but also he must do the same for the fine motor sequences necessary to execute them. On the typewriter the motor patterns are, comparatively speaking, much simpler. Certainly they are much more limited and repetitive. Acceptable results may be achieved with use of only one finger and at a very slow speed, if necessary.

3. A third reason some patients may fail in test response to demonstrate their actual level of function is concerned with adults who are presented tasks they regard as childish. The adult often reacts to this by rejecting the task. This is then misinterpreted as indicating that the patient cannot (instead of will not) accomplish it.

4. A fourth possible reason for invalid test results may be the deterrent the patient sees in the tester's attitude. Preservation of tester objectivity does not necessarily demand a blank face which the patient may interpret as indifference. A smiling face accompanying the task presentation does not provide the patient with the answer. It may, however, help him to do his best. Human beings on the whole find difficulty in responding to behavior they interpret as indifference and disinterest.

5. A fifth reason may be the presence of too much pressure, especially pressure to perform quickly. Many brain-damaged patients who have recovered have expatiated on this topic. They are well-agreed that they need more time than is usually given them. Many testers are unaware of the subtle signs of impatience they display to the patients. Sometimes with these slow patients, the cue is presented too soon, inhibiting the original response the patient was processing, and also reducing the patient's score to that of a cued response.

6. Many factors other than the patient's ability need to be taken into consideration in interpreting test results: the patient's vision, hearing, fatigue, hunger, comfort, emotions, and experiences immediately preceding the test, to mention a few. The tester must be aware of the patient's needs, alert to indications of discomfort that may affect the test results.

It may be appropriate to ask (1) what the test is intended to elicit from the patient, his highest level of function or his lowest, (2) why this test is being administered, (3) what data are sought, and (4) what applicable information can be acquired.

The principal occasions for testing are admission and discharge. Tests on those occasions are meant to answer the questions: Should the patient be admitted/discharged, and why? The simplest answer for admission tests concerns another question: Can this patient be helped? The simplest answer on discharge contains the question: Has the patient been helped to the limit of the resources available? If these criteria are held firmly in mind in choosing specific tests from the large number available, testing will be both adequate and relevant.

Differential testing is largely centered about diagnosis, prognosis, and treatment progress, both daily and in lengthier terms. Here, too, there are numerous well validated assessment tools available for choice. The real value of tests lies in their proper *selection* to provide the needed information on which to base decisions concerning treatment for that patient.

When the patients are known to be speechless, the choice of appropriate tests is confined to those providing a response mode of which the patient is capable. A false assumption, however, frequently aborts the value of the test at this point. The tester assumes that the test can be administered in the auditory mode, despite the fact that the patient's ability to receive in this channel has not been established. Informal testing of both receptive and expressive modes is in order, but this may not be the most desirable initial project.

Optimum treatment planning accrues from testing only when the patient provides his or her best responses. The patient may be inhibited from this by factors previously mentioned. Many of these can be reduced by establishment of familiarity and rapport with the testing clinician. In a friendly and relaxed atmosphere with a person with whom the patient has already established a relationship, the patient's responses may be much closer to the true level. Nonstandardized approaches may be used informally to establish such a relationship prior to formal testing.

Receptive language may be assessed by a series of requests for specific actions within a familiar context. Later, formal tests may be chosen in of the results. Similarly, optimum expressive modes may be explored in a nonstress atmosphere through simple tasks that provide information concerning conceptual level, manual motor ability, shape, size and color recognition, as well as attention span. The following ladder can be used, not only for informal testing, but also for planning activities in treatment sessions. The tasks would require the patient to:

1. accept or reject the clinician's choice
2. sort pictures, objects, forms to match a model
3. point to one (of many) that matches a model
4. sort without a model
5. match like with like
6. reject one different from the group
7. arrange a series in order
8. verbalize to any of the above, if possible

Observation of the patient's method of attack on the nonverbal tasks can provide very helpful clinical information indicating specific acceptable approaches to the individual patient in treatment.

For patient admission to the Amer-Ind Code program, the clinician will wish to know whether or not the patient can use any skills from the preceding list to match objects with pictures, to match clinician behavior with action picture, and/or to imitate clinician gesture. The Amer-Ind Scale (see pages 97–107) will also suggest testing activities for this early assessment. To date, the best prognostic indicators have proved to be (1) attention by means of eye contact, (2) imitation of clinician movement, especially of the hands, (3) attempts to present self-generated gestures, and (4) use of the index finger to point to desired objects or needs.

While its picture content is not too well suited for use with the adult, the Peabody Picture Vocabulary Test has been utilized in some studies to provide a standardized base. With brain-damaged patients, however, its pictures are probably too highly symbolic to provide a secure score. Also, its method of presentation by both speech pathologists and psychologists may need to be modified for these patients. The pictures may need to be framed to be recognized: the four pictures on each page may need to be presented serially by masking the other three each time, and requiring an accept or reject response only from the patient. In using standard tests with congenitally brain-damaged patients, it is well to consider that some of the stimulus material may be outside their experience and so affect their ability to respond appropriately.

One of the most useful tests with the speechless patient has been the Leiter International Scale, in the Arthur adaptation. This is a completely nonverbal, nonlinguistic test, organized by its author and intended by its adapter for use with patients without *language*. It correlates highly with other intelligence tests. It also provides many cues to the testee's approaches to problems. The most valuable asset of the test lies in this latter aspect. In the test the individual patient uses highly individual methods of solving the problems presented. Each of the patient's attacks demonstrates a way to start that patient's treatment in concept development, and consequently whether to choose Amer-Ind Code or speech as a major goal. The speech clinician should understand the test thoroughly, but in the opinion of the writers, *observation* of an experienced tester administering the Leiter provides the most valuable information for the speech pathologist. The latter is then free to observe and document the patient responses for the specific use of them in treatment planning.

The Leiter is nonverbal, nonlinguistic, nonauditory. It is entirely visual, tactile, and kinetic. The instructions are given only in demonstration. It is not time bound. It can be administered serially, over a period of days. It indicates the patient's reasoning, observation, problem-solving tactics, and processing methods.

Speechless aphasic patients who are referred for Amer-Ind Code have usually been assessed by one of the many excellent tests in this field. Those in the projects reported in this text have test scores reported variously for the PICA (Porch), the SAS (Sklar), and the ALPS (Keenan) tests. As yet, no reliable correlation has been discovered between the patient's success or failure in Amer-Ind and his or her test scores. This may lie entirely in the fact that the tests are linguistically oriented and Amer-Ind Code is not. The tests do not assess nonlinguistic processing, even in the gesture tasks, since instructions are in many instances in the auditory mode.

Most tests proposed for use with brain-damaged patients begin at too high a point in any viable scale. Instruments that can test much lower levels of operation are very much needed. Some cautions are in order in creating them. Pointing is not always a reliable mode with brain-damaged patients. These patients are action-oriented. Action should be used in the tests, both as input and output. The effects of gestural input should be evaluated with use of both auditory and gestural code stimuli. Picture stimuli should be more carefully evaluated in terms of symbolic components and levels. Not all pictures are equivalent. Reality is the criteria. Color photographs are the closest to the actual objects. Concreteness decreases as information level decreases. The symbolic ladder might be considered to begin as soon as the real object is replaced by the color photograph. The black and white photograph is next on the ladder then the drawing with great detail (but not as much as the photograph), then the line drawing. Any reduction of information or distortion of reality prevents the brain-damaged patient from reacting optimally.

In addition to distortion, the brain damaged patient is easily subject to distraction. This reduces attention and concentration. These factors must be controlled in both testing and treatment situations, if they are to be productive.

Apraxic patients may be tested on any of the well-known tests available. They may also be evaluated usefully on a scale where the same tasks are presented with a graduated response to differential stimuli. An experimental form appears with the other test forms in this text. The surgical patients admitted to the code program may be included in the clinical schedule without specific tests other than those indicated by the individual deficit.

It is suggested that progress reports on Amer-Ind be organized in terms of the Amer-Ind Scale on pp. 97–107 of this text. For recording of daily task success, the Tally-Graph, developed by Macalyne Fristoe, and included in the text, is highly recommended. It provides a quick method of task notation and summary. Use of its totals on a weekly, monthly, or quarterly basis can accommodate report protocols of most clinics.

A thorough audiological evaluation of the speechless brain-damaged patient should occur early among admission tests to rule out organic hearing loss or to have such loss receive any indicated attention. The audiological battery should be administered by a clinician familiar with the hard-to-test patient who is incapable of voluntary responses. A tympanogram is suggested for check on middle ear pathology.

Evaluation of attention span, manual motorics, and capacity for imitation are, of course, indicated and valuable in providing information needed when making a clinical decision for code programming for a particular patient.

SKELLY ACTION TEST OF AUDITORY RECEPTION OF LANGUAGE

Many speechless individuals have been recorded as achieving only extremely low scores on some of the standard tests such as the Peabody and the Carrow. These scores would seem to indicate that these patients do not process language stimuli presented in the auditory channel. Yet some of them, especially those classified in the severe or profound range, also appear to *behave* appropriately in response to spoken directives.

It is important in making decisions concerning programming in Amer-Ind, to consider possible logical explanations of this apparent contradiction. One might be experiential deprivation, lack of opportunity to experience the actions or objects depicted in the tests. A second may lie in the test pictures, which may be too highly symbolic for the particular impaired testee. There is also a third possibility, that spoken directives to the patients are accompanied by gestures that are recognized easily by the patients, who are of course reacting to these rather than to the words.

The Action Test proposed here has proved useful in identifying patients who do respond in behavior to auditory language directives when the requests concern familiar actions with familiar objects in the individual's environment. For those who do not so respond, the test provides a gesture section with the same directives executed by the clinician in Amer-Ind. The test items in section A appear on current data to be valid and reliable. Sections B, C, D, and E on progressively higher levels, are still under investigation.

PREPARATION

The tester should make the acquaintance of the testee prior to administration of the test. Preferably there should be daily encounters over several days. The test should be administered in a room that the testee has previously visited at least once. All objects included in the test should have been utilized in a previous visit by the tester in view of the testee. The test should be conducted in the same friendly, informal manner as the previous encounters.

On a table or other surface in the test room, there should be an open box of tissues, a pitcher or other container of drinking water, and some paper cups. Under or beside the table should be a waste basket. In the top drawer of the tester's desk there should be several felt pens and some paper. (If there is no desk, the pens and paper should be in a box and the spoken directions suitably altered.) There should be a chair beside the tester's desk and another chair beside the other table (or elsewhere in the room).

The tester should be seated, the door open, and the overhead light turned off. A light on the desk is on.

The test should be recorded by describing as exactly as possible the actions of the testee. It should be scored at 5 percent per item, with the *five* assigned if execution of the task is as directed. If the task is initiated but not correctly completed, assign *four*; if the action is performed but not with the directed object, assign *three*; if the object is manipulated but not in the directed action, assign *two*; if the eyes of the testee are directed to the object but no action is taken, assign *one*. If there is no response, assign *zero*. (The tester should make requests of the testee, not issue orders.)

The test should be conducted like a friendly conversation with the testee's responses in action as his contribution to the interchange. The tester should smile and use suitable behaviors as when requesting a friend to do some favors. The responses of the testee to "Hello" and "Goodbye" should not be scored, but should be noted on the score sheet.

When the testee appears at the door, the tester should stop what he is doing at his desk, smile, and speak.

1. Hello! Come in.

[*As soon as the testee makes a forward movement, the tester speaks again.*]

2. Turn on the light!

[*If testee does not find the light switch, tester may point to it. If no testee action results, tester goes to light, turns it on, saying "Here it is!" and returns to desk.*]

3. Shut the door, please.

[*Seated at desk.*]

4. Where's my kleenex?

[*If testee points to or looks at kleenex, proceed. If he does not, tester indicates it.*]
5. Give me a kleenex.

[*If testee does not respond, tester takes one and uses it.*]
6. Do you want one? Take one.
7. Would you like a drink of water?

[*If testee responds no, substitute for 8: "Pour me one, will you?"; For 9: "Hand it to me, please."*]
8. Pour two cups, will you?
9. Give me one, please.
10. Sit beside my desk.

[*If he does not do it, indicate chair.*]
11. Open the top drawer.

[*If testee does not, tester does.*]
12. Pick a pen.

[*If testee does not, tester gives one.*]
13. Give me one.

[*If testee does not, tester takes one.*]
14. Take a piece of paper.

[*If testee does not, tester gives him one.*]
15. I want a piece.

[*Takes it, if testee does not act.*]
16. Let's draw a man, a woman, and a house.

[*If testee does, tester draws his own without showing it. If testee does not draw, tester makes quick sketch, shows it saying, "Something like this" and then puts the sketch in drawer.*]
17. Fold your paper.

[*If testee does not, tester does.*]
18. Give it to me.

[*If testee does not, tester takes it.*]
19. Please throw the dirty cups in the waste basket.

[*If testee does not, tester does.*]
20. Time to go now. Goodbye.

[*If testee does not rise, tester does, and escorts testee to door.*]

It is very important to the integrity of test results that the tester make *no gestures* of any kind except those specifically indicated in the test directions. This includes *looking* at the indicated test object.

If the results of this test appear to indicate lack of auditory comprehension on the part of the testee, a signal version of the test should be administered about two or three days later for comparison of behavior results.

Results of both are, of course, compared also with audiometric results.

If the patient exhibits a high score, the additional segments of this test may be administered, testing higher levels of language processing.

ACTION TEST OF AMER-IND SIGNAL COMPREHENSION
(See instructions on auditory version pp. 81–82)

1. HELLO (103)   COME IN (47)

2. PUSH (169)   (Point to wall switch and ceiling light.)

3. SHUT (188)   (Point to door.)

4. QUESTION (171)   (Point to nose, look around room.)

5. YOU (236)   GIVE (92)   ME (111)

6. QUESTION (171)   YOU (236)   GET (91)   ONE (149A)

7. QUESTION (171)   YOU (236)   DRINK (69)

8. YOU (236)   POUR (166)   TWO (149B)

9. YOU (236)   GIVE (92)   ME (111)   ONE (149A)

10. YOU (236)   SIT (189)   NEAR (144)   ME (111)

11. YOU (236)   OPEN (154)   TOP (218)   BOX (34)

12. YOU (236)   GET (91)   WRITE (235)   OBJECT (151)

13. GIVE (92)   ME (111)   ONE (149A)

14. GET (90)   SECOND (149B)   WRITE (235)   OBJECT (151)

15. GIVE (92)   ME (111)

16. WRITE (235)   MAN (124)   CAMERA (picture) (39)

17. SHUT (188)   WRITE (235)   OBJECT (151)

18. GIVE (92)   ME (111)

19. THROW AWAY (75)   DRINK (69)   OBJECT (151)

20. TIME (216)   YOU (236)   WALK (227)   GOODBYE (94)

SKELLY ACTION TEST OF AUDITORY RECEPTION OF LANGUAGE

SATAR–FORM A

DATE: _____

TESTEE: _____

UNIT: _____

TESTER: _____

SCORES:

A___ B___ C___ D___ E___

TOTAL: _____

(DIVIDE BY 5 = _____ %)

Directions: Overhead light turned off.
Kleenex on cabinet.
Drinking water and 2 cups on
   cabinet.
In drawer (or box on desk) 3 felt pens
   or crayons, some pieces of paper.
Waste basket.

	Task As Directed.	Initiated But Not Completed	Action Performed Not With Directed Object.	Object Manipulated	Eyes Directed To Object No Action.	No Response.
	5	4	3	2	1	0
1. Hello.						
2. Turn on the light.						
3. Shut the door, please.						
4. Where's my kleenex?						
5. Give me a kleenex.						
6. Do you want one? Take one.						
7. Would you like a drink of water?						
8. Pour 2 cups, will you?						
9. Give me one, please.						
10. Sit beside my desk.						
11. Open the box. (drawer)						
12. Pick a pen.						
13. Give me one.						
14. Take a piece of paper.						
15. I want a piece.						
16. Let's draw a man.						
17. Fold your paper.						
18. Give it to me.						
19. Please throw the dirty cups in the wastebasket.						
20. Time for you to go now. Goodbye.						

TOTAL SCORE _____

SKELLY ACTION TEST OF AUDITORY RECEPTION OF LANGUAGE

SATAR—FORM B (COTTAGE OR LIVING QUARTERS)

DATE:_____

TESTEE: _____

UNIT: _____

TESTER: _____

SCORES:

A___B___C___D___E____

TOTAL: _____

(DIVIDE BY 5= _____ %)

Directions: (Some spoon food ready)
Also two spoons, plates, and paper
napkins.

	Task As Directed.	Initiated But Not Completed	Action Performed Not With Directed Object.	Object Manipulated	Eyes Directed To Object No Action.	No Response.
	5	4	3	2	1	0
21. Hello! Ready to eat?						
22. Have a chair.						
23. Where's your spoon? (both eat)						
24. Would you like more?						
25. Take your plate to the _____ (sink, table, service window)						
26. Push in your chair (under table).						
27. Wipe the table (with paper napkin).						
28. Go get a towel (for your hands).						
29. Knock on the door (bathroom).						
30. Let's wash our hands. (Testee should do it first).						
31. Dry yours.						
32. Hand me the towel.						
33. Get your jacket.						
34. Let's go outside.						
35. Catch the ball.						
36. Throw it to me.						
37. Time to go back. You lead the way.						
38. Wipe your shoes. (On door mat).						
39. Open the door.						
40. Hang up your jacket. See you later.						

TOTAL SCORE _____

SKELLY ACTION TEST OF AUDITORY RECEPTION OF LANGUAGE

SATAR–FORM C

DATE: _____

TESTEE: _____

UNIT: _____

TESTER: _____

SCORES:

A___ B___ C___ D___ E___

TOTAL: _____

(DIVIDE BY 5 = _____ %)

(Wet wipes ready) also 3 pictures (for coloring and 3 crayons) and tape for wall. Waste basket is placed at a distance from the desk (table).

	Task As Directed.	Initiated But Not Completed	Action Performed Not With Directed Object	Object Manipulated	Eyes Directed To Object No Action.	No Response.
	5	4	3	2	1	0
41. Glad to see you. Come in.						
42. Ready to work? Are your hands clean?						
43. Get the wipes.						
44. Wipe your hands clean. (wet wipe)						
45. Throw the wipe in the wastebasket.						
46. Please put these pictures on the table (pictures to be colored)						
47. Where are the crayons?						
48. Have a seat.						
49. Pick a crayon.						
50. Let me pick one.						
51. You choose a picture.						
52. Give me one.						
53. Let's color our pictures. You start first.						
54. Shall we hang yours up?						
55. Give me the tape to fasten them.						
56. Where shall we put them?						
57. You hold the pictures on the wall while I fasten them.						
58. Put the tape back on the table.						
59. Put the crayons in the box.						
60. Put the box back on the cabinet. Time to go. Goodbye.						

TOTAL SCORE _____

SKELLY ACTION TEST OF AUDITORY RECEPTION OF LANGUAGE

SATAR–FORM D

DATE: _____

TESTEE: _____

UNIT: _____

TESTER: _____

SCORES:

A___ B___ C___ D___ E___

TOTAL: _____

(DIVIDE BY 5 = _____ %)

Ceiling light is off.
Needed: Sink, soap and soap dish or container, towel, toothbrush, paste, (paper) cup, comb.

	Task As Directed.	Initiated But not Completed	Action Performed Not With Directed Object.	Object Manipulated	Eyes Directed To Object No Action.	No Response.
	5	4	3	2	1	0
61. Hello. Let's clean up. Lead the way to the bathroom.						
62. Where is the light?						
63. Press the switch.						
64. Go to the sink.						
65. Turn on the water.						
66. Where is the soap?						
67. Wash your hands.						
68. Turn off the water.						
69. Where is the towel?						
70. Dry your hands.						
71. Look around.						
72. Find your toothbrush.						
73. Give me the toothpaste. (tester spreads toothpaste)						
74. Brush your teeth.						
75. Rinse the brush.						
76. Put the toothbrush away.						
77. Where is your comb?						
78. Comb your hair.						
79. Put the comb in your pocket.						
80. Time to go. Turn off the light.						

TOTAL SCORE _____

SKELLY ACTION TEST OF AUDITORY RECEPTION OF LANGUAGE

SATAR–FORM E

DATE:_____

TESTEE: _____

UNIT: _____

TESTER:_____

SCORES:

A___B___C___D___E___

TOTAL: _____

(DIVIDE BY 5 = _____ %)

Window curtains closed. Patient chair at distance from desk (or table). On clinic storage cabinet: Mirror, bowl, red box with bags of popcorn in it, each with 12 pieces of popcorn; wet wipes, kleenex.

	Task As Directed.	Initiated But Not Completed	Action Performed Not With Directed Object.	Object Manipulated	Eyes Directed To Object No Action.	No Response.
	5	4	3	2	1	0
81. Hello go to the (cabinet-table).						
82. Please bring me the mirror from the (cabinet-table).						
83. Polish it with a kleenex.						
84. Pull up a chair and sit down. (Both look in mirror.)						
85. Point to yourself in the mirror.						
86. Point to me in the mirror.						
87. Take the mirror back.						
88. Now bring me a bowl from the cabinet.						
89. Open the red box on the cabinet.						
90. Take one bag of popcorn out of the box						
91. Empty the bag into the bowl.						
92. Clean your hands with a wet wipe.						
93. You may have ten pieces.						
94. Please pass me the bowl of popcorn. (Clinician takes remaining pieces.)						
95. Wipe the bowl out with kleenex.						
96. Now wipe your hands with kleenex.						
97. Put the bowl back on the cabinet (table).						
98. Where's the clock?						
99. It's time to go. Put your chair away.						
100. Close the door on your way out.						

TOTAL SCORE _____

THE SKELLY COMPARATIVE APRAXIA TEST:
ORAL AND MANUAL

There are several standard tests for oral, oral-verbal, and manual (limb) apraxia. Those of Darley and of Goodglass and Kaplan especially explore a wide range of patient behaviors on which to base diagnosis and treatments in the customary channels.

In making therapeutic decisions related to the Amer-Ind program, a much shorter oral and manual apraxia test was devised for several reasons. For many of the patients under consideration, brevity was desirable in the early evaluation process, with lengthier tests postponed for administration later when indicated. The prime intent in the Skelly Comparative Apraxia Test (SCAT) was to compare the patient's behaviors orally and manually on the same five actions in terms of the effect of successive stimuli: (1) auditory command, (2) visual imitation face-to-face, (3) visual imitation at a mirror, and (4) appropriate reality objects. The tasks also provide opportunity to note any differential effects of touch and taste in item three, and any reflexive responses to smell or touch in eight, light in item nine, and noise in item ten. The total test provides forty possible opportunities for observation of the patient's use and control of his hands under a variety of conditions. Observations on differential response on the same task with different stimuli assist the clinician in making the decision to recommend the patient for the Amer-Ind program, either as a prime communication mode in itself, or as a possible facilitator for oral speech. The different effects of different stimuli on the same task provide a basis for decisions on therapeutic tasks and stimuli with which to effect desirable results.

PREPARATION

The tester should make the acquaintance of the testee prior to administration of the test, in a friendly and informal manner and setting. The tester requires preliminary information concerning the patient's favorite drink and food snack and, if possible, the status of the patient's vision and hearing.

Materials required for the test include: a stick of candy (diet if necessary), a glass, a bottle or can of favorite drink, cookies or other favorite food snack, small portion of jelly, box of safety matches, disposable toothbrush, paste for toothbrush, and a sink within reach. A lamp with a bright light and a switch, and an instrument capable of producing a loud, unpleasant noise (radio, TV, or tape recorder) are also needed. A small bottle of ammonia smelling salts or a feather or other long, pliant, tickling instrument, and a mirror are also required.

ADMINISTRATION

The clinician first seeks to elicit the required task response by presenting a verbal command. If the response is completely satisfactory at this stimulus level, there is no need to repeat the item further. If the response is not completely satisfactory, the clinician then presents silently the demonstration for imitation face-to-face. This should be followed by similar demonstration for imitation in a mirror. Unless at least one of the preceding methods has produced completely satisfactory response, the fourth step with a reality stimulus is administered.

The patient's responses indicate how well or how poorly he or she is able to invoke a voluntary response to a stimulus, auditory or visual; how well the patient responds face-to-face in imitation, as opposed to confrontation, in the mirror; and whether or not there is an observable difference in the patient's responses to the reality objects and whether or not there is any reflexive response to touch, smell, light, and noise.

Responses to the reality objects in the manual section can vary. The patient may (1) use his hands to bring the drink or food to his mouth; (2) push the ammonia bottle away from his nose with his hands; (3) turn out the bright lights or cover the eyes with the hands to shut it out; (4) point to the source of the noise or cover the ears with the hands. Any other response may be interpreted by the tester, in terms of whether or not it involves a voluntary, purposeful use of the hands.

This is not a readily scorable test, but rather one for use to confirm other diagnostics or to question them. For use with the Amer-Ind program, its

APRAXIA TEST

	Auditory command	Imitation face to face	Imitation at mirror	Response to reality object	
ORAL					
1. Stick out tongue	___	___	___	___	Candy sucker to lick
2. Pucker lips	___	___	___	___	Straw for favorite drink
3. Lick lips	___	___	___	___	Jelly on lip margins
4. Puff out cheeks	___	___	___	___	Lighted match to blow
5. Show teeth	___	___	___	___	Toothbrush with paste on at sink
MANUAL					
6. Show thirsty	___	___	___	___	Favorite drink within reach
7. Show hungry	___	___	___	___	Favorite snack within reach
*8. Show bad smell	___	___	___	___	Ammonia bottle under nose
9. Show stop	___	___	___	___	Bright light within reach
10. Show quiet	___	___	___	___	Loud noise on radio, TV or recorder, out of reach

*Alternative to No. 8: Tickle patient's nose with feather

PATIENT BACKGROUND AND TASTES

Patient name: _____   Date: _____

Address: _____   Hospital #: _____

Phone: _____   Ward: _____

Family contact: _____   Outpt: _____

Address: _____   Physician: _____

Phone: _____   Pt. DOB: _____

Brief statement of medical problem:

Education:

Employent:

Future plans or hopes:

Responsibilities to family:

Attitudes toward rehabilitation:

Patient is	Gregarious	Loner
Likes	Large parties	Just a few friends
Likes to	Talk	Read
	Play loud games	Play silent games
	Listen to loud music	Listen to HiFi
	Play musical instrument	Watch TV
	Travel	Draw/paint
	Garden	Work with tools

Favorite sport: Favorite music:

Favorite reading: Hobby:

Any other information which will assist clinician to formulate a signal repertoire to fit the patient's needs and interests:

chief value lies in differentiating manual apraxia, which may negate code. On the other hand, effective hand response indicates favorable potential for code. Positive oral results may negate prior diagnosis or question it, and may indicate potential for verbalization. Negative oral and positive manual responses indicate a candidate for Amer-Ind.

ANALYSIS OF PATIENT TASK STRATEGIES
(on the Leiter International Scale)

Many times observation of the method or methods patients use in attempting to accomplish test (or treatment) tasks provides information for treatment planning considerably beyond that yielded by the formal test scores alone. This is especially true of nonverbal, nonlinguistic tests such as the Leiter International Scale. This scale allows the speechless patient to demonstrate intelligence components by behavioral responses that cannot be used on verbal, linguistically organized tests of intelligence. During its administration, it also allows the clinician to observe the individual patient's strategies for problem solving as each test task is presented. An analysis of the patient's preferred strategies provides useful information in planning initial treatment tasks in terms of the patient's successful methods.

The analysis form that follows can also be used for similar recording of patient strategies on treatment tasks. The results of summation allow the clinician to guide the patient into using the most successful approaches and to dissuade him from the unsuccessful methods.

ANALYSIS OF PATIENT TASK STRATEGIES
LEITER INTERNATIONAL SCALE

Patient _____ Date: _____

Hosp. #: _____

Observation of Patient Responses and Methods of Task Attack (circle applicable terms; provide others where applicable)

ATTACK
    Quick attack   Slow

COMPLETION
    Fast Completion   Slow

SELF-CORRECTION
    Corrected mistakes   unassisted   Quickly
                                assisted   Slowly

DEMONSTRATION
    Learned by demonstration: (number of trials)
    Quickly   Slowly   Not at all

CUES
    Color cued responses are   better
                                    poorer   than black and white
    Shape cued responses are   better
                                    poorer   than picture/color

NUMBERS
    Numerical responses are   better
                                  poorer   than non-numerical

DISTORTIONS
    Patient distorted responses by:
    Inversion   Consistency   Rotation   Inconsistency   Shape
    Color   Numbers

ATTITUDINAL BEHAVIORS
> Attitudes and behavior when corrected on responses:
> Rejection   Applied   Departed   Acceptance   Ignored
> Ceased to respond   Became emotional
> Did patient seek clinician approval of completed task?
> Was he indifferent to it?

PATIENT ORDER OF ATTACK ON TASK:
> Random order
> Seeks stall for nearest block
> Places block in stall in order of stall proximity
> Seeks block for first stall
> Places blocks in stall order
> Begins with middle stall
> Begins with middle block
> Works to right, then to left
> Works to left, then to right
> Works from left to right
> Works from right to left
> Alternates from center
> Uses visual scan to locate appropriate stall
> Uses manual scan, matching
> Makes corrections in progress

If last block is obviously incorrect due to prior error
describe how patient proceeded to solve problem:
> (use reverse side of form if necessary)

Did patient request clinician help?
> Demand it?   Reject it?

When error was indicated, did patient
> Perseverate in prior response?
> Make random incorrect changes?
> Change one stall at a time experimentally?
> Withdraw all blocks and begin again?
> Withdraw incorrect blocks and place correctly?

Did fatigue appear:
> Gradually?   Suddenly?

Enter additional comments, if any, on reverse side.

TALLY-GRAPH

Developed by Macalyne Fristoe, Ph. D., Purdue University, based on ideas by Richard R. Saunders and Kathy Koplik, Kansas Neurological Institute. Reproduced by permission of Dr. Fristoe.

Refer to attached TALLY-GRAPH as examples of recording of Steps 1-4.

Step 1. Enter name of Client and name of clinician.
Step 2. Enter an abbreviated statement of the specific task; or *code* letters or numbers identifying it.
Step 3. Enter date on slanted line above column to be used.
Step 4. Draw a line below the number representing chosen criterion.
Step 5. Present first trial. If response is CORRECT, circle number of that trial. If response is INCORRECT, put slash through the 1. (Since the response on the first trial was INCORRECT, the 1 is marked with a slash.)

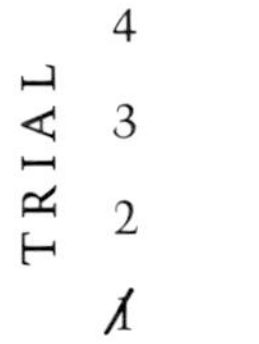

4
3
2
1̸

TRIAL

Step 6. Present second trial. Mark the 2 CORRECT or INCORRECT. (Since it was CORRECT, the 2 is marked with a circle.)

3
②
1̸
0̸

TRIAL

Step 7. Continue as above through the 10th trial (number 0 at the top of the column.) Check that you have underlined your criterion.

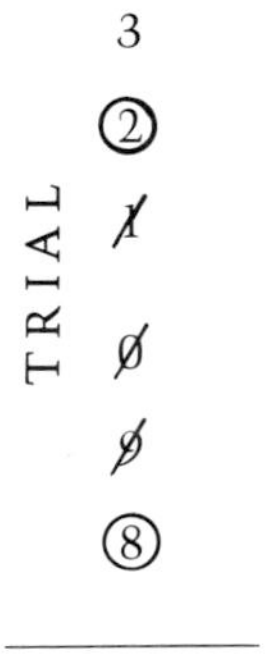

0̸
⑧

1̸
0̸
⑤
④
3̸
②
1̸

TRIAL

Step 8. Count the correct responses in that column (circled numbers). There are 4 correct responses.

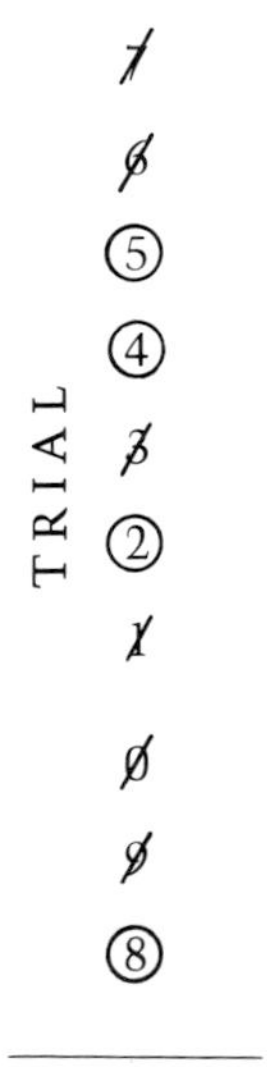

0̸
0̸
⑧

Step 9. Draw a box around the number that represents correct score. (In the first column, there were 4 correct, so the box is drawn around the number 4.)

Step 10. Shade the box lightly.

Step 11. If the box is above the criterion line, draw a vertical line to the right of that column and move to the next task. If not, repeat present task for 10 more trials. (Box is not above criterion, so first task is to be repeated.)

Step 12. The TALLY-GRAPH shows the client's performance on each trial, the number of trials presented, the percentage correct, and the success in meeting criterion. It also graphs progress over blocks of trials.

A TALLY-GRAPH base can be selected to suit the task needs (10, 15, 20 trials per block or some multiple of these numbers).

TALLY-GRAPH can be used to keep track of several clients or several types of behavior of one client simultaneously. Just use a separate line of blocks for each.

EXAMPLE TALLY-GRAPH (Base 10)

Client ____Jane Loan____   Clinician ____Tom Daw____

Date: 3-14-79

																%
0̸	0̸	0̸	0̸	⓪	⓪	0̸	⓪	0	0	0	0	0	0	0	0	100
9̸	9̸	9̸	⑨	⑨	9̸	⑨	⑨	9	9	9	9	9	9	9	9	90
⑧	8̸	⑧	⑧	⑧	8̸	8̸	[⑧]	8	8	8	8	8	8	8	8	80
7̸	7̸	7̸	7̸	[7]	⑦	[⑦]	⑦	7	7	7	7	7	7	7	7	70
6̸	6̸	⑥	[⑥]	⑥	6̸	⑥	⑥	6	6	6	6	6	6	6	6	60
⑤	⑤	⑤	⑤	5̸	[5]	⑤	5̸	5	5	5	5	5	5	5	5	50
[④]	[④]	[4]	4̸	④	4̸	4̸	④	4	4	4	4	4	4	4	4	40
3̸	3̸	3̸	3̸	③	③	③	3̸	3	3	3	3	3	3	3	3	30
②	②	2̸	②	②	②	②	②	2	2	2	2	2	2	2	2	20
1̸	①	①	①	1̸	①	①	①	1	1	1	1	1	1	1	1	10

Task: Retrieve 5 signals SIT-EAT-DRINK-WASH-WALK (object stimulus)

TALLY-GRAPH (Base 10)

Client _____   Clinician _____

| | | | | | | | | | | | | | | | | | | | %
|---|---|---|---|---|---|---|---|---|---|---|---|---|---|---|---|---|---|---|---|---|
| 0 | 0 | 0 | 0 | 0 | 0 | 0 | 0 | 0 | 0 | 0 | 0 | 0 | 0 | 0 | 0 | 0 | 0 | 0 | 0 | 100 |
| 9 | 9 | 9 | 9 | 9 | 9 | 9 | 9 | 9 | 9 | 9 | 9 | 9 | 9 | 9 | 9 | 9 | 9 | 9 | 9 | 90 |
| 8 | 8 | 8 | 8 | 8 | 8 | 8 | 8 | 8 | 8 | 8 | 8 | 8 | 8 | 8 | 8 | 8 | 8 | 8 | 8 | 80 |
| 7 | 7 | 7 | 7 | 7 | 7 | 7 | 7 | 7 | 7 | 7 | 7 | 7 | 7 | 7 | 7 | 7 | 7 | 7 | 7 | 70 |
| 6 | 6 | 6 | 6 | 6 | 6 | 6 | 6 | 6 | 6 | 6 | 6 | 6 | 6 | 6 | 6 | 6 | 6 | 6 | 6 | 60 |
| 5 | 5 | 5 | 5 | 5 | 5 | 5 | 5 | 5 | 5 | 5 | 5 | 5 | 5 | 5 | 5 | 5 | 5 | 5 | 5 | 50 |
| 4 | 4 | 4 | 4 | 4 | 4 | 4 | 4 | 4 | 4 | 4 | 4 | 4 | 4 | 4 | 4 | 4 | 4 | 4 | 4 | 40 |
| 3 | 3 | 3 | 3 | 3 | 3 | 3 | 3 | 3 | 3 | 3 | 3 | 3 | 3 | 3 | 3 | 3 | 3 | 3 | 3 | 30 |
| 2 | 2 | 2 | 2 | 2 | 2 | 2 | 2 | 2 | 2 | 2 | 2 | 2 | 2 | 2 | 2 | 2 | 2 | 2 | 2 | 20 |
| 1 | 1 | 1 | 1 | 1 | 1 | 1 | 1 | 1 | 1 | 1 | 1 | 1 | 1 | 1 | 1 | 1 | 1 | 1 | 1 | 10 |

																				%
0	0	0	0	0	0	0	0	0	0	0	0	0	0	0	0	0	0	0	0	100
9	9	9	9	9	9	9	9	9	9	9	9	9	9	9	9	9	9	9	9	90
8	8	8	8	8	8	8	8	8	8	8	8	8	8	8	8	8	8	8	8	80
7	7	7	7	7	7	7	7	7	7	7	7	7	7	7	7	7	7	7	7	70
6	6	6	6	6	6	6	6	6	6	6	6	6	6	6	6	6	6	6	6	60
5	5	5	5	5	5	5	5	5	5	5	5	5	5	5	5	5	5	5	5	50
4	4	4	4	4	4	4	4	4	4	4	4	4	4	4	4	4	4	4	4	40
3	3	3	3	3	3	3	3	3	3	3	3	3	3	3	3	3	3	3	3	30
2	2	2	2	2	2	2	2	2	2	2	2	2	2	2	2	2	2	2	2	20
1	1	1	1	1	1	1	1	1	1	1	1	1	1	1	1	1	1	1	1	10

AMER-IND SCALE OF PROGRESS

The purpose of the Amer-Ind Scale is to record as briefly and meaningfully as possible the results of treatments by certain methods at certain levels of acquisition, execution, and transmission by the patient. Within each of these levels the scale indicates the type of stimulus that was used when the recorded response occurred. These stimulus steps are arranged in a rising level of symbolism. Amer-Ind Code is, of course, very concretely based with a low level of symbolism. It may be of great importance for some of the brain-damaged patients exposed to it to examine the patient's progress, if any, from concreteness to higher symbolization in the patient's communicative functioning.

While the Amer-Ind Scale is based on levels, and steps within those levels, it is not viewed as unidirectional. The symbolic levels expressed in the steps parallel each other across all the levels. However, the steps are not identical in each level. It is, therefore, both possible and probable that the majority of patients will operate on more than one level. This will depend in each case on many factors related to the individual. Patients can, therefore, be scored on more than one level simultaneously. A patient can also pass over some steps, or even levels, without need for treatment tasks in that level. Some objectives may be accomplished adventitiously.

Since Amer-Ind is not a language, but rather a code or signal system, its use-measurement has not been planned in linguistic terms. It is proposed here in a basic communication definition: *successful transmission of a message.* Acquisition success is related to learning theory, based on need.

Our American culture today (and consequently our supported research) is largely quantity-oriented. We become fixated in evaluation on *how much.* It is questionable whether this is an appropriate appraisal of code acquisition or use with severely-impaired patients. Qualitative evaluation may be more relevant, although not as easy to achieve. The extent to which any acquired signals serve the patient's daily life needs, and also those of the patient's family, may be a more valid criterion. Certainly it is the most important *human* criterion of success with the system.

The scale, nevertheless, endeavors to show quantitative gains in terms of the number of signals in use, as well as the qualitative level at which they serve the patient's communication. The individual's abilities are probably best expressed at any moment by bracketing the highest level-step and the lowest level-step, and by indicating the number of signals employed in each. This shows succinctly *the range in which the individual is functioning.*

This range can be graphed easily. The step-level range from zero to ninety-nine lends itself to facile percentage calculation. The basic repertoire of fifty signals can also be quickly and easily converted to percentage. The top level-step at which the patient functions, even with only one signal, indicates the potential ceiling for all signals acquired. This ceiling may elevate as the patient progresses. An early ceiling may be a favorable prognostic.

It may well be that further attention to repertoire growth in itself is not of primary importance. Fifty signals, with their possible agglutinates, provide an extensive communicative tool. (There are now 250 signals in the clinically tested repertoire.) All the concepts expressed by the basic thousand most used words in English are covered. As Part III of this text demonstrates, for each concept label (of the 250 signals), there is an average of ten additional words in English included. This is equivalent to a 2500 English word vocabulary.

If the first fifty signals are characterized as *basic* and the other two hundred as *extended* repertoire, gains can be expressed in meaningful terms for all types of patients. The zero to ninety-nine rating of the steps can be used for fast daily entry of status for reporting purposes, while the response-stimulus abbreviations are also entered in the patient treatment folder for planning purposes.

The scale attempts to encourage the positive and prevent the negative by equating verbal and gestural stimuli, especially in the early levels. This shows the clinician as a signaler as well as a talker. The present scale is an extension of a briefer earlier version, which concentrated on patient needs and wishes as motivating factors. While these have been continued as part of the current approach, the total scale has been greatly extended at both ends. It now comprises ten levels, with a total of ninety-nine steps up from zero. The ten levels are divided into four groups: pre-use, transition, use and transfer.

There are four pre-use levels:
  I. Minimum Response
  II. Recognition
  III. Execution
       Imitation
       Replication
       Socialization
  IV. Retrieval
There is one level between pre-use and use levels:
  V. Transition (to use)
There are three use levels:
  VI. Self-initiated signal for:
       Need satisfaction
       Wish satisfaction
       Information acquisition
  VII. Conversation
  VIII. Propositional equivalence
There are two transfer levels: (for patients capable of oral verbal out-put)
  IX. Facilitation of verbalization
  X. Verbalization support
Within these levels there are steps in which the visual and auditory stimuli components move from concrete (1) acting-out of the uses of things, and (2) actual presence of object-things, through several steps upward in symbolization. This is explored through (3) reality photographs in color, (4) without color, (5) artist's drawings in color with selective detail omitted, (6) without color, (7) line drawings presenting a minimum of information, (8) illustrations of high visual symbolism (in text), and (9) auditory stimulus with the high symbolism of words.

AMER-IND SCALE

Level I		Stimulation for Minimal Response	
Step	Notation	Response	Stimulus
0	00/all	zero	all modes
1	GG/0	unreliable gesture	none
	PP/0	unreliable phonation	none
2	EC-/g	eye contact intermittent	gesture
	EC-/v	eye contact intermittent	verbal
3	GG/g	inconsistent gesture	gesture
	GG/v	inconsistent gesture	verbal
4	PP/g	uninflected phonation	gesture
	PP/v	uninflected phonation	verbal
5	P/g	inflected phonation	gesture
	P/v	inflected phonation	verbal
6	EC/g	eye contact sustained	gesture
	EC/v	eye contact sustained	verbal
7	H/g	head movement: yes; no	gesture
	H/v	head movement: yes; no	verbal
8	Pn/g	points with index finger	gesture
	Pn/v	points with index finger	verbal
9	A/g	acts appropriately for task	gesture
	A/v	acts appropriately for task	verbal
10	G/g	uses self-created gesture	gesture
	G/v	uses self-created gesture	verbal

Note: If subject is able to perform with facilitation, add as appropriate: k for kinetic, t for tactile. Tactile and kinetic facilitation aid in shaping ineffective gestures to their code equivalents. Step numerals may replace notation for recording purposes.

Failure of a patient to move up the symbolic steps does not prevent that patient from moving up the levels of signal use. The steps indicate the present symbolic competence at that use level. When the patient is able to function at a higher step on even one of the signals in his or her personal repertoire, the potential for improvement is indicated. The patient can probably elevate all the signals to this level.

Specific tasks, designed by the clinician as appropriate to the individual patient at each level in the total treatment plan, are assumed as stimulating each step in the progress sequence, until a ceiling is reached.

From accumulated data recorded by the scale, more knowledge may accrue concerning acquisition, execution, and transmission of Amer-Ind by patients, especially through analysis of explored and reported productive components and programmings. This can provide a base with which to adjust goals and subgoals realistically for each patient, distinguish effective from ineffective clinical tasks, and identify any prognostic factors. This will enable the clinician to choose patients more effectively and consequently improve both evaluation and treatment.

DISCUSSION OF LEVEL I: STIMULATION FOR MINIMAL RESPONSE

The zero base is used because there is a need to register such a base where it is appropriate. The first four numerical steps are listed to provide some methods of recording even very slow, very minute degrees of progress toward testability. It should be noted that in zero response all possible modes of stimulation have been presented without effect. The patient should probably be checked periodically for any change that may justify retest. Those in 2, 3, and 4 may be able to profit from a schedule of brief periods of stimulation at frequent intervals during each day. This might be programmed for administration by other qualified personnel. Patients in Steps 5 and 6 should be definitely placed on a stimulation program. Those in 7 should have attempts made to shift head movement to hand signals and those in 8 should have some attempts at shaping. Those in 9 and 10 are ready to be integrated in a signal program.

Since many patients placing at level I may have auditory deficits, both auditory and visual stimulators (verbal and gestural) have been equated in the scale. From steps 7 through 10, code treatment might begin on signal recognition, especially on signals that might be classified as need signals for the particular patient.

The notational abbreviations are organized with the *patient response* preceding the slash (/) and the clinician stimulus following it. The abbreviations are usually composed of first letters of the descriptive phrases of

AMER-IND SCALE

Level II		Signal Recognition	
Step	Notation	Response	Stimulus Clinician Signals One
11	Pn/S__a	pointing to choice ...	of 3 actions
12	Pn/S__ob	pointing to choice ...	3 objects
13	Pn/S__ph__a	pointing to choice ...	3 action photos
14	Pn/S__ph__ob	pointing to choice ...	3 object photos
15	Pn/S__px__a	pointing to choice ...	3 action pix
16	Pn/S__px__ob	pointing to choice ...	3 object pix
17	Pn/S__dr__a	pointing to choice ...	3 action drawings
18	Pn/S__dr__ob	pointing to choice ...	3 object drawings
19	Pn/S__il	pointing to choice ...	3 signal illustrations
		of 3 signal illustrations, matches 2, discards 1 ...	When presented
20	M__il/a		2 actions
21	M__il/ob		2 objects
22	M__il/ph__a		2 action photos
23	M__il/ph__ob		2 object photos
24	M__il/px__a		2 action pix
25	M__il/px__ob		2 object pix
26	M__il/dr__a		2 action drawings
27	M__il/dr__ob		2 object drawings

(ey): On 11 thru 19, when subject is unable to use index pointing, but can make choice of displays placed some distance apart, by *sustained eye focus*.
(hd): similarly for *head nod*.
When clinician can facilitate from eye or head to index, (t): Tactile; (k): Kinetic.

responses and stimuli. The word **photo** indicates color photograph, while **pix** means black and white print.

The step numerals may be used as a notation. Their application as scores is under clinical investigation.

DISCUSSION OF LEVEL II: SIGNAL RECOGNITION

Treatment that associates and demonstrates signals by concrete methods for conceptualization and generalization should precede scaling of the level. Level II, step 11 presents some problems in presentation. Ideally, three persons should each present a different action. If the signal to be identified is

AMER-IND SCALE

Level III		Signal Execution	
Step	Notation	Response	Stimulus
28	SI/Ssoc:tk	imitation (facilitated)	clinician held social signal
29	SI/Ssoc	imitation	clinician held social signal
30	SI/Sm:tk	imitation (facilitated)	signal at mirror
31	SI/Sm	imitation	signal at mirror
32	SI/Sf:tk	imitation (facilitated)	signal face to face
33	SI/Sf	imitation	signal face to face
34	SR/Ssoc:tk	replication (facilitated)	signal removed signal social
35	SR/Ssoc	replication	signal removed signal social
36	SR/Sm:tk	replication (facilitated)	mirror removed signal pattern
37	SR/Sm	replication	mirror removed signal pattern
38	SR/Sf:tk	replication (facilitated)	face to face signal pattern
39	SR/Sf	replication	face to face signal pattern
40	Ssoc/Ssoc:tk	Responds (facilitated)	(2 plus) social signal
41	Ssoc/S soc:	Responds	(2 plus) social signal
42	Ssoc/V:tk	Responds (facilitated)	verbal social
43	Ssoc/V	Responds	verbal social
44	S/Sil:tk	Signals (facilitated)	signal illustration
45	S/Sil	signals	signal illustration
46	S/V:tk	signals (facilitated)	verbal concept label
47	S/V:tk	signals	verbal concept label
48	Sag/pix	signals agglutination	pix
49	Sag/V	signals agglutination	verbal

EAT, one of the three persons should be eating, another perhaps drinking, and a third washing. When the clinician signals EAT, the patient points to the person who is eating. As an alternative, the clinician might present three actions serially, then one signal. The clinician then may repeat the three actions with the patient pointing *whenever* correct action recurs. On this repetition, signaled action could be rotated positionally.

Materials for all the levels need to be accumulated by the clinician for treatment and consequently would be available for scaling. The ideal situation would be to have a kit with all these materials for the fifty basic signals. Many of the excellent picture and photographic materials already on the market commercially can be adapted. Selected daily-life objects and specially designed photographic and art work are under clinical investigation, directed toward standardization of a clinical kit.

Many magazine pictures are photographic. It is usually possible to locate a similar nonphotographic picture with reduced information among standard clinic cards. Most clinics usually have treatment kits including black and white line drawings adaptable to this task level.

In steps 20 through 27, the intent is to assess the patient's ability to recognize a two-dimensional, static picture as equal to the signal that is three-dimensional and kinetic. This also is probably a favorable prognostic and can regulate speed of treatment progression.

When the patient can recognize a signal, it should be programmed into the next session for execution.

DISCUSSION OF LEVEL III: SIGNAL EXECUTION

Treatment on motoric patterning should precede level III tasks where appropriate. Tactile and kinetic shaping of the signals are valid approaches. Approximations of the precise signal should be accepted and utilized until suitable shaping can be accomplished. Where the patient is motorically unable to achieve precision, adapted imprecise signaling should be accepted and rewarded, but the shaping program should be continued if greater precision is a realistic objective.

Attempts to condition the patient to automatic execution of social signaling should occur at this level.

Imitation, in the context of the scale, means that when the clinician presents the signal for the patient and holds the pattern (or repeats the pattern), the patient is matching something visible to him.

Replication means that the pattern is presented and then removed before the patient reproduces it. He must rely here on short-term memory.

Responds means that the patient attempts some kind of gesture response to the social signal presented to him in a social context. His gesture may then be shaped to the coded signal.

Concept label means use of the English word so designated for the signal in the repertoire in Part III.

Agglutination means putting together two or more signals to convey a concept not inherent in any one of the signals so used. As soon as the patient can execute any signal, retrieval of it from memory should be attempted at the next session.

AMER-IND SCALE

Level IV		Signal Retrieval	
Step	Notation	Response	Stimulus
50	Ssoc/cl	Social signal routinely	clinician presence
51	S/cl__a	appropriate signal	clinical action
52	S/cl__ob	appropriate signal (add object signal)	object
53	S/ph__a	appropriate signal	photo__action
54	S/ph__ob	appropriate signal (add object signal)	photo__object
55	S/px__a	appropriate signal	pix__action
56	S/px__ob	appropriate signal (add object signal)	pix__object
57	S/dr__a	appropriate signal	drawing__action
58	S/dr__ob	appropriate signal (add object signal)	drawing__object
59	S/il__a	appropriate signal	illustration
60	S/il__ob	appropriate signal (add object signal)	illustration
61	S/v__a	appropriate signal	verbal__action
62	S/v__ob	appropriate signal (add object signal)	verbal__object

If signaler requires facilitation, signal: t or k is added.

DISCUSSION OF LEVEL IV: SIGNAL RETRIEVAL

Two objectives are included at this level. The first is automating recall of the signal for execution. For motorically impaired patients, both tactile and kinetic assistance is given as required. The highest aim is, of course, shaping it to the code. Where this appears unrealistic, the objective is stabilizing the patient's version of the signal, provided this is the nearest he can approximate the precise signal of the repertoire. The second objective is to have the patient establish a reliable difference between action signals and object signals, where this is necessary for clarification in transmission (see the repertoire in Part III for OBJECT). As soon as a patient is able to retrieve a signal transitional use of it should be included in the next treatment plan.

DISCUSSION OF LEVEL V: TRANSITION TO USE

This level expects the patient to use social signals stimulated by the presence of an appropriate *person*. The aim is to extend this from the protected environment of the clinic to other locations and persons. It also includes extension of the message beyond replication of the specific social signals presented to the patient by the other person. The first extension to persons is within the clinic, in order to include staff members other than the treating clinician. The second extension includes other patients and visitors. The third extension brings this social signal outside the clinic to the patient's other environments. There will probably need to be a related person

AMER-IND SCALE

Level V		Signal Use	Transition to Use
Step	Notation	Response	Stimulus
63	TSsoc/cl	Makes social signals not limited to replication	clinician presence or greeting
64	TSsco/st	Makes social signals not limited to replication	staff presence or greeting
65	TSsoc/oth	Makes social signals not limited to replication	others presence or greeting
66	TSsoc/out	Makes social signals not limited to replication	outside clinic
67	TSL/choice	Makes appropriate signal for item: I like. . . .	one of items offered
68	TS/Q1g TS/Qlv	Answers in code	questions on one preassigned topic
69	TS/Q3g TS/Q3v	Answers in code	questions on three preassigned topics
70	TS/Qg TS/Qv	Answers in code	questions on unassigned topic
71	TSag/Q	uses agglution any of above 6	questions

reporting on this when it concerns home, stores, church, etc. The actual use of this step may occur earlier than is here posited.

Step 67 is intended to include this extended environment, also, with use of choice in all daily situations where it is appropriate. At this level, however, it is expected that the cue will be a concrete one. This means the patient is offered a choice of concrete objects or demonstrated actions. The choice at this point is not intended to include hypothetical choosing, a very much higher level of symbolism. When a patient is able to use a signal repertoire (no matter how small) at this level, that patient should be encouraged to extend it to level VI.

DISCUSSION OF LEVEL VI: SIGNAL USE: SELF-INITIATED

The intent here is to use the motivational drive of *need* to assist the patient in self-initiating the use of signals so far acquired. It is very important that the patient's early efforts should be adequately rewarded by success in serving various needs. More and more responsibility should be transferred to

AMER-IND SCALE

Level VI		Signal Use	Self-Initiated	
Step	Notation	Response	Stimulus	
72	*Ssoc/cl	Initiates social signal	with clinician	
73	*Ssoc/st	Initiates social signal	staff	
74	*Ssoc/oth	Initiates social signal	others	
75	*S/Ncl	initiates appropriate signal	with clinician	
76	*S/Nst	initiates appropriate signal	staff	to
77	*S/Nfam	initiates appropriate signal	family	express
78	*S/Noth	initiates appropriate signal	others	need
79	*S/Wcl	initiates approp. signals	with clinician	
80	*S/Wst	initiates approp. signals	staff	to
81	*S/Wfam	initiates approp. signals	family	express
82	*S/Woth	initiates approp. signals	others	wishes
83	*S/Ycl	initiates approp. signals	with clinician	to
84	*S/Yst	initiates approp. signals	staff	acquire
85	*S/Y fam	initiates approp. signals	family	infor-
86	*S/Y oth	initiates approp. signals	others	mation

*Indicates that the signal is self-initiated.

the patient for initiating the communicative encounter. Preparation for this can begin early in the clinic program with simple social routine activities.

The scale is organized in relation to four human contact groups. The last of these, "others," may be a source for additional specific task assignments to friends, mail carrier, salespeople, etc., as appropriate to the individual patient. It may be advisable to make preparation in advance with some of these persons to assure initial success, and thus prevent discouragement. This is a very big challenge to the signaling patient. If the normally speaking person will imagine the most difficult communication incident he has ever experienced and then extrapolate it to speechlessness, that person may have some small empathy for the signaling patient trying to use this system for the first time with a stranger. Consider the problems a normal speaker encounters when alone in a foreign country whose language is unfamiliar and where no one understands the traveler's language.

Consideration of the patient's pretraumatic personality and behavior should dictate whether or not such tasks should even be suggested at this level. While the patient might be encouraged to attempt them, it should be made clear that the decision is the patient's so that he or she experiences no sense of threat or failure, if the decision is negative.

DISCUSSION LEVEL VII: SIGNAL USE: SPONTANEOUS CONVERSATION

At this level, the patient is self-directive and like all communicating humans, responds to a stimulus consisting of the presence of other persons. The asterisk (*) is used to indicate this type of behavior.

There are some people who seldom initiate conversation with others, but do respond well when the other person makes the first overture. With

AMER-IND SCALE

Level VII		Signal Use	Spontaneous Conversation
Step	Notation	Response	Stimulus
87	*SCPsoc/oth	routinely offers social signal	in presence of others
88	*SCP/cl	initiates, freely participates	clinician
89	*SCP/st	initiates, freely participates	staff
90	*SCP/fam	initiates, freely participates	family
91	*SCP/oth	initiates, freely participates	others
92	*SCP/out	initiates, freely participates	outside clinic

SCP is signaled conversational participation.

a patient who has such a history, this level may be attributed to that patient if the quality of his or her conversation appears to justify it. However, some distinction should be made. This may be indicated by using the same step figure, but omitting the asterisk (*).

It is well to consider whether or not level VII may, for a specific patient, be the highest level achievable. If so, every effort should be made to perfect it as far as possible.

AMER-IND SCALE

Level VIII		Signal Use	Equivalent to Propositional
Step	Notation	Response	Stimulus
93	*SE	uses signal to communicate at level equivalent to propositional speech	
94	*SEag	also creates agglutinations	

DISCUSSION OF LEVEL VIII: SIGNAL USE: EQUIVALENT TO PROPOSITIONAL SPEECH

It is difficult to define one mode of communication in terms of another. Consequently, many people reject the proposal that signaling can be used at the propositional level. If *propositional* is interpreted to mean that the signaling must follow the grammatical and linguistic rules of a language then, of course, it is impossible for Amer-Ind to qualify. If by propositional level we mean that the individual signaler is able to convey most ideas clearly to others with no more redundancy or explanation than most of us use when we converse, then this level is possible to the expert signaler. It is even feasible for the inexpert signaler, provided the signaler exercises great persistence and the viewers exercise equal patience.

This level is an admirable goal for those patients who may never be able to achieve oral verbalization.

AMER-IND SCALE

Level IX		Signal Use	Oral Speech Facilitation
Step	Notation	Response	Stimulus
95	*SF 10	signal facilitates oral verbalization 10–19% of the time	
96	*SF 20	20%–29%	
97	*SF 30	30%–39%	
98	*SF 40	40%–49%	

DISCUSSION OF LEVEL IX: SIGNAL USE: ORAL SPEECH FACILITATION

From the clinical data available at present, it appears that use of signal facilitates oral verbalization for some patients. This is well substantiated for oral–verbal apraxics, and is becoming more frequent with some aphasics. It is not wise to establish this as a feasible goal until the patient, not the clinician, introduces it in treatment. Giving a patient false hopes of oral verbalization is to be avoided. It may be an unrealistic goal, and failure to achieve it may discourage the patient from using the code for communication.

AMER-IND SCALE

Level X		Signal Use	Verbal Support
Step	Notation	Response	Stimulus
99	*V	verbalizes 50% or more of the time, with or without signal facilitation	

Note: If the signaler continues in the Amer-Ind program at the levels VIII, IX, and X, the same notation but without the * (asterisk) may be used if he requires stimulus to operate at this level. The * signifies that the patient does not require such stimulation and is ready for discharge or for transfer to a program emphasizing verbal skills.

DISCUSSION OF LEVEL X: SIGNAL USE: VERBAL SUPPORT

When the patient's verbalization exceeds his or her signaling (at the 50 percent level or higher) the patient is functioning at level X. From this point onward, the true goal is to transfer him entirely to the verbal mode. His ability to use code reliably as a trigger should be evaluated. When he has enough confidence in his or her own ability to support the verbal, the patient may even be shifted to a completely verbal program for improvement of language and speech. Such patients should, however, be encouraged to maintain their code expertise, so that it is available as a facilitator when they wish to use it.

Clinical Signaling

6

CHARACTERISTICS

NONLINGUISTIC

Before a clinical program in Amer-Ind is undertaken, some basic concepts that underlie theory and application should be considered. There are certain relevant aspects of Amer-Ind that must be accepted by the speechless patient who is a candidate for this alternative mode of communication. It may be even more important that these aspects be recognized by the professional clinician who is to induct the patient into the system.

It appears to be extremely difficult for persons who know no other communicative mode than a linguistic one to realize that there are other valuable methods of concept transfer. The idea persists that the nonverbal method must be inferior. Actually, in some frames of reference, the nonlinguistic modes may be more effective. This linguistic bias causes persons holding it to insist in describing American Indian code and Amer-Ind in linguistic terms and, even more erroneously, on shaping them into a linguistic structure to which they are not suited. This error may be due to prior knowledge of one of the manual systems developed for the deaf, systems that are usually linguistically structured.

Amer-Ind is not a language. It does not have a linguistic base. It is rather a code or a signal system. It has no structure dictated by rules. It has no grammar. It should not be described by nor forced to conform to the rules of English grammar, or of any other language.

Amer-Ind should not be interpreted by exact translation. The fundamental basis of Amer-Ind lies in its direct, visual, kinetic relationship to concepts. A signal conveys an idea, not a word. There is no single word in any language that is *the correct* word. Any signal can have a wide range of meaning within a broad concept. Specific interpretation is determined by the context. The signal listed in the Repertoire with the concept label CRY is equally applicable to *sad, tears, weep, depressed* or any other word expressing this general idea. These need not be synonyms, in the lexical sense.

It is also possible for several signalers to convey a specific concept with each using a different signal. As an example, the basic concept of negation can be expressed by signals bearing concept labels, NO, REJECT, STOP or even DEFY. The general concept of affirmation can be expressed by signals with the concept labels AGREE, ALIKE, or OK.

CONCEPT ORIENTED

Concepts are conveyed by the signaler to the viewer by means of hand position and movement. This produces what may be described as kinetic pictographs of ideas. These may be joined in various sequences to convey lengthier, broader, more complicated, or more general ideas. Or they can be reduced to specifics by additional signals indicating limits, thus narrowing the concept to the particular.

ACTION ORIENTED

Amer-Ind is action oriented, rather than nominally organized. The signals usually demonstrate an action, a use, or a function. They can also be interpreted as the associated person or object. The interpretation is determined by the context. If there is a possibility of misunderstanding, an added signal is used to indicate that it is the object. A forward thrust of the flat hand, palm up, is used for this purpose, meaning "thing I can hold." This is considered a clarifying signal, however, and is not added routinely. Similarly, the signal for PERSON is added for clarification when the signaler is referring to the *performer* of an action. For example, DRIVE + OBJECT means *automobile*, while DRIVE + PERSON means *driver*.

REALITY ORIENTED

The signals convey concepts *highly related to reality*. It may enable people of other cultures to view this process more clearly if some classification is made of the signals in nonlinguistic terms and some style factors in their use are described. It is inappropriate to use such terms as *noun, verb, parts of speech, sentence,* etc. Amer-Ind conveys its messages through a string of related signaled concepts. The signals may be categorized as: Actions, Actors, and Descriptors. The Actors may be divided into persons, animals, and objects. The Descriptors may be divided into relators, locators, timers, and identifiers.

TELEGRAPHIC

Reality terms are more consistent with a nongrammatical, telegraphic style. Inherent in the style are two principles: (1) superior style is achieved by encoding the message in the fewest possible number of signals; (2) this is enhanced by expressing the broad prime concept first, followed by the restrictors that narrow it. These are not rules, but rather logical arrangements to enable the viewer to follow the thinking of the signaler. To achieve competency in Amer-Ind, the signaler must learn to think telegraphically. It does not serve the purpose for the signaler to think in his own language and then translate this into code. The signaler should strive, rather, to think visually in action and then to have the hands represent the action. The resulting signal communication is much briefer than its linguistic interpretation.

TRANSMISSION

TRANSPOSITION

The process of encoding in signals is called *transposition*. One transposes thoughts into the briefest form for encoding, execution, and transmission at successful levels. Some examples of transposition (from English) are:

Spoken English	Transposed for Code
How are you?	QUESTION YOU WALK
What is your name?	QUESTION YOU TALK YOU
Almost all people who see Amer-Ind understand it easily.	ALL PERSON SEE HAND TALK KNOW EASY
Let us limit comments to brief statements so we may adjourn promptly for lunch.	CHOP TALK TIME NEAR WALK EAT

CLARIFICATION

A number of methods have been developed to assist signalers who experience difficulty in transmitting messages. These clarification techniques include the flat hand thrust, which was previously mentioned, to distinguish object from action. There is also a time clarifier, since action signals are always interpreted in the present tense unless modified. To place the action otherwise, the signal for FUTURE or the signal for PAST is added.

Four other adaptations for clarification enable the signaler to elaborate beyond the briefest form whenever it is either necessary or desirable to do so. (1) **Rate control** enables the signaler to achieve greater precision at a slower pace, as well as to insert or lengthen pauses between signal strings. (2) An **alternative** signal may approach the concept from another point of view. A somewhat synonomous signal may be substituted. For instance, if NO is not understood, substitute REJECT.

The alternative clarification is more helpful than may at first appear. There is no single signal specific to any concept, except numbers. Almost any other idea may be expressed by one or more of several signals. Amer-Ind is action oriented; therefore, objects can always be restated in terms of their uses, which may vary. Persons may always be related to their customary or distinctive behaviors. (3) An **additive** signal may extend the message thus making it clearer with greater detail. A general topic, a place, or a time reference may be used. Explanations of use, reason, method, description, or personnel involved may assist. (4) **Negative–affirmative contrast** emphasizes what the concept *is* by indicating what it is *not*. For example if the signal QUIET is interpreted as "cease noise" when signaler means "I can't talk," it can be clarified by signaling I MOUTH TALK NO, HAND TALK YES. Confirmatory feedback from the viewer to the signaler might be regarded as another clarification. The viewer speaks or acts the interpretation of each concept as it is signaled.

It is highly inadvisable for the viewers to pretend to understand when they do not. It is much more helpful to the signaler if the viewers are frank and state that they do not understand. If necessary, a viewer may signal: YOU HAND TALK FAST . . . I NO SEE. Alternative messages may be: I NO SEE . . . HAND TALK DIFFERENT or ADD MORE. This cues the signaler to clarify.

AGGLUTINATION

The principle of agglutination allows limitless extension of the repertoire. Technically it means the invention of new ways to express a concept for which one definite signal does not exist. The most common is a string of signals which, taken together, transmit the new idea. There is, of course, no one correct agglutination for an idea. There are usually several possibilities. The Signal Index (pp. 469–483) lists about 250 agglutinations with reference to the component illustrations and descriptions in the repertoire. A brief list of samples will illustrate the process: *Library* is SHELTER plus READ; *bookstore* is SHELTER plus READ plus MONEY; *girl* is WOMAN plus LITTLE; *Taxi* is DRIVE plus MONEY; *television* is BOX plus LOOK plus HEAR; *grocery store* is SHELTER plus EAT plus MONEY; *restaurant* is SHELTER plus EAT plus MONEY plus SIT. (It is not necessary to use *plus* signal (ADD) unless viewer misunderstands the implicit relation.)

Consider the four samples involving SHELTER as the most general concept. The second signal differentiates the type of shelter into two categories, that related to reading and that related to eating. *Bookstore* is further differentiated by adding the signal for MONEY. *Restaurant* and *grocery store* both involve shelter, eating, and money, but the latter is differentiated by SIT. The order suggested is logical but not mandatory. It has been demonstrated as contributing to efficient transmission of meaning.

EXECUTION

Amer-Ind signals may be described by their manner of execution: *static, kinetic, repetitive.* When a signal is static, its concept is transmitted by viewing a held hand position, as in ADD. A kinetic signal conveys the concept through a specific movement, as in ABOVE. A repetitive signal conveys a concept by repeating a specified movement three times, as in ANGRY.

In a number of instances, the manner of execution is the differentiating feature among several related signals. An excellent example of this occurs with BRAIN which is static, KNOW which is kinetic, and SMART which is repetitive. All three signals use the basic pointing of the index finger at the temple.

There are specific American Indian *criteria for effective signaling* for efficient communication. These are as applicable today to clinical use as they were centuries ago when they derived from experience. These are: (1) *Precision*, (2) *Consistency*, and (3) *Completion*. Positioning and movement must be precise. Precision implies economy of motion. This implies limits on variation in execution. Carelessness must be avoided. *Extraneous gestures* or random movements must be suppressed. It is helpful in avoiding unconscious use of such distracting additions if the signaler habituates himself to resumption of a neutral hand position at the end of a signal or signal string. This rest position can be that of simply allowing the hands to drop lightly to the lap, to the knees, to the sides, or even to the arms of an armchair. Unless this is included in the early sessions, the signaler frequently indulges in a series of meaningless adjunctive hand maneuvers which only serve as interference to transmission. Clinicians also need to direct some attention to acquisition of the hand rest or neutral position habit.

For consistency, the same signal or signals must always be used for the same meaning, once the latter has been established. This precept implies that self-generated gestures will be shaped to the code. This is very necessary if proliferation of dialects is to be avoided. Dialects produce degeneration of both meaning and understanding. They cause loss of the primary asset of Amer-Ind, the easy recognition of the concept by the untrained viewer. If approval is given to the beginner in code for invention of personal signals, the result will be a private code which is then useless for communication except with the few who, because of environmental contact, will learn it. Invention should be praised, but the self-developed movements must be firmly shaped to the code.

Signals must not be abbreviated. They must be executed completely each time they are used. Many times among groups of signalers who are familiar with each other and each other's signaling there is a tendency to elide portions of the movement basic to the concept. Such abbreviation leads to loss of concrete reference, and finally to an arbitrary form from which no meaning can be *directly* derived. The arbitrary signal is as symbolic as language, and therefore much less useful to the brain-damaged patient. Since the unique advantage of Amer-Ind lies in its high level of interpretation by the untrained viewer, the signaler who uses elliptical signaling with his familiar associates at the same time reduces his transmission to those who are not family or friends.

In addition to the three criteria for effective signaling, precision, consistency and completion, there is of course, another skill which should be constantly improved. The efficient signaler must also be adept at the use of clarification, if and when this is required by the situation or the person.

Even when the signaler is quite skilled, some problems in communication occur with specific viewers. The latter must have two qualifications to contribute to the communicative moment, motivation and observation. The viewer must wish to communicate with the signaler, and he must have a modicum of visual imagination with which to receive meaning through the visual and kinetic modes used in code.

Application by the signaler of the criteria for effective signaling enables the viewer to perform his part as interpreter of the code at a higher level. The precision of the signaler enables the viewer to interpret more speedily. Consistency of the signals provides greater ease of interpretation for the viewer. Completion of the signal contributes to the accuracy of the interpretation. These, with any necessary clarification, provide communicative satisfaction to both participants in the signaled message.

ACQUISITION

Because Amer-Ind has been easily interpreted by untrained viewers, many persons have concluded that it may be just as easily acquired and executed by the uninstructed signaler. This of course is an erroneous conclusion. The more expert the signaler, the clearer the communication of the message. The signaler definitely must know the coded signals and their concept meanings, and limitations. He must be able to execute them with competence accruing from extensive, successful, communicative use of them.

Clinical sessions using Amer-Ind should not be undertaken by clinicians uninstructed in Amer-Ind. Neither should clinical research be based on inexpert signaling. Besides erroneous results, there is great potential for harm to patients in such procedures.

It is suggested that those who wish to use Amer-Ind acquire it from an experienced, knowledgeable signaler. After acquisition of such expertise, the new signaler may be qualified to use it with patients. A year of such clinical practice with patients is suggested as a prelude to research design, as well as attempts to teach the code to other professionals in rehabilitation.

REPERTOIRE

DESCRIPTION

The current clinically tested signal repertoire consists of 250 concept labels. Since each concept embraces several English words, the repertoire has an English vocabulary equivalence of about 2500 words. This is also extended by agglutination, relative to the imagination and invention of those using it.

Of the clinical repertoire, only 20 percent of the signals require two hands for execution. A very large proportion of these can be adapted quite easily to one-hand execution. The few for which one-hand adaptation is somewhat difficult have had alternatives created and clinically tested.

In the best interests of the hemiplegic patient, it is suggested that clinicians habituate themselves to the use of the left hand for single-hand signaling. This gives the patient a correct model that does not require reversal for imitation. It reassures the patient that left-hand use is both possible and normally acceptable.

There are a few frames of reference that require special attention for effective execution. These include arithmetic, direction, time, questions, and probably the uses that have been designated as social signals.

ARITHMETIC: NUMBERS, COUNTING

Simple counting is done with the fingers. The illustrations present clear instruction for this activity. There are also signals illustrated for the four basic arithmetical processes: ADD, REJECT, MULTIPLY, and DIVIDE. To express "2 plus 2 equals 4," one signals: TWO ADD TWO SAME FOUR. To express the idea of "total" when more than two numbers are added, the signal ALL is used.

There are two general arm movements that are useful in quick methods of arithmetic. The drop of the wrist (illustration 238) also means ADD. A three-panel illustration demonstrates TEN WRIST DROP ONE as a method of expressing ELEVEN. A five-frame illustration indicates ELEVEN with one hand: FIVE WRIST DROP FIVE WRIST DROP ONE. There are two ways to signal TWENTY. With two hands, the signaler can show TWO MULTIPLY TEN. With one hand the signaler can show TWO ELBOW DROP (ill. 237) ZERO as TWENTY. The elbow drop between numerals indicates that the numeral signaled first has moved to the adjacent column (the tens column). Similarly, TWENTY-FIVE can be signaled TWO ELBOW DROP FIVE. Contrast FIVE WRIST DROP FIVE with FIVE ELBOW DROP FIVE. The first equals TEN, the second FIFTY-FIVE.

To express a fraction, the signal for DIVIDE is signaled first, followed by the appropriate numbers. To signal ONE HALF, use DIVIDE ONE TWO. It is customary to position the two numbers differently to assist the eye of the viewer. This is illustrated in the repertoire section.

DIRECTION

In indicating direction, the signaler should think of himself as a map. On all maps, east is depicted at the left of the map. (Of course the map reader viewing it sees this on his right.) Confusion results if these signals are attempted with two hands. The signaler will remember and execute *direction* properly if he will habituate himself to the fully extended left arm with index finger pointing as EAST. Consequently, by bending the elbow so that the index points in the exact opposite direction, he is then signaling WEST. Apparently viewers have no problems, it is only signalers who confuse the directions. NORTH of course is pointing upward, and SOUTH downward.

In traditional American Indian code, distance was expressed in terms of days required to walk or ride on the journey. Clinically there has been no problem in conveying miles, although there is no specific signal for this concept. The signaler uses DISTANT followed by the numeral for the miles. It has been quite consistently interpreted as miles.

TIME

Use of PAST and FUTURE have already been explained in relation to action signals. Other expressions of time relationships cover a wide variety of signals. The most commonly used is that for DAY, which is actually the signal for SUN. The distinction is one of position. When the *sun* is indicated specifically, the signal is executed over the head. For DAY it is made in any other position. To avoid confusion, it should be mentioned here that this same signal, executed with a slight jerky movement, is interpreted as OK, meaning *well, good, fine, agree, approve,* etc. It may be of interest to those studying Amer-Ind to know that to the American Indian the OK signal says "the sun shines" and that therefore everything is fine, or OK.

In ancient code, the SUN signal was swept in a half circle from left to right with the arm to indicate the passage of a day. Today, the DAY signal is simply made as a static position. If there is confusion, the sweep can be used as a clarifier to indicate the *passage* of a day.

The DAY signal is combined with the signals of direction to express particular divisions of the day. MORNING is expressed by positioning the arm for EAST, and then making the DAY signal with thumb and index in circle. Similarly AFTERNOON is signaled to the WEST. The time of day called *evening* in English can be expressed by executing the signal for AFTERNOON and then dropping the sun, as it were, that is, breaking the thumb–index circle into a flat hand, palm down. *Night* is usually signaled as SLEEP TIME. Today, the hours of the clock are indicated with numerals, following the signal for TIME. To distinguish DAY from NOON, the latter is usually executed at the centerline of the body, the former at the side.

Week is expressed simply as DAY SEVEN (seven fingers elevated at once). The days are indicated by numbers also nowadays, although originally, like the months, they had names. *Saturday* is DAY SEVENTH, fingers elevated one-by-one until they total seven. All names are difficult to signal, so numbers have been used for the purpose generally, and usually successfully. The concept MONTH is expressed by the new moon. Calculation problems can result however upon occasion since the moon cycle is only twenty-eight days, so YEAR is usually signaled as MONTH ALL.

The seasons may be denoted as *Spring*: TIME HOT LITTLE; *Summer*: TIME HOT; *Fall*: TIME COLD LITTLE; and *Winter*: TIME COLD. Clarification could include TIME BIG COLD. Originally in American Indian Code, the concept of TIME was expressed by showing the sweeping of the sun across the sky. Today everyone wears the sun on his wrist, so the modern signal for TIME is the touching of the index finger of one hand to the wrist of the other.

QUESTIONS

Interrogatives are a special category in code. The signal for QUESTION precedes the signaling of the specific query. This signal may be interpreted as any of the interrogative words of English: *who, when, where, why, what* and *how,* as well as *which.* The specific meaning is usually identified by the context. Whenever this fails, however, there are clarifications that serve, as follows:

who = QUESTION PERSON
when = QUESTION TIME
where = QUESTION HERE (place)
why = QUESTION THINK (reason)
what = QUESTION OBJECT
how = QUESTION WORK (method)
which = QUESTION FIRST SECOND
how much = QUESTION MONEY

SOCIAL SIGNALS

A number of references are made in the text under various topics to what is usually called *social* signaling. This includes all signals for the casual and somewhat routine remarks most human beings make in brief, social encounters. The primary social signals, of course, are HELLO and GOODBYE. The first could easily be titled *greeting*. Actually it is the American Indian signal for *peace*. The holding up of the weapon hand empty of weapon signified that the signaler came in peace, or wished for peace, or desired to be a friend. The signal for FRIEND was the next step, of course. The clasp was at the wrist rather than at the palm. There is an interesting primitive reason for this. It is difficult to remove one's hand from the present-day hand clasp if the other person is strong and determined to hold. But the wrist clasp can be easily broken by simply revolving the wrist quickly. The palm-to-palm clasp was permitted only to friends of long standing who were fully trusted. Incidentally, the American Indian hand shake (wrist clasp) is a great boon to arthritic persons, for whom the ordinary hand shake can be quite a painful experience.

The usual social query following greeting is: "How are you?" In Amer-Ind this is signaled: QUESTION YOU WALK. The usual reply is: OK. A variation on greeting among friends is the signaled version of the usual spoken welcome to a friend: LOOK YOU HEART ME DANCE. ("To see you makes my heart happy.") The customary reply is SAME ME. If the signaler means to be enthusiastic in this reply, he can precede the SAME ME with ALL.

Routine comments on the weather or the news and other casual conversation with a friend or acquaintance can also be called social signaling. These offer opportunities for the clinician to establish routine social signal patterns for the patient which can be repeated with various people in different settings. Thus, an early social signaling program can provide the patient the agreeable sensation of participating. If these signals are used routinely by all those around him, the patient soon imitates them and uses them meaningfully, often without further instruction. It is easy to indoctrinate persons in the clinic environment, merely through example, to add the signals when they speak social comments. This can be very rewarding and also stimulating to the speechless person attempting to learn and use code.

Adjustments to the clinic environment can be programmed in this same way to offer opportunity for repeated use of the same signal string in a reality situation. Deliberate disarrangement of the customary background by the clinician can provide stimulus to the patient to elevate the social repertoire to a higher level in an effort to adjust the change.

PLEASE and THANKS are probably the next most common social signals after HELLO and GOODBYE that the new signaler wishes to acquire. It may be interesting to the signal learner and also help in remembering the signal to know the basic meaning of each. PLEASE is modeled after PRAY. In other words, PLEASE means *I pray you*. Incidentally, the early English phrase was also *I pray thee*.

These explanations indicate how important it is in interpreting code to be observant of the *action* the hands are portraying, rather than trying to decide what *word* the signaler has in mind, which often leads the viewer into error. Social signals have meaning from a long history of human conduct. If the viewer will let the hands talk, social signals can lead eventually to expert interpretation of all signals.

Clinicians and others in association with the signaling patient should always appropriately use as many social signals as each situation accommodates. As quickly as possible the responsibility should be transferred to the patient for initiating the social communication encounter. It may be necessary to deny the usual reward until the patient does so. With the brain-injured patient, this reward should be as concrete as possible, especially in the early stages of signal acquisition: the cup of coffee, with or without cream, with or without sugar, as he likes it. Mistakes should be made deliberately so that he will be motivated to use his signal to correct them. The coffee might be withheld until he initiates a request for it. He should be encouraged in every way to *use* signals at the level at which the clinician believes he is at that moment capable.

The signaling patient can in this way achieve an early sense of social integration. This will provide motivation for extending the repertoire and its use.

In the group session, each patient might be encouraged to behave as at a party. He should greet each of the others, offering comments to each newcomer upon arrival. The patients might be rotated in the responsibility of a host, thus preparing for such occasions in their homes. It cannot be sufficiently emphasized that this should be in a reality context, rather than in a school-room fashion. The situation should be manipulated by the clinician so that the task elicits the signal response.

As an adjunct to social signaling, many signals associated with arrival and departure can be repeated frequently in a situational context. These include COME [in], SIT, STAND, WALK, EAT, DRINK, etc.

ADAPTATION TO ONE HAND ONLY

In Part III, the adaptation of number signals for the left hand only is clearly illustrated and has already been discussed. Exclusive of the number signals, there are in the clinical repertoire 236 other signals. Of these 131 are normally executed by one hand only, either the left or the right. Of the remaining 105 signals, 94 can be quite easily adapted for one-hand execution. Some of these signals have already been discussed.

Adaptations can be achieved by application of one of the following methods:

1. Substitute fingers of the left hand for the two hands, as in BIG or LITTLE, which can then be executed by extending or bringing together the thumb and index of the left hand.
2. Substitute the inert hand, one of the legs, or some other near-by surface as in ALIKE where the left index is brought to touch the inert index of the right hand.
3. Substitute sequential for simultaneous movement, as in ARROGANT, by showing the large head with left hand at left side of head, and then showing it at right side.
4. Substituting a drawing in space, as in ADD or MULTIPLY where the left index finger draws the signal sequentially in the air.
5. Establishing a base with the left hand, and then using left hand to provide movement from that base, as in ABOVE or UNDER.

There are eleven signals that do not yield themselves to the above adaptations. In many instances, however, the concept involved can be expressed in some other signal or string of signals. This is probably the best solution to this problem.

BOAT—Can be signaled as SHELTER WALK ON WATER.

BREAK & MEND—Can be signaled in each case by using the inert hand in a special way, indicating by index pointing that something has been inserted under the inert hand, and then proceeding with the left hand movements of breaking or putting together.

DOOR—Can be shown as vertical by holding the left hand in the usual position for DOOR, and then using it to show OPEN/SHUT either on the inert hand or on the leg.

ENTER—Can be adapted by shaping the inert hand to the proper form, and then proceeding as usual, or the concept may be expressed by combining WALK and IN, using the inert hand for the IN.

FENCE—Can be adapted extending the left arm forward with elbow flexed and wrist flexed with finger tips touching right arm, thus shaping an enclosure. This can be clarified by using BOX HOLD ANIMAL.

HANG—Can be adapted by sequential movement, using the straight index to show that which holds, and then using it suitably bent, to show the hanger. It may be clarified by pointing to a picture on the wall, or by using the signaler's left hand to show a throttling of his own throat.

HELP—Can sometimes be adapted by using the inert hand for the interlace, and by adding a slight tremor and an assist from facial expression of distress.

JUSTICE—Can be adapted by substituting the signal for MAYBE but using it at a very slow pace, and bringing it into level equilibrium.

PEEL—Can be adapted by indicating that the inert hand is holding something, and then executing the peeling motion appropriately.

WRAP—Can be adapted by first showing a BOX and then proceeding with left hand to wrap as usual.

Clinical Planning

CLINICAL DECISIONS

MOTIVATION

Amer-Ind has been clinically supported as a useful communication system on either a temporary or permanent basis for several types of speechless patients. The patients will not learn or use it, however, if they are not properly motivated to accept its communicative strengths. Some patients, particularly those who retain normal cerebral functioning and also their mastery of language, may view the system as abnormal or demeaning. Certainly, the code is not the exact equivalent of their premorbid level of speech functioning. However, neither is their current speechlessness nor its alternatives: random gestures that produce only further frustration, or lengthy written communiques that often go completely or partially unread.

With patients whose impairments are due to cerebral insult, the clinician is often faced with concomitant physical problems. Relevant to Amer-Ind, the chief of these is hemiplegia. Other motor impairments may involve the arms and hands. Some adaptation is then necessary in signaling.

It is of prime importance that patients be motivated to accept the system, or they will not be interested in expending the necessary effort to acquire it. Initial sessions should establish the use and acceptability of code by the general populace. Many professions and occupations have definite manual communication systems, including television, radio, sailors, construction workers, sports referees, etc. The patient must be made aware that these are very similar to the mode suggested for him. Television, magazines and newspaper illustrations and even visits from members of signaling professions may be used to illustrate this.

Providing immediate positive re-inforcement for any meaningful signals patients use also motivates them. This is particularly true if the signals are effective in fulfilling needs or wishes. It also enhances acceptance of code if patients observe the clinicians using it, even with persons who can speak.

Each patient's interests, personality, disability, and motoric capacity differ. Adapting clinical tasks to the individual patient's mental, physical and communicative capacities and structuring them around daily life needs facilitates both acquisition and use of code. For some patients with cognitive problems, concretizing the clinical procedures with real, manipulable objects will improve motivation by providing a higher level of success than more symbolic approaches.

The problems encountered in transition from signal recognition and retrieval to signal use are more easily remedied if the patients have had actual, life-like reinforcement of their initial attempts at code. This type of positive feedback should be an integral part of the initial clinical procedures. If patients have found the signaling to be a rewarding experience from the start, they will probably be motivated to expand its use beyond expression of basic needs.

SESSIONS

Type

Primarily, the type of session will be determined by the current stage of the patient's code acquisition and use. Whether this should be conducted on an individual or group basis depends on the particular patient. Probably a combination of the two provides the best overall program for the majority of patients.

There are advantages and disadvantages associated with each method. The individual session permits focus on the problems of the one patient. It is a valid approach with those who are severely handicapped physically. The time necessary for tactile and kinetic methods prohibits the group session for this kind of physical assistance at the level required. This is also true of those brain-damaged patients with whom the concretizing of concepts must be accomplished as part of the code session. The severely brain-damaged patient is usually either highly distractible or difficult to arouse to attention. In either case, individual clinical treatment is required, at least in the beginning of the program. The patient who is shy, retiring or over sensitive to the handicap is usually in need of private sessions in the early stages, also.

Some group sessions for all, even those who are unable or unwilling to participate, can pay large dividends. The group provides an accepting social unit and thus a receptive audience for code, even when it is very imperfect. It provides a supportive occasion for patients to learn that a number of other persons have the same problems. Group signaling provides patients with a wide variety of patterns, many repetitions, and both the successes and failures of others against which to measure their own.

The group situation also provides a number of situations in which patients can use signals to control the actions of others. The professional using code to the group can also demonstrate the communicative quality of signals in controlling the behavior of others.

When patients reach the level of signal use, group sessions provide more interests, more topics to discuss, more ideas to be elaborated, more occasions for using clarification. Generally speaking, group sessions are more interesting and motivating to the patients in precipitating more frequent use of signals.

The group meetings can also provide signal skill maintenance for those patients who have reached their full potential in code and who are no longer on the active treatment schedule. These patients usually need periodic stimulation, feedback, and encouragement from the clinician. Unless such supportive sessions are provided, their code skills tend to deteriorate. If such discharged patients return on a regular basis for group sessions, this not only assists them to sustain their own communicative level, but their presence provides support to the other group members in many ways.

Including family or friends in the group sessions is a helpful method of involving the patient's associates in the therapeutic process. A visitor's day can be a most stimulating occasion for the group and provide new frames of reference in which to use signals acquired in previous sessions.

On the other hand, in group sessions, individual patients may not have even one signaling experience at certain times. The clinician must be aware of those who merely attend, and draw them into the conversation. However, although it is highly desirable that each participate, it is equally possible that much can be achieved by observation.

Recently, many programs have been developed to enable impaired persons to accomplish additional improvement in planned independent sessions. This can be carried out in signaling by using TV cassette tapes.

Many patients can profit from seeing themselves on the tape. They can also, in many instances, improve both their understanding and execution of signaling by viewing TV tapes of expert signalers.

In the final analysis, the clinician must decide which patients are to be included in group sessions, and when the introduction is to occur. For the latter occasion, it is well to explain to patients that at first they are permitted to be "visitors," with nothing required of them, except courtesy. Social signals can be included here. If they feel comfortable at this kind of session, they are more likely to wish to continue in the group at a higher level of participation.

Frequency and Duration

Patient tolerance of the frequency and duration is, of course, the first criterion in deciding the details of scheduling. As in many other instances, it is possible to reduce both to the point of uselessness. Clinical experience supports the logical conclusion that concentrated effort is most productive. Daily sessions are most desirable. When possible, more than one session per day provides repetition without exhaustion.

Some individuals are able to concentrate and remain productive for a sixty minute period, while others reach the point of diminishing returns in a shorter time. Certainly when the patient can tolerate only brief sessions, they should occur with greater frequency. Every effort should be devoted to extending the short sessions. Many times a patient can tolerate two 10 or 15 minute periods, if they are separated by even a brief rest period. In this case, the patient might, especially if an in-patient, be scheduled both morning and afternoon for this double exposure. Then the ten minute segments can be gradually increased, five minutes at a time. The rest periods at first may need to exceed the treatment periods, but they can be reduced slowly. It may be wise, no matter what increase occurs in time span of attention, to divide the treatment session into two parts, with a relaxation period between, even if the latter is only five minutes.

In the early stages of treatment, it is very important to have as many sessions weekly as it is possible to arrange. As the patient progresses, these may be reduced. For out-patients, families may have difficulty in making more than two trips per week. Instead of accepting this as a valid reason for scheduling at this somewhat abortive level, other means of bringing the patient to the clinic should be explored. Many cities and towns now have service groups of different types willing to provide this kind of transport. Usually it is without fee, although sometimes it involves the cost of gasoline.

Many times members of the extended family are willing to share the trips if they are asked to do so on an infrequent, but regular basis. It may be that more of them would be interested in this contribution if they were involved in the sessions. It is quite important that all persons in the patient's environment become acquainted with the signals. If learning sessions for family and friends were scheduled, perhaps by TV cassette, while the patient is attending the clinic sessions two objectives could be served. Transport is provided the patient, and the group of persons in his environment responding to his signals is increased. Many relatives and friends are more than willing to make one trip every month, or even every two weeks, especially if there is something interesting to do while they wait. Ten such drivers, on a two week schedule, can provide daily transport for the patient.

REVIEW

The planning of adequate repertoire review tasks is a challenge to the clinician, especially when adult patients are concerned. Review should *never* be a drill demand for signal matching to an English word spoken by the clinician. The situation in signal acquisition is not at all similar to that of vocabulary learning in a foreign language. It is far from helpful to have the speechless patient forced to associate a signal with any *one* word, even when it is the concept label used in the repertoire for convenience. It is well to remember that what is meant here is the convenience of the viewer, who is not the patient! Just as in early acquisition of the signal, the *concrete referent* which represents the concept is more helpful. The drill approach is more likely to precipitate "signomia" than the meaningful signal, or to result in a conditioned response in code equivalent to parrot speech.

Review is more usefully as well as more successfully accomplished in a *situational* frame of reference, with as much reality orientation as it is possible to achieve. The presence of concrete referents is very helpful in enabling the patient to retrieve the associated signals. For example, if the review topic is furniture, the patient task might be to identify furniture in the clinic which is like or different from that in his home. Such a session might profit from use of a lounge resembling a living room, instead of being held in the clinic. Open end questions from the clinician allow the patient more degrees of freedom in reply than specific demands. Cueing can provide a semblance of conversational give and take, leading the patient to add details that extend his contribution beyond the minimal response.

When the patient has produced successful signal response to pictures in the sessions, review may encompass pictures as stimuli. Invitations to comment on a picture appears to have a much lower threat value than the demand to produce a signal to match the clinician's spoken word. This task is more suitable in several ways than the spoken word stimulus. The picture allows the patient to signal his *concept* of the picture, it is opened ended, it is in the visual mode.

In early reviews it is quite acceptable for the clinician to do the signaling, with the patients merely replicating each. Kinesis is an important contributor to signal storage and retrieval. This type of review has also the advantage that it again presents well-executed signals as models, providing reminders of concise, consistent, and complete execution.

Review of a group of signals related to a specific topic may be desirable before tasks involving signal reply to questions, role playing, and topic conversations. This has the additional value that immediately after the review, the patient is engaged in additional activities or tasks which call for retrieval of the signals in a different situational context. It is important for patient progress that the patient be very comfortable with the situation, the task and the results. Pressures will reduce his level of contribution.

If video equipment is available, it can provide excellent observational review. The patient, clinician, or group can be filmed on tape, and the tape used for many purposes, both review and critique. The making of situational cassettes can provide valuable clinical material for signal acquisition and review. These are more interesting, more appropriate and more useful materials than the mere taping of signal lists. They show the signals in use (a reality context) rather than in a drill or schoolroom frame of reference.

When agglutinations have been added to the clinical tasks, then review of this technique is appropriate. This can indicate situations where the agglutinations can be extended. In group sessions, for instance, this might bring the suggestion that each person contribute a different agglutination for the particular concept. It may even be used in a game context: how many different ways can that be signaled? Or who can think of another way to signal the same idea? Here again the task is open ended. The patient does not need to retrieve one exact signal. This experience contributes considerably to the patient's ability to make alternate choices when he has difficulty in retrieving a specific signal he wishes to use. This type of experience also convinces him that signaling is flexible, and shows him how to use its flexibility.

PATIENT SELF-CRITICISM

It is very difficult for human beings to see themselves as others see them. Yet this ability to view one's actions objectively has a high correlation with success in many areas. Signaling is one of them. Signalers intend their hand positions and movements to match the model. They usually do not succeed without considerable feedback. In the early stages of signal acquisition, personal kinetic feedback is usually not sufficient. The patients need visual feedback from videotapes or mirrors.

The patients' imitation usually improves when the clinician models both a precise version and the patients' imprecise ones. Then the patients are asked to reproduce their own imprecise attempt, which the clinician then shapes both tactually and kinetically into precision. This procedure allows patients to feel their own imperfect and then more precise signals. Use of a mirror in which the patient may also see the results may further facilitate improvement. The mirror should be sequential to the first kinetic, however, not simultaneous with it.

These tasks may be used to the same purpose in group sessions, and even in family/friend group sessions. It is sometimes very stimulating to signaling patients to discover that their signals are more precise than those of their normally speaking family and friends. With certain individual patients in group sessions, it may be profitable to pair them for the critical tasks of signal improvement.

The use of the videotapes made by patients has the great advantage of requiring patients to attend to only one task at a time. While they are making the videotape of their signals, they concentrate on execution. While viewing the tapes, they can devote their attention wholly to criticism of their own execution.

Even if patients cannot profit from these tasks in terms of modifying their deviant signals, it is a worthy clinical activity. The objective may be, not only modification of the deviance, but the positive message to each patient that even the imperfect signal *does* communicate.

MODALITY OF INPUT

In the situation where a person with a special expertise is proposing to share it with others, it is usually important that the expert show clearly that he or she knows how to do it, not just talk about it! The clinician therefore should use as much code as possible in communication with patients. The question whether signals or speech or both should be used exclusively by the clinician has several possible answers. They depend somewhat on the individual characteristics and needs of the particular patient or patients in the sessions. There is no doubt however of the value of code in-put to the patients.

With speechless patients who have intact cognition and intact receptive language through the auditory channel, of course, spoken language should be used by the clinician for signal descriptions and directives, explanations and critiques. But the code itself can best be elicited from the patients through demonstration and use by the clinician, even with speechless patients who understand spoken language.

The methods of teaching foreign languages as a communication tool give some insights on the problem and our assumptions concerning procedures. Can French be taught at the useful communication level with the instruction given only in English? Is it not necessary in the acquisition of any skill that it be seen/heard by the novice with expert users demonstrating? Is it not also necessary for the novice to use it, rather than have it verbally presented?

Field study results in Amer-Ind indicate that use of code in-put by the clinician, especially to brain-injured patients, is vital. This means use of signals for communication, not limiting signaling to demonstration. Signal modeling should occur through use in actual clinical situations.

All patients attempting to acquire code should see it used by accomplished signalers for real communication. This shows them clearly that it is a viable, respectable mode. It presents precise models for imitation in a normal adult manner. It illustrates telegraphic style and transposition. It adds to the patient's repertoire.

There is considerable support from the field data for use of one in-put modality at a time, and that the first one should be code. It appears that, if and when auditory input is added, many patients of all syndromes find it distracting when presented simultaneously with signals. It assists many patients to have the two presented sequentially: code followed by auditory interpretation of the message.

A large number of normal persons have difficulty with simultaneous input from two quite different systems. An example of this occurs at international conventions when the presenter in one language is simultaneously interpreted in another. Some distraction results for the listeners and this is augmented when they understand both languages. There are many other reasons obvious to speech pathologists for use of one mode at a time, especially with signaling. Those who are listening to a speaker habitually focus the eyes on the speaker's face. Consequently, when attending to a signaler for the first time, they continue the habit of facial focus and so miss the message the hands are presenting. If there is no auditory stimulus, the hands are much more likely to receive the full attention of the viewer. Consequently, rewarding message transmission is much more likely to occur.

As a concomitant part of the patient's program, it should be the professional's charge to bring this facial focus habit to the attention of the patient's family and friends. Hospital and nursing home personnel should also be alerted. The signaler might well be advised to lift his hands toward the face level when first beginning a signaled message.

Clinician input is not limited to inculcation of the code. Responses and re-actions of any kind are part of the gestalt. These may include reinforcement through appropriate facial expressions, head nods, tactile rewards and a generally receptive attitude toward the patient's early attempts at code. This reveals that signaling is accepted as truly communicative.

The professional must be highly alert to the smallest indication that the patient is producing a signaling attempt, however minimal or imperfect, so that the fact that a message is in transit may at least be acknowledged. Even abortive attempts to signal should be rewarded in the early stages of the program. Others in the signaler's life situation must be similarly instructed, so that they will not inadvertently destroy the signaler's motivation by careless comments or reactions to the first inadequate attempts. Encouraging reactions to early signaling attempts may be much more important to ultimate code output than any other factor.

The clinician is a vital part of any therapeutic technique. How he or she describes procedures to be undertaken influences attitudes toward both the technique and the patient with whom the technique is to be used. Both attitudes are conveyed to the patient, either overtly or covertly. The clinician's self-image affects treatment, planning, and results.

Should professional communicologists be designated as behavioral modifiers rather than as teachers? And should those with whom they deal in communication rehabilitation be designated as "clients" or "patients" rather than "students." This is especially relevant when adults are concerned. This aspect of rehabilitation communication deserves much more attention than it has received to date. There is little doubt that such semantics play a large role in therapeutics. What the practitioners allow themselves to be called in any profession and what they call themselves are both highly related to professional and client attitudes toward the profession. These also affect the attitudes of professionals toward themselves, their profession, and their own professional behavior, but most important of all, toward those patients who entrust themselves to the professional's care. Terms which imply an unacceptable stance or relationship may be responsible largely for the rejection by many adults of the speech services they need.

The individual clinician's attitude as a person as well as a professional is a vital factor in patient progress. There is definite input from this which influences results in numerous ways, some of them very subtle. This is largely ignored in both therapeutic reports and in research studies and their results. Just as patients are individuals, so are the professionals who deal with their problems.

While current efforts to establish criteria with which to assess clinical efforts have resulted in some useful methods with which to judge clinical competence, there is still much more to do before the criteria will be definitive. Even when that is achieved, divergences in individual backgrounds, philosophies, education and experience produce numerous and varied differences in clinical behavior with patients. The professional's theoretical biases affect clinical performance in many ways, also. Life style and personality are determinants of professional performance that are seldom considered. They, too, modify the input to the patient as well as affect the way in which the patient accepts and applies techniques proposed for rehabilitation.

Any assumption that every properly qualified professional will have the same level of expertise in a particular technique is unjustified. This factor must always be considered, not only in evaluating results, but also in the assignment of patients with particular deficits. The clinician's positive attitude and enthusiasm for the task are definitely strong influences on the results obtained with patients. This phase of input merits more study.

GOALS

The choice of goals in the initial stages of clinical programming for a patient seriously affects the entire result. Modest goals are more likely to be fulfilled and are less likely to discourage the patient by the enormity of the undertaking. Goals can easily be elevated as progress occurs. This is stimulating and rewarding to the patient. It is traumatic to lower them due to lack of progress.

Effective planning then depends on the realistic choice of the general goal, and a clear understanding with the patient and family of its extent. Upon this goal depends the efficient division of the goal into subgoals usually related to estimated time segments. Each subgoal is plotted then in terms of objectives, which in a well-planned series lead to the fulfillment of the subgoal. The objectives each have predetermined criteria. Each objective is expressed in terms of a series of tasks, which when completed lead to the successful accomplishment of the objective. The tasks should be quantitatively scorable. Acceptable scores for criteria satisfaction should be stated in advance; patients are not expected to achieve perfection. Each trial on each task should be scored and plotted in a consistent manner so that the patient's progress may be measured both against the patient's own base and earlier scores as well as against those of other comparable patients.

Examples of goals, objectives and tasks are listed in the sections concerned with programming for specific patterns of deficit. The objectives and tasks are based on a ladder of difficulty which is schematized in the Amer-Ind Scale.

Several considerations concerning goal choice, however, deserve some discussion before the scale is applied to both planning and recording progress. It should be constantly emphasized that progress in *use* levels is much more important to the patients than mere extension of the size of their signal repertoires. The levels of the scale represent objectives. The true goal is *use*. It is usually considered desirable to extend the size of one's vocabulary, but actually it is the use of it that is the most valid criterion of success.

If the patient can execute even one signal, the next objective and its tasks should involve use of that signal appropriately. The patient should be encouraged to do this with the first signal, even while simultaneously acquiring others. Emphasis on meaningful use of the first few signals should not wait upon mastery of a greater number. Each acquired signal should be plotted to move up the levels through recognition, imitation, replication, retrieval, transition, initiation, etc. The levels are objectives which indicate the tasks for daily sessions. Use is the first subgoal; communication is the final goal.

How communication is defined has relevance to goal success. Communication is not limited to language. The mathematician uses numbers, the musician tone and pattern, the painter color and shape, the architect form, the dancer movement. All communicate eloquently. The actor uses the body as much or even more than voice and speech. That superb master of mime, Charles Chaplin, has always been acknowledged as a superlative communicator. One of the professional scales used by actors to rate other actors is how long they can hold an audience *without speaking.*

Customary human communication uses hearing, voice, speech and language. It is quite possible, however, to achieve quite adequate communication using vision, hands, position and movement. When face and body contribute to the hand meanings, another Chaplin is possible.

Many people have a decidedly negative reaction to manual communication. They express or convey silently a derogatory opinion of any method other than the usual, which they categorize as normal. A clinician with this attitude will unconsciously convey to the patient who is a potential user of code that a hand-talk system is inferior, and thereby abort the goal of successful signaling use by reducing or destroying the patient's motivation for its acquisition.

A parallel is available in the negative attitudes of some persons toward use of an electrolarynx by a laryngectomized patient. In both cases, there is an unwarranted assumption that the patients are capable of and will develop the normal mode.

When the major goal of treatment is rehabilitation at a level the patient may never achieve, this unrealistic aim may actually prevent the more limited progress of which the patient is capable in code. The gradual elevation of the major goal, as the patient progresses through the planned objectives, has been well-supported as a more effective procedure. To put it simply, small successes build toward larger future successes, but early failure breeds further failure.

If the initial goal for the speechless patient is code for expression of basic needs, the patient can feel successful when this is achieved, even with a limited number of signals and though the patient may proceed no further. However, if this initial goal is verbalization, the patient feels only defeat when only signals for needs are achieved. The actual result of the clinical program is the same in each case, but the unrealistic goal turned success into failure! In the reverse situation, where an initial low goal is exceeded, the patient feels in both steps, successful. To propose a grossly unrealistic goal is then not only clinically unwise, but rather cruel, which is certainly unprofessional and unethical. With the speechless patient, the initial goal should be modest.

When two modes of possible progress, code and speech, are potential, the advantages and disadvantages of pursuing both simultaneously should be assessed. That in which the patient has the best chance of achieving some early rewarding success is patently the mode to be explored first. When the clinical emphasis is constantly on the more difficult, speech, the patient is discouraged from regarding even minor successes in code as having value.

Use of code does not in any way prevent development later of speech. For the laryngectomee, use of the electrolarynx does not prevent eventual esophageal voice. Actually preoperative use of the instrument contributes to later use of esophageal voice, since it improves the articulation and, consequently, intelligibility. Similarly, hand talk has been supported as facilitating any latent capacity for verbalization in many patients. This will occur, however, only when such patients develop the hand signals. They will do this *only when they respect code for its own values!* If they regard it as a somewhat lowly and even despicable means toward the desired end of speech, their progress in signaling will be impaired, and consequently they may fail to use it at the level that facilitates speech. If they fail to achieve speech after being conditioned to expect it, they are then discontented with signals. Sometimes then, even when they are able to use signals well for communication, they do not do so. They have been led to believe that the *mode* is more to be valued than the *message*.

Low-level goals should not be despised when they are appropriate. Two signals are better than none. Two signals may lead to two more. Not enough study has been completed on patients rated as severely impaired. The major effect of most prognostic studies appears to be the relegation of many patients to the hopeless category. All clinical effort is then concentrated on those with favorable prognoses. Currently, Federal interest in rehabilitation focuses on those at the lower end of the prognostic list. Perhaps it is time to ask: are they hopeless because they have been abandoned? Would the application of greater persistence and imagination change the hopelessness to achievement? Especially if the initial goal is modest. It can always be extended with success.

Within the present century the lighter-than-air balloon was regarded as the only possible vehicle for air travel. The prognosis for success with heavier-than-air machines was very unfavorable. Those who suggested that this could be achieved were regarded as somewhat unstable! Had the latter ceased to persist, imagine, or invest, where would be the 747? supersonic speed? the moon shots? the new useful satellites? Early air-age goals were modest, but they were also expandable.

Human expertise is not limited to things. It can be applied to humans.

ENVIRONMENTAL REINFORCEMENT

If the clinician escorts the patient to and from the clinic and ward, many signals can be demonstrated concretely to describe what both clinician and patient are doing, seeing, and encountering on the way. Persons met on the trip can be included in these environmental contacts.

Time is one of the most difficult concepts to demonstrate in a strictly clinical situation. But it is easily illustrated in the escort frame of reference. The other personnel in the patient's environment can be alerted to use of the TIME signal where appropriate, also. This includes the nurse who presents medicine, the ward attendant who presents the food tray. Time can be included in the clinic sessions as time to rest, time to go, and so on, with frequent reference to the clock and watches.

Any of the human beings in the patients' lives can assist them in extending their new communicative mode by precipitating occasions for them to use it productively. These must be adapted to the patients' degree of competence, of course. Personnel around them should show that they *expect* the patients to use the signals they are able to execute in order to convey their needs to those serving them, when the patients' clinician have indicated that they are able to do this.

Conversely, their family, friends, nurses, and others, must discontinue gradually the perfect service rendered the very sick or those unable to communicate. Many speechless patients, by the time they are referred to the speech clinic, have all their daily needs so well served by loving family members and friends, that they have no very pressing need to develop either speech or code.

Of course, withdrawal of service should be at first tentative, and continue to be gradual. One of the less important need services should be delayed in attempt to precipitate signaling. By gradual stages, the patients should be expected to produce the signals they have acquired to control the actions of those around them in respect to the patients' needs and wishes. The automatic provision of all needs and wishes should cease when the patients are able to signal for them. The patients should be required to initiate the need request at their current potential. The frequency of communicative situations requiring patient response is highly related to patient progress.

Both clinicians and families should recognize that *self-initiation* of signals is a critically important advance for the patient. They should show that they regard it highly by providing favorable reinforcement for every attempt. Actually, for a patient who has been unable to communicate, this is a significant achievement. For many patients, this may be the highest possible goal. Unless they receive positive feedback from their human environment concerning the *value* of this level of signaling they may become discouraged and consequently regress. Human environmental support at this stage is more important than at any other.

The patients should then be encouraged in every possible way to shift to the conversational level of code. Every instance in which they *volunteer* the slightest comment should be highly rewarded and appreciated by all those in contact with them. However, if a particular patient prior to trauma was not a talkative person, his or her reticence should be respected now.

The three great motivating forces of need, wish and desire for information should be utilized to assist the patients to extend their communicative efforts beyond their immediate human contacts. To promote the patients' advance to conversational level, as well as bolster their self-esteem, activities should be planned to demonstrate in reality-situations their ability to signal outside their homes. Some patients are very reluctant to attempt this. Some of their fears may be alleviated if proper pilot situations are arranged.

The choice of a setting where limited talking is necessary is appropriate for the first trial. The objective may be minimal communication with a stranger. The experience should subject the patients to a short enough sample that they will be willing to try a second time, no matter what the result of the first. A brief visit to the public library to borrow a map, a pictorial history or other illustrated book that the patient may be interested in examining may serve. The signal repertoire for this occasion may be rehearsed priorly several times, and essayed when the patients are ready. The clinician may prepare the librarian in advance, so there will be understanding of the problem and cooperation with the project. Prior sessions based on pictorial materials may assist the patients' ease.

A number of libraries show moving pictures at stated times. Attendance at one of these might offer the occasion for a second visit necessitating minimal performance from the patients. The place and personnel will then be familiar from the first visit. The conversational topic will be limited also, so signal review and rehearsal would again be appropriate. The conversation may be limited to questions concerning the movie, the length of time of the showing, when it begins, who wrote it, who are the stars.

Similar situational experiences can be planned at church or temple. Participation of the religious leader and other parishioners may be solicited in advance. The barber shop can offer opportunities where cooperation will probably be easily obtained.

A visit to the bank, post office, or drugstore is usually brief and the necessary conversation centers on limited topics. Almost any neighborhood setting can be utilized after some experience with the situations listed.

Each of these expeditions provides material for use of the patient's signal repertoire in a reality framework. If the patient's escort on these occasions is a family member or a friend, the patient can then reuse the repertoire to recount possible experiences to family and the clinician. At this time, additional repertoire for the next occasion may be either reviewed or acquired as indicated.

Many patients may be unwilling to undergo these suggested trips. If so, each can be reassured that contacts at home with family and friends actually constitute the major portion of any individual's communicative behavior. Whether or not to press the patient for further signal use in an expanded environment should depend on the importance to the individual and his or her family of such extended communicative activity.

Weekend projects might be arranged for the signaling patient with interested friends or relatives. A friend of the patient's might take him or her to a ball game. They might arrange to meet another friend after the game with whom the game could then be discussed, with the patient encouraged to participate in signals. On returning home, the patient can again be stimulated to use the signals to tell the family about the experience. Many other projects of this kind can be developed from the patient's individual interests. These are what can convince the signaler that signals can really be used on a conversational level.

It is highly important to involve family and friends in the patient's program. This is especially important for those who come to the clinic infrequently. Counselling the families with complete and detailed advice on supportive projects equips them to understand the communicative problem and to provide continuing support to the patients in addition to their sessions at the clinic.

VERBAL FACILITATION

In all recorded cases in which the patient, while signaling, spontaneously produced some verbal output, no matter how limited the first effort, great progress in verbalization has resulted through continuation of the clinical emphasis on improving both verbal skills and performance in Amer-Ind. In those cases where the *clinician*, attempting to hasten this process, initiated the facilitation before the patient produced spontaneous verbalization with signaling, the results have not been as encouraging. At present, it appears highly advisable to wait until the patient himself produces some verbalization accompanying his signals, before entering facilitation as a goal. There appears to be a readiness factor as yet not too well identified.

In these earliest verbalizations with code, there is usually some percentage of error. Clinical experience over the past five years indicates that when this early verbalization is in contradiction to the signals which it accompanies, the signals carry the intended message. In this case, the patient should be supplied the concept label for the signals. The patient's verbal attempts should be encouraged if they are intelligible and appropriate.

Use of signaling may also be a verbal facilitator in that it helps the patient to control unintelligible flows of jargon in many aphasia cases. Use of code directs the patient's attention to the hand and its positions and movements which provide intelligible communication. Suppression of jargon may be a first necessary step toward use of signals communicatively. The signals then later facilitate intelligible verbalization. Although the patient may be concentrating on production of the signals for the concepts, signaling seems to clear the verbal channel so that the patient can execute the appropriate, intelligible verbal response more accurately.

There are special problems at this level for those patients who have organic hearing problems or other auditory reception deficits. This brain-damaged population may also be limited in verbal facilitation. Every possible encouragement should be provided for the verbal output to increase, but the signaling expertise of these patients should be maintained as an alternative as well as a supportive mode.

When the patient's verbalization exceeds his or her signaling, the true goal is to transfer the patient to the verbal mode. Some patients at this point may even be shifted to an entirely verbal program to improve speech and language. However, in each case, the individual's expertise in using code as a verbalization trigger should be evaluated carefully. The patient's syndrome also may affect decisions here. The surgical patient's competence in esophageal voice or compensatory phonetics may be a deciding factor in continued use of code as verbal support.

If for any reason a patient is still somewhat dependent on signals, that patient should continue in signal sessions in order not to lose this communicative competence. The patient should be given the assurance that either mode is acceptable (to prevent any opinion that signaling is necessarily inferior). Such a patient may need to rely on code many times, and should be encouraged to use it frequently enough to maintain a level of expertise. Unused skills frequently fade.

If attempts at transfer result in loss of a viable system without providing the more desired substitute, they are lamentable. They are equally so if, when the transfer occurs, the patient abandons the system that has already demonstrated its usefulness.

It may be important to emphasize here again that not all patients who acquire competence in code can use it to facilitate verbal output. Until valid and reliable prognosticators are available to distinguish the two groups, it is imperative that patients entered in code programs have the initial goal set in terms of *signal expertise*, rather than verbal facilitation.

The goal can always be shifted when the patient's behaviors indicate that this change of emphasis may be productive.

Clinical Programming

8

DESIGNING A PROGRAM

Decide upon a realistic goal for the total program for the individual patient. It should state clearly and briefly what is to be expected as a result of the proposed program. Divide the goal into appropriate subgoals, which if accomplished will implement the total goal. The subgoals are usually associated with time segments, but not necessarily segments of equal length. For each subgoal, list a sequence of objective stages that will accomplish the subgoal. Each objective is composed of a series of tasks which, if completed in order and repeated frequently enough, will achieve the objective. The tasks must all be measurable. The tasks must be so clearly stated that success or failure is observable, not a matter of subjective opinion.

Criteria for the acceptable accomplishment of the objectives must be stated in the program. Perfection is not expected of anyone, so criteria are usually set at about 75 or 80 percent. Satisfaction of criteria for each objective must precede advancement to the following objective. Criteria for satisfaction of the subgoals and the major goal must also be stated in the program. This includes criterion for termination.

Accomplishment of tasks must be noted daily and cumulatively until criteria is reached on each. Monthly or quarterly reevaluation of the programming can be used to adapt goals, subgoals, objectives, and tasks, if necessary. It is wise to set lower, realistic, reasonable goals and subgoals which might be exceeded than to set those which might be so high that they build failure into the project.

For effective Amer-Ind Code programming, the task situations must be as life-like as possible. They must be purposeful. Much repetition must be integrated in the tasks, but it is more valuable if it is placed in a variety of relationships or settings. However, the first four times a segment is presented, execution must be exactly the same. After these are successful, variety may be achieved in a number of ways. This may be accomplished by introduction of one of the signals the clinician wishes the patient to habituate, such as pointing with the index finger to any visible object, or the use of the social signal THANKS. Variety can be attained by changing the food or drink item daily, where it appears in the program. Inducting other personnel in the patient's environment into knowledge and use of the specific signals the patient has acquired reinforces their acquisition and use by the patient, especially if this serves the patient's needs or allows the patient to control the actions of staff personnel. Use of the programmed signals with this variety of personnel assists in generalizing the concept for the patient, also.

A model program may be reduced or enlarged to suit the abilities and needs of the individual patient. Each segment suggested may be divided into smaller portions, if necessary, suited to the individual attention and retention spans. For those who progress more rapidly, additional signals may be added, if desired or needed. Each patient should be encouraged to proceed at his own pace. Programmed successes can be greatly reinforced by being transferred to another location with another person or persons present who will act, signal, and react appropriately. This type of situational repetition advances competence, as well as generalization. It is also very rewarding to the patient. There is opportunity here for interdisciplinary cooperation with physical therapy, occupational therapy, educational programs, and any other activities in which the patient is involved. Families, friends, other associates and contacts may be similarly involved.

Each clinician can develop programs for specific patients. Certainly no one is bound to use the exact signal order presented in the model. It is certainly not either the perfect or the only signal order that may be profitable. The patient's abilities, needs, and interests are the proper bases for choice.

Successes should always be reinforced, but not necessarily materially. It is unwise to have the rewards always related to food, although this may be advisable at the beginning. With some patients it may need to be continued. However, other types of reward should be substituted as quickly as possible. Rewards should also be varied when possible. The most valuable is, of course, that which is built in to the situation, and occurs as a result of the patient's action. The reward should always be relevant to the task, if at all possible. This is especially true when concept development is also involved. For many patients the friendly human reactions between people may be the most valuable rewards, such as a smile, a hand or shoulder pat, an approving nod, the hand movements meaning applause.

PROGRAM POPULATIONS

Amer-Ind Code has demonstrated its usefulness as a therapeutic tool with a number of patients whose speech impairments are due to a wide variety of causes. The rationale for treatment design in these cases has historically been based on differential diagnosis by syndromes. The success and failure experiences with varying approaches in Amer-Ind to date appear to indicate that a treatment plan for a specific patient may be more profitably related to that individual's pattern of competences and impairments. While a general pattern of deficits may usually be associated with a particular syndrome, pattern and syndrome are not synonymous. Nor are relationships between pattern and syndrome invariable. The same pattern may appear in different syndromes; there may be variant patterns of deficit for different individuals within the same syndrome.

In communication disorders it is inappropriate to treat the syndrome. The speech clinician is limited to the behavior exhibited by each speechless patient as a unique human being rather than as a unit in a syndrome class. For the patient to receive maximum benefit from a personalized approach with Amer-Ind Code, it is helpful to divide the potential patient population on the basis of the individual patient's capacity for the auditory reception of language. The individual can either process language received through the auditory channel within normal limits or display generalized or specific deficits in this competence. For the purpose of the Amer-Ind Code program, normal limits may be defined as the ability to receive and respond to, with appropriate behavior, a variety of simple spoken directives.

This group with intact auditory comprehension of language would probably include patients with (1) severe dysphonia, (2) severe dysarthria that renders speech unintelligible, (3) oral–verbal apraxia when the deficit does not significantly affect processing of spoken language, and (4) surgical deficits such as total glossectomy, total laryngectomy, and laryngectomized total glossectomy.

Many adult aphasics classified as mild to moderate in involvement may retain some speech. If their auditory reception of language is adequate, most of these may be approached through the customary avenues of speech and language rehabilitation. In those cases, however, where although the auditory reception of language is apparent the prognosis for speech recovery is not favorable, Amer-Ind Code may be used as a communication mode, and introduced to these patients also by means of the following program.

INTACT AUDITORY COMPREHENSION OF LANGUAGE

TREATMENT PROGRAM A

The following treatment outline can apply to any patient who is speechless or functionally unintelligible, but who retains (1) normal symbolism, (2) intact auditory reception of language, and (3) adequate manual motoric competence. Treatment strategies have been designed to develop skills in the acquisition and use of Amer-Ind Code following the hierarchy of the Amer-Ind Scale previously presented.

It is impossible to discuss all the uncertainties that might confront a clinician when dealing with a patient. Therefore the outline is presented in general terms and is applicable to the majority of this group of patients. Naturally, suitable adjustments will need to be made in establishing the ultimate goal in each case, and in posing reasonable subgoals, objectives, and tasks when applying the program to each individual patient. Some modifications differentiating the approaches to the oral–verbal apraxic patient appear at the end of the outline.

Goal. Use of signals at a level equivalent to propositional speech.

Subgoal. Acquisition of readiness (pre-use) skills in Amer-Ind: motivation, recognition, execution, and retrieval.

Objective 1. Establish signaling as an acceptable method of communication for everyone in certain situations and to varying degrees.

Tasks. When introducing Amer-Ind to these patients the clinician's first and most important objective is to demonstrate that this method of communication is normal, acceptable, and truly useful. It is presented as an alternative method of communication that in some instances, may not be as effective as writing or talking, but in other instances, is even more effective. To develop this attitude the clinician proceeds with the following tasks:

1. Clinician explores with the patient specific users of signals:
   a. sports referees, umpires;
   b. TV Camera operators;
   c. traffic officers;
   d. signalers on aircraft carriers;
   e. the deaf who use manual sign.
2. Clinician explores with the patient everyone's personal use of gestures:
   a. turn signals while driving;
   b. greetings;
   c. handshake;
   d. hug;
   e. pat on the back;
   f. inadvertent gestures usually accompanying verbalizations such as head shake, finger snapping, finger pointing, gestures for "come here," finger over mouth for "quiet," and so on.
3. Clinician discusses the rationale for use of signals.
   a. Gesture in various professions: Explain how signaling is more effective than verbal speech in some instances such as when the voice cannot convey the message due to noise (construction workers); distance (sports referees, aircraft signalers, traffic police officers); or the need for quiet (TV camera operators, etc.).
   b. General use of signals: Mention that it is often used independent of verbalization in everyday life because in some way it transmits a meaning that cannot easily be put into words. An embrace, a pat on

the back, a handshake are examples. Even the gestures that accompany verbalization somehow enhance the thought transmission. Gesturing is natural, not inferior. Most people use it when they are in a foreign country whose language they do not speak.

    c. Deaf sign: Discuss how it is an alternative method of communication for those who are deaf.

4. Clinician introduces American Indian Hand Talk.
    a. Its development: as a means of cross language communication.
    b. Its rationale: idiomatic, skeletal, realistic, guessable.
    c. Its differences from modern clinical use of Amer-Ind:
        (1) Signals not used in today's culture are deleted from Amer-Ind. Examples: BUFFALO, ANIMAL SKINS, FLINT;
        (2) Signals have been added, based on the original rationale, to convey modern concepts. Examples: FLY (an airplane), DRIVE (a car);
        (3) Some signals are now executed in a smaller more limited range than they were originally. Examples: MAN, SUN

5. Clinician discusses the use of Amer-Ind for this patient. (Expand this area to particularize it to individual patient's needs and goals.)
    a. To the patient whose verbalizations are unintelligible, explain that use of signals is an easily and quickly learned alternate method of communication. These signals can be used immediately to convey basic information without the need of intelligible speech. As the patient's speech intelligibility improves, the signals will supplement verbal transmission and signal use will diminish as the oral mode becomes more reliable.
    b. To the patient who writes, explain that the signal is quicker and that it maintains eye contact. Writing withdraws one from the other person, whereas signaling is more interactive in communication.

Assigned Patient Tasks

1. Patients recall any use of signals they have recently observed. Discuss the following:
    a. Circumstances of its use;
    b. its effectiveness
2. Patients execute the most common signal they have observed. Clinician can use this opportunity to assess patients' motor skills and to stabilize their signals to consistency and precision.
3. Patients who can use writing are to begin a daily log of all written communication. This is to be dated and kept faithfully. From this the clinician can ascertain a need vocabulary, assess the individual patient's quantity of communication (perhaps indicative of the desire to communicate), and determine the amount of communication being transferred to code (as written communication diminishes).
4. Patients continue observing the use of signals in others' communication.
5. Patients are instructed to make a conscious effort to use the signals discussed and successfully executed in their communication encounters.

Criteria. If at the onset of treatment, the patient is using some signals spontaneously, the objective of motivation is easily established. The fact that the patient is attempting to communicate in this manner indicates an awareness of the usefulness of signaling and an acceptance of it.

A patient's motivation cannot be objectively measured as an entity of its own, but there are several behaviors that the clinician can assess as indicators of the patient's attitude: (1) regular attendance at treatment sessions, (2) promptness of arrival, (3) attention and cooperation, (4) self-initiated contribution to the treatment session, and (5) performance of assigned tasks. Specific to the Code program, the criteria is the clinician's subjective assessment of the patient's attitude and performance of the assigned tasks. If the patient fails to attempt the five tasks presented, perhaps additional time should be spent on this objective. The patient may not be totally convinced that signaling is useful but must be at least willing to cooperate in this clinical endeavor. It may be profitable for the clinician to take a walk with the patient outside of the clinic environment and help the patient to recognize the use of signals by others. Watching a football or hockey game on TV may also achieve this recognition. Seeing signals used naturally and productively by normally speaking adults should be emphasized. If the patient rejects signaling as an alternate method of communication after all motivation techniques have been exhausted, it is doubtful that pursuing the rest of the Amer-Ind program will be profitable.

It is likely that this group of patients will move through the next several treatment objectives rather quickly. It is important, however, to determine and/or develop the individual patient's skills at each level before moving on to more extensive use of signals. Failure of a patient to utilize code to full capacity and to the extent necessary to achieve propositional usage may be due to inadequate presentation and development of one of these early levels of treatment.

After the patient has progressed through the preuse levels of treatment it becomes rather difficult to establish objectively measurable criteria for assessment of the desired objectives. This is a proposed treatment program designed to place the patient in as many realistic situations as possible in order to stimulate and develop the use of signals as a communication mode. Particularly at the transition level and beyond, it does not lend itself to a format of a predetermined number of stimulus presentations to which the patient gives a response that can be qualitatively measured by a rigid standard. There is no prescribed test that the patient passes or fails to determine advancement or retention at a particular objective. This approach yields little information regarding the patient's reaction to or self-initiated action in communication situations. The number of attempts the patient makes to communicate, what stimulated these attempts, and how successful the patient was in transmitting a message seem to be the important factors in assessing use level of signaling skills. As a result, the clinician must be observant of subtle changes in patient behavior as the patient interacts with staff members, other patients, hospital personnel, and family. Does the patient now initiate social greetings when entering the clinic? If approached by another patient or another patient's family, how does the individual react? Has the clinician observed the patient stopping another clinician to offer a comment? Has the patient begun to approach other patients, initiating contact via a signaled message?

The answer to these questions and others like them are often the best measure of patient progress in Amer-Ind. The whole intent of the program is to give the speechless patient a useful communication mode. The program has succeeded if the patient *uses* it in real-life situations and has failed if the patient does not use it in *any* way, or in *any* situation. It does not matter how well the patient may recognize the code, execute it, and retrieve it in a treatment session designed to elicit a mechanical response apart from realistic usage.

Observing and assessing the patient's willingness to communicate and success in doing so is facilitated by the involvement of significant others in the patient's environment. Communication situations should be well structured throughout the course of treatment to involve the patient's family, other clinic staff, relevant hospital personnel, and the patient's community associates (barber, neighbor, etc.). The clinician should attempt to receive reliable feedback from these parties regarding the patient's interactions with them.

Objective 2. Achieve signal recognition.

Tasks.

1. Clinician and patient discuss several pictures of activities. These should be easily identified activities such as eating, drinking, driving, sleeping, and walking. The patient shows awareness of what is happening in the picture by writing, by attempts at verbalization, or by pointing correctly after clinician's verbal description. The clinician points out the critical distinctive features of the activity and how these features are transmitted with hand positioning or movement to a viewer. The rationale is to show the patient what the clinician's hand position or movement is portraying in the picture. If the patient is unable to do this using pictures, real activities and real objects should be demonstrated. The signals should then be related to these reality activities and objects. Treatment suggestions for achieving recognition through concrete approaches using reality objects, activities, and situations are presented later in this chapter.
2. Clinician presents patient with a signal for a picture not presented in Task 1. Patient must identify the activity by pointing to the accurate picture. Clinician presents signals for objects and descriptors and patient must identify the appropriate picture.
3. Clinician presents a signal and the patient must match it to the appropriate illustration of the signal.
4. Clinician presents a statement or command in signals and the patient must respond with appropriate behavior. These presentations need not be delivered in a confronting, drill-type session, but can be casually worked into the treatment sessions.

Assigned Patient Tasks.

1. If videotaping equipment is available, the patient views a prepared tape of a series of signals demonstrated, explained, and identified.
2. Patient can add to his or her signal recognition repertoire by matching a set of action, object, or descriptor pictures to their corresponding signal illustrations.

Criteria. Since few patients in this category will have conceptualization problems, the criteria for progressing is rather stringent. The patient must be able to recognize, by pointing to the appropriate picture of the activity, the signals in his or her basic signal repertoire (approx. 50) when executed by a skilled clinician. This repertoire is structured to include highly usable signals that meet the patient's daily life-need situations. As a result, the patient should certainly be able to demonstrate a recognition of these signals by matching them to their corresponding pictures before emphasis is placed on signal execution.

Objective 3. Achieve signal execution

Tasks.

1. Clinician presents a signal and holds it. The patient is instructed to imitate. If the patient is unable to imitate the signal, the clinician explores the patient's ability to imitate the signal at a mirror and/or face-to-face. Tactile and kinetic facilitation may also be needed for the patient to produce the signal accurately.
2. Clinician presents a single signal and then removes the stimulus and the patient is to replicate it. Again, this should be done at the patient's level of functioning, that is: mirror or face-to-face or with facilitation if necessary.
3. Continue in this manner with agglutinations.
4. Clinician presents the illustration for a signal and the patient is to execute it. If the patient is unable to do this, the clinician explains and demonstrates. Patient then replicates the clinician's signal and then executes the signal again, following the presentation of the signal illustration.

At this time the emphasis of treatment is on completeness, precision, and accuracy of the motoric response. It is unlikely that the surgically involved patients, as a group, will experience motoric patterning and execution problems, therefore, the bulk of this stage of treatment is concerned with demonstrating the motoric patterns for the signals relevant to the patient's communication needs at the time. Use of video tapes expedites this stage of treatment. Video recording the patient executing the signals and using this material for self-criticism and improvement of performance is invaluable. Such things as accurate start and stop position, complete rather than abbreviated signaling, suppression of random hand movement by establishing the use of the rest position, modifying and shaping the patient's executions to conform with the codified system of signals should be stressed during this stage of the treatment program.

Assigned Patient Tasks.

1. Patient practices executing the signals by replicating the clinician. This is videorecorded. The patient is then asked to exercise self-criticism of the execution.

2. Patient practices signaling using the signal illustrations as a stimulus. Patient is to watch own productions in a mirror and assess it for completeness, consistency, and precision.
3. If the patient needs an auditory cue of the concept label accompanying the signal illustration the Language Master can be utilized. Patient hears the concept label while looking at the signal illustration. Patient executes the signal before a mirror and judges execution.

Criteria. The patient meets the criteria of this objective if he is able to replicate the signals in his basic need repertoire. If each signaling attempt is successful only with tactile or kinetic facilitation, the patient needs continued work in execution skills. The patient must be able to execute the basic signals completely, consistently and precisely with only occasional need for facilitation. The patient should also be developing control of extraneous hand movements and meaningless pointing.

Objective 4. Achieve signal retrieval.

Tasks.

1. Clinician presents patient with pictures of actions, objects, descriptors and the patient is to recall and execute the appropriate signal. These signals should have been demonstrated to the patient during a previous treatment session.
2. Clinician presents an auditory stimulus and the patient executes an appropriate signal.

Assigned Patient Tasks.

1. If the patient is writing most of his communication, he is to analyze one day's (or several days) written communication. He is instructed to write down all the concepts he conveyed by writing for which he can now recall appropriate signals. This written material can serve as a basis for future treatment sessions involving not only retrieval exercises but precision of signal execution as well.

Criteria. The patient is judged to be functioning adequately at this level if the appropriate signals can be retrieved for at least 75 percent of the basic signal repertoire (approx. 50). If the patient falls below this criteria, additional work is needed before the major thrust of treatment progresses to the next objective of treatment. However, the patient should be advanced in the treatment program to facilitate higher level usage of those signals retrieved. For example: if the patient can retrieve only the signals for PAIN, HOT, NO, OK, EAT, SLEEP, clinical effort should be made to develop the patient's use of these signals in the transition to use stage and in self-initiated usage. In other words, the patient's progress should not be delayed in total because this criteria has not been met, but is an indication that the patient's general level of functioning could profit from greater emphasis on retrieval skills.

Subgoal 2. Acquisition of transition of signals from pre-use level to use level

Objective 5. Achieve transition to signal use.

Tasks.

1. From the onset of treatment in Amer-Ind the clinician should be using signals naturally, and in varying degrees in communication encounters with others in the clinic. This should be done at times whens the patient can readily observe that signaling as natural, spontaneous, and useful as a communication mode. These signals include the appropriate use of HELLO, GOODBYE, THANKS, PLEASE, OK, AGREE (*yes*), NO, MAYBE, COME, I, QUIET, YOU, HOT, COLD, EASY, and other signals that may be used repeatedly in the clinic routine. By frequent observation of these signals in real use by normally speaking adults and without the need for direct instruction, the patient should now begin to use them spontaneously in short, casual interchanges with others.

2. Clinician questions patient on a preassigned topic. Patient is to respond with a single signal. (Agglutinations are not demanded). For example: The patient and clinician both read a short newspaper article. The clinician then asks for specific information contained in the article. If the patient is unable to convey the concept in signal the answer may be pointed out in the printed text. Then the clinician demonstrates how this concept could be signaled. Questions should be carefully structured so that they can be answered with one signal with which the patient is already familiar. For example: Was the article about a person or an idea? When did it happen? Yesterday or long ago? Did the story happen here or some place far away? Was it generally a happy story or a sad story?

3. Clinician questions patient on several different preassigned topics. Questions are now structured to elicit more spontaneous signaling. For instance the choice of signals is not contained in the question as it usually was in the previous task. For example: What sport was this story about? When was the game played? What was the score? Was there a particular star of the game? Where was the game played? Again if the patient is unable to signal appropriately the clinician identifies the answer and demonstrates how this could be transmitted in signals.

4. Clinician continues in the above format but adds questions which draw on the patient's own experience of the topic. For example: continuing the above questioning the clinician may add: Did you follow the game? Did you watch it on TV, listen on the radio, or hear a news report about it? Is this particular sport one of your favorites? Why?

5. The patient now selects a topic and attempts to convey various concepts about it to the clinician. The clinician guides the conversation through questioning techniques. At this time the particular emphasis of treatment can vary from session to session. A great deal of time might be spent practicing precision, completeness, and accuracy of the execution of signals used. Signal phrasing and rest position can be emphasized and illustrated. Building the signal repertoire to include concepts which the patient is attempting to communicate can be included.

6. Through careful questioning, the clinician encourages the development and use of agglutinations to express more complex concepts.

Assigned Patient Tasks.

1. Patient is to prepare in advance to communicate (in code) specific ideas about an assigned topic.
2. Patient is to prepare to communicate (in code) specific information to the clinician on a topic the patient chooses.
3. Patient is to prepare in signals answers to questions asked at home or in the hospital.

Criteria. The patient is now observed by the clinician to use signaled social greetings upon arrival and departure from the clinic. These signaling attempts are precipitated by the presence of familiar, supportive persons. The signaling is not limited to replication. The patient is also observed to be using some of the familiar signals presented to him through use rather than by direct demonstration. Therefore, the patient should now be observed signaling such concepts as MAYBE, HOT, EASY, OK, etc. The patient should also be able to convey three ideas about a topic unknown to the clinician. The family or hospital personnel report at least one incident in which the patient answered questions successfully using signals. These responses should be signals other than the social signals of those very common signals habituated through clinician use (signals discussed in Task 1).

Subgoal 3. Acquisition of signals at the use levels of self-initiated use, spontaneous conversation, and use equivalent to propositional speech.

Objective 6. Achieve self-initiated signal use.

Tasks. At this level the treatment program becomes less obviously structured. The clinician has a well-defined treatment objective and tasks but the session is more like a spontaneously available situation in which the patient is stimulated by his need, wish, or desire for information to initiate the use of signals. Therefore:

1. Clinician provides a situation in which the patient expresses a need. For example: The clinician asks the patient to stay longer when he has the car pick-up appointment. The patient needs to explain why the session must terminate on time.
2. Clinician provides a situation in which the patient expresses wishes. For example: The clinician provides some condition the patient does not like such as, too bright a light, too cold a room, TV or radio too loud. The patient wishes to change the undesirable condition and must express this in signals.
3. Clinician provides a situation in which the patient must ask for information. The clinician provides inadequate or incorrect information about the next clinic appointment. (Says to come on Saturday or a holiday) or on the patient's next assignment (clinician repeats an old assignment done well and on which the patient knows no additional work is needed).

Assigned Patient Tasks. These situations must be well-structured so that the cooperating hospital personnel are aware of what the patient is attempting to communicate and can respond with positive reinforcement.

1. The patient is instructed to ask the ward secretary, in signals, for some specific information: May I walk outside? May I go to the cafeteria? Is my doctor here? Has my wife called? Is it time for medicine? Several questions should be practiced so that the patient can choose one which will be appropriate to the situation at the specific time.
2. Accompanied by the clinician, the patient goes to the gift shop to ask the price of a specific item for future purchase.

Additional structured communication situations may include the following:

In the clinic environment:

1. On special occasions (birthdays, anniversaries, etc.) another patient or clinic staff member is instructed to question the patient about the event. Questioning is designed to elicit signals to identify the event, to establish time (dates), number of years, etc.
2. Patient is scheduled at an irregular time. Other clinic staff are instructed to question patient: Is this your regular time? What time are you scheduled for today? Why was your schedule changed? How long is your session?
3. The clinician presents the patient with a particular task but does not supply all the necessary equipment. Patient must ask, in signals, for what is needed: pencil, book, mirror, etc.
4. The patient is directed to ask another staff member for something which is needed by the clinician: a pencil, book, Language Master, etc.

In the home environment:

1. Use of TV—The situation is structured so that the volume is too soft or too loud, wrong channel, poor picture, etc. Patient must use signals to indicate to family members what adjustments should be made. If patient is mobile enough to adjust the TV himself, family member should question the patient about what he is doing and why. The patient is to respond with the appropriate signals.
2. Use of the telephone—If the wife wears glasses she might say "I don't have my glasses, could you tell me this phone number while I dial?" This gives the patient practice in the use of number signals.
3. Grooming—If the patient needs some assistance in grooming, the family is instructed not to supply the comb, shaver, makeup, etc., automatically. The patient must use the appropriate signal to indicate the needs.
4. Eating—Many situations can be structured around this activity.
   a. The family deliberately gives the patient a cold cup of coffee for breakfast to elicit such signals as BAD, MORE, COLD, REJECT, and the like. If these signals are not spontaneous, the family directs leading questions to the patient to elicit them.
   b. The family asks specific questions about the meal to elicit signals. "Do you want something to drink? Would you like dessert?"

Criteria. The patient is judged to have achieved this objective if the appropriate use of signaling is initiated to acquire information in at least one structured situation in the clinic environment and in the home or hospital environment.

Objective 7. Achieve spontaneous conversational use of signals.

Tasks. At this point, the patients should have experienced enough success in structured use of signals that the mere presence of an interested person will stimulate them to converse beyond routine social interchanges, and to signal in response to direct questions and the presence of needs, wishes, and the desire for information. Hopefully, then, the patient will begin almost automatically to initiate conversation with familiar, supportive associates when provided with an accepting atmosphere. The task of the clinician is to continue to provide, through direct intervention or counseling, an atmosphere conducive to signaling in the clinic, the hospital ward, and/or the home. Specific tasks to achieve rewarding and positively reinforcing conversational situations include practice in the following:

1. Suppression of extraneous hand movement
2. Habituation of the use of the rest position
3. Execution of complete (non-abbreviated), precise, and accurate signals
4. Clarification techniques such as: rate control, use of additive signals, alternative signals, negative/affirmative contrast, confirmatory feedback

Assigned Patient Tasks.

1. Patient is asked to initiate a conversation with another clinician or family member and concentrate on one particular aspect of signaling. For example: during a short interchange the patient (a) is to be aware of any extraneous hand movement which may interfere with the transmission of the signaled message, (b) to pay special attention to feedback from the viewer and (c) to make suitable adjustments in signal execution.
2. The patient is encouraged to participate in family discussions. With the cooperation of family members, the patient can be drawn into conversations and encouraged to signal comments.

Criteria. In meeting this objective, the patient must routinely initiate social interchanges. The patient must also initiate transmission of a message in response to open-ended questioning by the clinician. For example, the clinician may ask, "How was your weekend?" This question should now elicit a more complex response than OK, BAD, MAYBE (so-so) which would be acceptable at an earlier stage of the program. In addition, the patient must begin to initiate communication without a direct question. For example: the patient arrives at the clinic and informs the clinician that he is sorry that the bus was late, or that he is happy that the family ate at a restaurant the previous evening. Hospital personnel and/or family report that the patient is beginning to use signals in this manner in the clinic or at home.

Objective 8. Achieve use of signals equivalent to propositional speech.

Tasks. The clinician's role becomes increasingly more passive as the patient now uses the code repertoire and skills in transmitting thoughts at a level equivalent to propositional speech.

1. Clinician continues to offer an opportunity to practice the signaling techniques.
2. Clinician continues to encourage the patient to use signals in the communication situations encountered.
3. Clinician continues to familiarize the family and the patient's close associates (if available) with the Amer-Ind program so that the patient receives supportive reinforcement beyond the clinic environment.
4. Clinician and the patient continue to explore the use of agglutinations to express more complex concepts.
5. Continued emphasis is placed on clarification techniques if the patient is still experiencing difficulty in this area.

Assigned Patient Tasks.

1. To maintain signaling skills, the patient is asked to periodically critique the most frequently used signals in terms of consistency, completeness, and precision.
2. To avoid carelessness in signaling, particularly when communicating with family members, the patient is asked to make a deliberate effort to execute each signal in the codified manner, suppressing extraneous hand movement and meaningless pointing.

Criteria. It will be fairly obvious when the patient meets the criteria of this objective. Naturally, no patient will function at this level at a criteria of 100 percent perfection. There will always be some minor points the clinician would like to resolve but there should not be any major deficit still existing in the use of signaling which significantly interferes with the transmission of the message. If major problems still exist, the patient should not have been advanced to this objective. It is quite possible that only a few patients will actually achieve it. After extensive treatment in each of the prior objectives, the clinician may find it necessary to determine that any one of the previous seven objectives is the optimum goal for that particular patient. Termination from the program may be realistic at any prior point. However, that decision should not be made too hastily. Perhaps a reexamination of the methods used in the very early stages of treatment is in order.

A patient who reaches this final objective, and the ultimate goal of treatment, is ready for termination from an active treatment schedule in Amer-Ind. The patient may be scheduled for periodic check-up sessions for maintenance of skills or to offer support to other patients in the Amer-Ind program.

Verbal Support. It is presupposed that any recent laryngectomee, glossectomee, or laryngectomee/glossectomee patient will be concurrently participating in a treatment program to develop intelligible verbal speech.

Apraxic patients may also be scheduled for treatment sessions focusing on verbal production skills and using a variety of techniques other than Amer-Ind Gestural Code. The gestural and the verbal approach need not conflict with patients who retain auditory reception of language. Use of gestures can satisfy the patient's pressing need to communicate before verbal skills become functional. If the patient finds gesturing to be a method of facilitating oral productions, this technique can be incorporated into treatment sessions emphasizing the oral mode. The dysphonic patient will concurrently receive instruction in vocal rehabilitation. In fact, depending on the rate of progress in the verbal mode, patients may reach the verbal support level of signal use without having progressed through each of the previously outlined objectives. If the patient's verbal output is such that it serves his or her communication needs most of the time, the patient may rely on signal use only to supplement or clarify verbalizations. However, signal use, even in this limited context, is profitable to the patient.

Although the use of Amer-Ind Code may be profitable for only a brief time postsurgically for some laryngectomees, others may find it a valuable communication method for an extended period of time depending on their postsurgical recovery and adequacy in the use of the electrolarynx or esophageal voice production.

Glossectomee rehabilitation is a lengthy program, sometimes extending over a year or more. The use of Amer-Ind can reestablish for the patient quick, easy communication with associates almost immediately after surgery. The use of Amer-Ind signals can be developed concurrently with a glossectomee rehabilitation program. As the patient becomes more proficient in use of the glossal compensations, the need for and use of code support will diminish.

The therapeutic challenge presented by the total laryngectomee/glossectomee patient is monumental. Although some patients have been rehabilitated to a functional level of intelligibility, their course of treatment is long, tedious, and sometimes frustrating. For these patients, use of an easily acquired, easily transmitted signal system provides a means of integrating the patient into the hospital, home, and neighborhood environment. Even when surgical patients regain an oral mode, they can retain code as an emergency mode when colds or edema interfere with phonation or articulation, or when batteries are depleted unexpectedly in assistive instrumentation. Signaling also serves as an alternative in noise and in crowds.

For patients whose surgical involvement or other contributing factors render a poor prognosis for rehabilitation of functional speech, Amer-Ind may be the patient's choice as a prime method of communication. The individual patient's potential for rehabilitation in the oral modality and that patient's rate of achieving intelligible speech determine his or her long-range treatment goal in Amer-Ind. If the patient's verbal intelligibility increases rapidly, the Amer-Ind program may not need to be completed. The patient may need to use signals only occasionally for verbal support. However, as a group, these patients can proceed through the Amer-Ind program at a fairly rapid rate and it is probable that they could reach the use of code at a level equivalent to propositional speech before the verbal modality becomes totally effective for communication.

ORAL–VERBAL APRAXIC PATIENT

Another group of patients who have benefited from the use of Amer-Ind are those patients termed oral–verbal apraxics. While these patients may demonstrate some impairment in other modalities, their major deficit is the inability to exercise voluntary control of the sequencing of motor synergies necessary to produce intelligible speech. For the purposes of the following treatment outline, those patients who also exhibit a severe manual apraxia are not included in this group.

The emphasis of treatment with this type of patient is use of signals to communicate in the individual's current life environment. Use of signals for self-expression is the goal, not necessarily verbal speech facilitated by signals. With some patients, facilitation has been a successful technique and certainly should be employed whenever patients are observed clinically to be responding to the Amer-Ind program in this way. However, undertaking a program in Amer-Ind with the severe oral–verbal apraxic solely for the purpose of achieving verbal output is not the intent of the Amer-Ind approach. Patients who retain most other language skills but cannot express themselves verbally deserve to be given a communication mode which in and of itself is intelligible and useful in a communication situation. The long-range goal of treatment for this group of patients is use of code as a primary method of communication, optimally at the propositional level. To attain this end, the general treatment outline presented previously can be utilized with only minor shifts in emphasis.

The goal, subgoals, and treatment objectives remain the same. However, the projected length of time required to progress through the program is longer for the severely apraxic patient. This group of patients does not include the patient who also has auditory-comprehension deficits that significantly interfere with the reception of spoken instructions. If the patient has severe involvement of auditory processing, that patient should be considered for one of the treatment outlines presented later in the chapter. A general depression of language functioning may be present with both auditory and visual linguistic/graphic skills mildly impaired. As a result, the treatment tasks involving lengthy spoken instructions such as in Objective 1 may have to be modified to include visual (picture) demonstration of use of signals.

Question/Answer tasks that center around a story read by the patient may be adapted to the use of photo-sequence cards. These cards present an activity in four stages and, in a sense, tell a simple story visually. The clinician can then proceed with the question/answer activity. Situation pictures and brief written stories accompanied by explanatory pictures may also be used for this activity.

Many of these patients write very little, or not at all. Reliance on the patient's written responses for treatment material is impractical. The clinician will need to make assessments of the patient's need repertoire and progress in signaling by other measures than a reduction in written responses. Generally, a closer contact with hospital personnel and family members is necessary to make these assessments. Because of the patient's physical impairments, other than speechlessness, the family or nursing staff may tend to speak to the patient less, do more for the patient automatically, expect the patient to be passive in communication, or even deny the patient the opportunity to make needs and wants known to them. Counseling those in charge of the patient's care with regard to the Amer-Ind program and encouraging them to direct questions to the patient, allowing the patient an opportunity to respond, thus including him or her in communication, becomes an important clinical task.

Many of the patients in this group may also be hemiplegic. As a result, more time should be allotted to achieving the signal execution objective. The hemiplegia does not significantly affect the patient's use of Amer-Ind. Only 20 percent of the signals in the repertoire are executed with both hands. Of these, many transmit intelligibly when executed by the hemiplegic patient using only one hand. This is the very simplest type of modification and does not require any direct therapeutic intervention. These signals are demonstrated by the clinician as if they were one-handed. Some signals, particularly those referring to spatial relationships, can be transmitted successfully if the hemiplegic patient is directed to use the inert hand, leg, or even a table top, if appropriate, as the static reference point. Some patients may exhibit difficulty with finger movement. In these cases, the signal is modified to use the whole hand or an arm movement to convey the concept. Specific adaptations are discussed elsewhere in the text.

If the oral apraxic patient has been speechless for a long period of time before beginning Amer-Ind, that patient may have developed a personal manual dialect. This gesturing is often random, inconsistent, imprecise, and incomplete. Often the patient will resort to vague pointing in an effort to communicate. As a result, the patient's use of these gestures does not serve as an acceptable mode of communication. The clinician's task is to shape and modify the patient's spontaneous efforts to conform as closely as possible to the manner of execution described in the signal repertoire in Part III. Transmission studies have shown that these coded signals do transmit at an 80 percent level of intelligibility or greater. Random pointing should be discouraged. The patient is to point only at concrete objects which are clearly in sight of the viewer.

If the patient cannot imitate the clinician's execution of a signal, the clinician should place the patient's hands in the accurate static position or should move them through the kinetic execution of the signal by manual facilitation. This is an important technique with some patients in this group and should be given an adequate amount of treatment time to achieve favorable results. The patient may also need to see the facilitation in a mirror.

The patient's physical involvements in general may necessitate a slower treatment pace. If the patient is confined to a wheelchair, attendance at the clinic sessions may be irregular. If the patient is unable to provide personal means of transportation, he or she must rely on escort service or family members for attendance. This physical confinement also makes it difficult to arrange the number and variety of communication situations necessary for greatest progress in Amer-Ind.

Oral Facilitation

For those patients who are attempting to verbalize while signaling, the Amer-Ind program may become dually effective. The treatment program now has two points of emphasis: (1) continued development of signals to the highest use level possible, and (2) use of signals to facilitate verbal production, optimally to the level of verbal support. Tasks to develop both points of emphasis proceed concurrently. However, the patient may achieve greater results at a faster rate in one than the other. For example, some patients may find Amer-Ind a facilitator for only a few verbalizations and even this may be inconsistent. They will have achieved only the lowest level of the oral facilitation objective. However, the use of signals as a primary communication mode may continue to improve toward the propositional objective. Other patients may have great success with Amer-Ind as a facilitator and therefore develop the verbal modality to a more functional level than they achieve with signals.

The question also arises as to when clinical emphasis should be placed on the patient's attempts to verbalize while signaling. The clinician should not press for verbalization, but wait until the patient offers verbalization spontaneously. Then if the patient knows the manner of execution of a signal and can retrieve it in response to a variety of stimuli, any attempts at verbalization should be encouraged. After executing the appropriate signal, the patient should then repeat the signal, now focusing on the verbalization. The clinician facilitates or modifies the verbalization in whatever manner is appropriate for the particular patient. The patient's attempts to verbalize with signals continue to be reinforced as the Amer-Ind program progresses. The patient should be encouraged to use signals first, then attempt the verbalization. If the patient progresses to appropriate verbalizations of one word or short phrase length, but needs cueing to achieve this, the use of signals can be very effective. The advantage of the patient's use of signals for self-cueing is obvious. The patient then does not have to rely on outside support. He becomes more self-directed in the communication situation. A verbal response which can be elicited only when facilitated by auditory stimulation, phonetic placement, or sentence completion cueing is not very functional when the patient is attempting to participate in a true communication interchange. The patient who can use the retrieval and execution of the signal as a method of self-cueing becomes an active communicator in the oral mode.

Verbal Support

The patient who responds favorably to Amer-Ind as a facilitator for verbal speech may progress in the oral mode to the point where signal usage becomes secondary and verbalization takes over as the prime mode of communication. If this occurs, the patient should certainly be continued in a treatment approach to develop oral skills and the Amer-Ind program should be terminated.

IMPAIRED AUDITORY RECEPTION OF LANGUAGE

The second broad group of speechless patients is comprised of those with serious impairment of the auditory processing of language. It is obvious that since these patients do not react in the normal manner to auditory stimuli the implementation of their therapeutic approaches must be quite different from that with the group already discussed (patients with intact language comprehension).

Amer-Ind Code can be profitably used by the clinician as an in-put mode. Many patients who do not respond appropriately to auditory stimuli often interpret accurately and respond appropriately to the codified gestures. These patients can also profit from a program that emphasizes Amer-Ind Code as a mode of communication *by* the patient, as well as *to* the patient.

Within this group of patients there are some additional important differences affecting the programming. The most significant is the level of the individual's symbolizing. Over the group a wide range of impairment may be observed. Some patients may be operating only at a reduced *concrete* level, apparently with limitation in associating with familiar environmental objects and their functions. Others may be able to perform at a slightly higher level on the symbolic scale, making conceptual association of familiar objects and their use in the environment, but unable to extend their associations beyond the familiar. Some are able to *generalize*, grouping dissimilar objects together on a basis of similar function.

Motoric differences may exist for some patients in this group. Minimal motoric command of at least one hand is desirable in mastering a manual system. Many patients have coped with limitation, however, especially when it has been amenable to tactual and/or kinetic facilitation, in which case even somewhat distorted signals have provided basic communication with a limited code repertoire.

Another dichotomy exists in the group of patients with impaired or no auditory reception of language between those who have had normal language functioning and lost it, and those who have never acquired it. Restoring a lost competence (rehabilitation) is a somewhat different process than establishing a competence that has never been acquired (habilitation).

Speechless patients diagnosed as brain-damaged are usually categorized under one of two broad syndromes: aphasia or mental retardation. These deficits can have a variety of etiologies. Aphasia is most frequently associated with cerebrovascular accidents (stroke) but there appears to be a rising incidence due to head injury in highway accidents. Developmental impairments are largely attributed to various hereditary anomalies or congenital deficiencies. The age levels affected and the degrees of impairment are wide and diverse: The elderly victimized by strokes; the developmental problems of the young; and the accident victims of all ages and severity of impairment.

For patients who have impaired auditory reception of language, the principles of progression through the Amer-Ind levels apply to programming. But many aspects of treatment differ. Sessions must be more structured, and content more repetitive. Repetitions may need to be more frequent, such as breaking up a 60-minute daily assignment into four sessions of fifteen minutes, each of which replicates the first. Increments will probably be smaller and may require more time, both in number of sessions and scheduling over months. The customary clinical pictures may not be effective, as almost all of them are at a symbolic level above the comprehension of those who are moderately or severely impaired in symbolism.

Patients with impaired symbolism and/or conceptualization require repeated demonstrations of the associated appropriate behaviors in regard to real-life objects to enable an understanding of meaning and the function of conceptual systems, such as Amer-Ind. This demonstration cannot be effective in a drill context. Drills may produce only meaningless, mimetic performances. The demonstrations must occur as part of an actual situation, or at least in a well-organized replication of a real-life situation. Although repetition is necessary both to initial understanding and to later use, this repetition must be achieved as it is in real life, by *recurrence of the situation,* with all its attendant associations and rewards.

Many professionals advocate multimodal stimulation and consequently use both auditory as well as Amer-Ind input to these patients. Experience to date with Amer-Ind Code appears to indicate that for the majority of the more highly impaired patients, simultaneous presentation in two modalities only provides a distraction. These patients tend to watch the clinician's mouth rather than the hands.

If and when patients have acquired meaningful signaling with Amer-Ind and at the same time have indicated in progress tests that their prognosis for speech acquisition has improved, it may then be advisable to consider adding the auditory modality for stimulation. Even under these highly favorable circumstances, the visual/kinetic aspects of code and the auditory stimulation of language should be sequential not simultaneous. Simultaneity can be processed easily by most normal communicators, but it presents, even under the best circumstances, some serious problems for brain-damaged patients.

Any of these persons may have additional neurological and/or physical problems that may dictate certain approaches and negate or limit others. Deficits in auditory, visual, kinetic, and tactual systems will indicate which channels may be profitably utilized for rehabilitation procedures. All of the variables must be assessed in terms of the individual patient and applied to modification and selectivity in use of the sample programming which follows.

This nonverbal, nonlinguistic approach is based on the demonstration of the meaning of human actions (behaviors) in relation to use of familiar environmental objects in prearranged sequences closely resembling ordinary situations in daily life. The approach is conducted entirely in demonstration behavior accompanied by the appropriate Amer-Ind signals.

Program B is directed primarily to the moderate to severe aphasic adult who lacks auditory reception of language. It is also usable with speechless patients lacking auditory reception of language and diagnosed as mildly or moderately mentally retarded, and when the prognosis for oral speech is unfavorable.

Approaches for severely and profoundly involved patients in both syndrome groups will be discussed later in Program C.

TREATMENT PROGRAM B

Goal. Patient use of fifty signals for basic social and need situations, to be acquired in 12–24 weeks with a minimum of five sessions per week of at least thirty minutes per session, or ten sessions per week of at least fifteen minutes each. Clinician input is limited to reality demonstration in a situational context, plus Amer-Ind signals. The signals to be acquired by the patient are usually introduced in groups of five, but this is certainly variable. At all times other signals relevant to the situation are used appropriately by all staff concerned. Initially, each signal segment has a stated objective from the Amer-Ind Scale. The patient may progress at different speeds with individual signals, however, using some of them very early at higher levels, while dealing with others at lower levels. Most patients will grasp the meaning of ten of the frequently used and repeated signals, merely through constant repetition in the appropriate situation by the clinic staff. Those acquired in this manner are referred to as "habituated" signals.

Habituated signals used in early demonstrations include: HELLO; GOODBYE; I; YOU; OK; REJECT (*throw away, no good*); THANKS; PLEASE; COME; WALK (*go*).

Other signals demonstrated in the first session and repeated frequently in the following sessions include: SIT; SEE; DRINK; QUESTION; NOISY; QUIET; POUR; WRITE; OBJECT; STIR; PHONE; BREAK; BOX (*TV*); TIME; FUTURE; CHOP (*terminate*).

Additional signals programmed for demonstration include: YES; NO; BIG; LITTLE; PAIN; PILL; RAIN; HOT; COLD; TALK; PHONE; DOCTOR (*boss*); SLEEP; WATER-CHAIR (*Toilet*); EAT; MORE; WRITE; MONEY; WATER; WASH; DRIVE; LOCK; MAN; WOMAN; SHELTER; RING (*wedding*); HELP; HEART; GIVE; GET; HAPPY; SAD; HEART (*like, feel*); ALL.

If the ten habituated signals are included, this program presents a total of sixty signals. Any of these may be replaced at the clinician's discretion if others will serve the particular patient's needs better. Clinicians are reminded that the above English words are merely **concept labels** used for retrieving the signal. Many other words are equally appropriate and meaningful for the concepts involved. These are listed with the related illustrations.

Objective 1. Demonstrate to patient in reality situation that many normally speaking adults use hand signals for normal communication under certain circumstances.

(The following abbreviations will be used in the program: C for clinician, P for patient, S for staff member, G for guest, and P2, P3, etc. for other patients in groups.)

TASK **A**

[*C meets P on arrival at clinic door.*]

C: HELLO—COME—YOU I WALK—(C leads P to session location)

C: YOU SIT—I SIT—

[*If necessary, assist P into chair, then sit. S appears at door*].

S: HELLO (to P)—HELLO—(to C)

C: HELLO—

S: QUESTION WRITE OBJECT—

[*C points to pencil on desk. S picks up pencil and shows broken point to C. C points to pencil sharpener*].

S: THANKS—

[*Sharpens pencil. Loud continuous noise occurs in corridor by prearrangement.*]

C: NOISY—YOU SEE—CHOP—

[*S looks out door.*]

S: CHOP NOISE—QUIET—

[*Noise stops.*]

C: OK—THANKS—

[*Phone rings by prearrangement, S answers.*]

S: (to C) PHONE—YOU—

C: NO—I PHONE TIME FUTURE—

[*S answers phone and hangs up.*]

S: QUESTION YOU DRINK (to C)

C: YES THANKS

[*S goes to sink, picks up paper cup and draws water and gives to C.*]

S: QUESTION YOU DRINK (to P)

[*Fills cup of water and gives to P.*]

C: (to S) QUESTION YOU DRINK

S: NO THANKS

C: DRINK CHOP—[*shows empty cup*]—REJECT PLEASE

[*Gives paper cup to S who throws it in waste basket.*]—THANKS s: GOODBYE (To C)

c: GOODBYE

s: GOODBYE (To P)

[*S leaves room.*]

c: (to P) QUESTION YOU DRINK CHOP—

[*C examines P's cup. If it is empty, signals* CHOP YES, *if not yet empty* CHOP NO YOU DRINK. *If* CHOP YES, *takes cup and signals* I REJECT. *If* NO, *waits till P finishes and then signals* CHOP—REJECT *and throws cup in wastebasket. In each case, C shows P the cup, full or empty as the appropriate signal is made.*]

[*If only* TASK A *is to be presented to P at this session, continue with the following.*]

c: TIME YOU WALK—I SEE YOU—TIME FUTURE—

[*Escorts P to clinic door.*]

c: GOODBYE—

[*If session is to continue with other tasks.*]

c: YOU—I—SEE HEAR BOX— (or CAMERA)

TASK B

[*If videotapes for this purpose are available, clinician shows P television monitor, identify-it by signal* SEE HEAR BOX, *tracing the box on front of monitor. Tape shows various professionals using gestures appropriately, such as sports referees, traffic police officers, construction crews, etc.*]

TASK C

[*Clinician shows P photographs of professionals using gestures typical of their work, such as police officer stopping traffic. If these are actual photos in color, this provides the best type of stimuli at this point.*

For some patients, these may be more effective if presented as projected slides which provide larger stimuli. Reduced lighting with slides also assists in focusing attention.]

TASK D

[*Pictures in color (preferably) obtained from magazines, depicting similar persons at work, (especially if they show the worker making a gesture) can then be compared with the clinician's demonstration showing the similarity between the work action and the Amer-Ind code signal that represents it.*]

TASK E

[*With collaboration of fellow workers, the clinician can stage a demonstration of workers in various parts of the hospital or clinic using gestures to communicate. These can include such simple, everyday occasions as:*
1. directing someone at a distance to COME *to you;*
2. pointing out to someone where something is located;

3. *look out the window to see something interesting;*
4. *pointing to the clock and then to the abdomen indicating that it is hungry time;*
5. *go away and don't bother me;*
6. *time to stop now.*

Task F

[*May be added to any of the prior tasks.*]

[*S appears at door of clinic session.*]

s: TIME BREAK

c: THANKS—(to P) YOU I WALK—TIME BREAK—DRINK

[*Escorts P to location of coffee break.*]

s: (to C) QUESTION YOU DRINK

c: YES THANKS

[*S prepares small paper cup of coffee for C.*]

s: QUESTION YOU POUR (points to cream pitcher)

s: QUESTION YOU STIR (points to sugar container)

[*C replies according to real wishes. S supplies cream, sugar or neither suitably, seeing that P is able to observe results of YES and NO replies. Then S signals to P and prepares his coffee accordingly. Head shakes or nods should be accepted from the patient, as well as finger pointing, but C and S should exhibit the thumbs up or down signal and call his attention to it. Should the P at any time in these tasks imitate a signal appropriately, he should of course be immediately rewarded.*]

Task G

[*At end of coffee break, S uses DRINK CHOP appropriately with P, takes empty cups, uses REJECT and throws them in waste basket. C and S use YES TIME CHOP and TIME YOU WALK appropriately to P as well as I SEE YOU FUTURE TIME. The P may be shown both clock and calendar. P may be given a formal appointment card to take to ward or home, accompanied again with signals I SEE YOU FUTURE TIME. P is then escorted to exit, with both C and S using GOODBYE.*]

Criteria for Accomplishment. P accepts signaling behavior and cooperates in indicated actions so far as he is able to do so, offers no objection to second appointment and returns as indicated with apparent willingness. The clinician must not assume that this demonstration has enabled P to use any of the demonstrated signals meaningfully, although a few may do so with some of the signals.

Some of the tasks may require a full session, depending on the attention span and activity tolerance of the individual patient. If so, the greeting segments, the coffee break segments and the next appointment farewell segments may be attached to any of them profitably. These in any case should become a regular part of every session with suitable change in objective of course.

Objective 2. Recognition of signal meaning by appropriate P 1 behavior.
Signal Group A: HELLO—DRINK—POUR—STIR—YES—NO—GOODBYE—.

[*C has arranged to have two other persons present at the coffee room, preferably P 2 who uses some signals, and also P 3 if possible, as well as S, who will adjust* YES *and* NO *responses so that both affirmative and negative are modelled following each question.*]

C: HELLO— [escorts P to coffee room] YOU I WALK—DRINK—.

[*On entry to coffee room, C greets each person with* HELLO. *If possible, all others should be led to greet P 1.*]

C: (to P 2) I DRINK—QUESTION YOU DRINK—

P 2: YES—I DRINK

C: (to S) QUESTION YOU DRINK

S: NO—I DRINK NO—

C: (to P 1) QUESTION YOU DRINK

[*P may respond with head movement. If so, C signals with thumb to match. If not, response should be facilitated, if possible. If no response, assume P will take coffee and move to addition of cream and/or sugar or neither. S demonstrate proper signals with C first, then with P 2, then proceed to P 1 for his sugar/cream or neither. C invites each to* SIT *as soon as served. As each is served, each sits. When all are seated, preferably around a coffee table on which the creamer and sugar containers are easily within reach of all, C proceeds to ask each as follows.*)

C: (to S) QUESTION YOU DRINK—POUR—STIR

S: I DRINK—POUR YES—STIR NO

[*S points to creamer and sugar container appropriately.*]

S: (to C) QUESTION YOU DRINK—

C: I DRINK—POUR NO—STIR NO—(to P 2) QUESTION YOU DRINK

P 2: I DRINK—POUR (yes or no)—STIR (yes or no)

[To P 1] QUESTION YOU DRINK [C may help P 1 to reply.]

[*P is regarded as fulfilling the objective if he points with the index to the* cream *and* sugar *appropriately when each is signaled, or if he refuses each appropriately. C then models proper reply in code for P 1, describing coffee properly. It may require several sessions before P is reliable in his response of* YES *or* NO *(head nods acceptable) on both* cream *and* sugar. *Progress to the next objective is then indicated.*]

The order in this programming of presenting the signals and the signal groups is not the only order. It is intended to demonstrate the situational method. Choice of signals and their grouping should be made by the clinician in the best interests of the individual patient. The location of treatment may also affect these choices and require certain changes. Specific signals may require earlier placement depending on the setting (hospital, outpatient clinic, health care facility, home visit, etc.).

After the initial sessions, more than one objective may be incorporated in any session. The patient may be expected to learn reality and situational meanings and associations for new signals, and at the same session to imitate those acquired at the previous day's session, also replicate those from the prior day, retrieve those acquired the previous week and initiate those already retrievable. It might be said that each signal is moved up the ladder of objectives. The patient is constantly encouraged to use each signal at the highest possible level and is provided the situational context that will effect this. When the patient is able to initiate signals for certain needs, these needs should not be served until the patient signals.

Objective 3. Imitation by patient of the signals HELLO DRINK POUR STIR YES NO GOODBYE.

TASK A
Patient imitates clinician's HELLO at clinic entrance while clinician maintains the signal in patient's view as a model. If patient does not succeed, clinician assists with tactual and kinetic facilitation. C maintains signal with left hand, while shaping P signal with right. C then lowers hand, and if P does not, C gently moves P's hand down.

TASK B   (used only if P did not succeed in A)
Repeat total A task exactly. No matter what P response has been at this point, do not repeat either A or B again at this time, but instead proceed to task C.

TASK C
C has arranged to meet S on way to clinic room. S GREETS C HELLO, C returns HELLO. S greets P HELLO. P is expected to imitate. If not, S facilitates. Repeat once, if first is not successful.

TASK D
One other stop is prearranged, possibly with secretary, with greetings again exchanged by both C and P, and facilitated if necessary.
Then C signals YOU I WALK—DRINK and escorts P to coffee room of clinic.

TASK E
C signals DRINK. P is expected to imitate. If P signals appropriately, P is rewarded with big smiles and a quick cup of coffee. If not, P is facilitated, then imitation trial is repeated once, also with facilitation if needed.

TASK F
C signals POUR—YES—NO. P is expected to choose and imitate. If P signals POUR, this should be rewarded with smile and approval, but cream should not be provided until P chooses YES or NO, similarly. When decision has been made, C models POUR YES (or POUR NO) and P is expected to imitate (or be facilitated) before cream is poured or withheld.

TASK G
Proceed with STIR as in F with POUR. C then signals SIT and all sit.

TASK **H**

C seeks signal agreement with P about C's coffee. C points to own cup—DRINK YES—. P is expected to imitate. Then C points to P's cup DRINK YES. P is expected to imitate. C points to own cup POUR (yes or no) P imitates. C points to P's cup, POUR—YES—NO. P imitates appropriate signal. Similarly, STIR is signaled for C and for P.

TASK **I**

C summarizes own drink: DRINK—POUR (yes/no) STIR (yes/no). C summarizes P's and P is expected to imitate.

Criteria for Accomplishment. Patient must successfully *imitate* the signals without facilitation at a single session.

If P does not meet this criteria by the third session, the sequence should be demonstrated again at the fourth session by having the C proceed with each step with the S for P to watch. Step by step the P should be led to imitate the actions just demonstrated by the C and S. The S should hold the signals each time as models for the P to imitate. In the imitation objective, the model should always be held in view for the P. When necessary, the P should have the hands shaped kinetically or tactually in the signal, and then asked to imitate without the facilitation. In any modeled sequence, facilitation should not be repeated on any one occasion more than the second time. It should not become drill.

Objective 4. Replication by the P of the signals.

The same tasks are performed but the P is expected to replicate the signals from short term memory after the models have been removed from his view.

Criteria for Accomplishment. Replication of the chosen signals on 80 percent of the trials in a particular session.

Objective 5. Retrieval.

The same sequence is performed, but the P is expected to retrieve the signals without a model, stimulated only by the appropriate situation, person or object as cues.

When the C meets the P, C merely smiles and expects the P to signal HELLO. When this is executed, the C responds with smile and HELLO. The C may cue this step on the first trial, if necessary by pointing at the P and signaling YOU. At a lower level, it may be cued by having the C turn away from the P and signal HELLO to the secretary, a passing staff member, or another patient or family member in waiting room.

The tasks on the other signals may follow the same pattern. The C may cue P by pouring self a cup of coffee and ignoring P. C may cue with cream and sugar by holding each up and signaling self YES or NO appropriately and acting accordingly with own cup.

Clinician may provide situational cue to trigger the signal. Other staff persons or other patients may enter and request coffee, with or without cream/sugar, all ignoring P until P signals HELLO; then signaling him HELLO—QUESTION YOU pointing to the coffee. On first attempt at retrieval,

C should, after P had tried and failed, become the friend in need, take P aside and show signal for DRINK. It may be even better if another patient does this, on arrangement from C.

When session is over, C may cue GOODBYE by blocking door, or holding handle until P executes GOODBYE.

Criteria for Accomplishment. P retrieves 80 percent of the signals in a single session, with at least two retrieved without cue.

Objective 6. Initiation of signals to serve social or need purposes.

One or two other signaling patients may be included in a small group session. Preferably one of these should be operating at a higher level than P 1. The latter is expected, as a social effort, to initiate HELLO to the others and either at this or successive sessions, to act as host by offering the coffee, etc. If no other signalling patients are available, the group may be composed of staff, family members, friends, etc. or other hospital personnel involved in P's treatment.

Successive sessions with choices from above groups may serve both as motivators and as practise sessions.

Criteria for Accomplishment. P is expected to execute relevant signals to 80% in the social situations involving self needs or needs of others.

Signal Group B. WALK (go) OK HOT COLD EAT.
(C meets P at clinic door, and waits for P to initiate.)

P: HELLO

C: HELLO—I OK—QUESTION YOU OK—OK YES—OK NO—

[*P is expected to respond with* YES *or* NO. *C facilitates if needed. Then C again models* I OK YES/NO *in consonance with P's reply. P is expected to imitate. Facilitate if needed.*]

[*C has previously arranged to encounter three persons in clinic as follows.*]

s1: HELLO (to P) who is expected to respond.

C: HELLO (to S1) QUESTION YOU WALK

s1: I OK THANKS (to P) QUESTION YOU WALK

P: is expected to respond either I OK or OK NO

s1: GOODBYE—SEE YOU TIME FUTURE (departs)

s2: [enters from nearby—(to C) HELLO—(to P) HELLO (to C)—QUESTION YOU WALK (S2 is wearing sweater).

C: I OK THANKS

s2: (to P)—QUESTION YOU WALK

P: is expected to respond
C: (to S2) QUESTION YOU WALK

s2: I NO OK—I HOT

c: C takes sweater from S2. HOT NO—QUESTION OK

s2: HOT NO—I OK THANKS GOODBYE (departs)

s3: (enters) HELLO to both C and P

P: HELLO

c: HELLO—QUESTION YOU WALK OK

s3: OK NO—I COLD
    C offers sweater. S3 puts it on.

C: QUESTION YOU COLD

s3: NO COLD—I OK—THANKS—GOODBYE (departs)

[*C escorts P to clinic room where at least three warm and three cold items are ready for demonstration, such as warm radiator and cold window, or cold air conditioner and warm window, pan of ice cubes and a hot water bottle, a refrigerator and a stove, a hot plate and an ice pack, etc.*
C touches alternately a hot and a cold item, and signals correctly. Leads P to touch them in order while C executes appropriate signal. Then presents the following tasks.]

TASK A
C repeats above sequence, identifying each item with correct signal. P is expected to touch the item and imitate the signal.

TASK B
C repeats sequence, touching items in different order, and signals HOT—QUESTION YES/NO—. P is expected to make appropriate YES/NO signal.

TASK C
C repeats sequence in different order and signals COLD—QUESTION YES/NO. P is expected to signal correctly.

TASK D
C touches each item, asks P to touch it and to execute correct signal when C signals QUESTION HOT/COLD

C: CHOP—TIME BREAK—

C escorts P to coffee room YOU I WALK—DRINK. *Cold soda or coke has been added to the drink list. C identifies it for P as* COLD, *then the coffee as* HOT. *Repeats this, having P touch soda, C signals* DRINK COLD. *Leads P to touch coffee, C gives signal* DRINK HOT.]

C: QUESTION YOU DRINK—HOT—COLD

[*If P points to his choice, C presents the correct signal and ask P to imitate it. Facilitates if needed. If facilitation is used, then repeat request for imitation, once, then give proper drink. Use* POUR *and* STIR WITH HOT. *C offers plate of small cookies, preferably of limited sweetness, such as oatmeal raisin. C signals* EAT. *P is re-*

quested to imitate. C: QUESTION YOU EAT *P is expected to respond with imitation of* EAT *or with* YES *or* NO. *If latter, C repeats* EAT YES *or* EAT NO *and expects P to imitate this. P is served accordingly.*]

C: I SIT—YOU SIT.

[*C then identifies own food and drink in signals.*]

C: DRINK HOT/COLD—EAT YES/NO—

[*Then identifies P's and P is expected to imitate. (All food and drink servings should be very small.) When P has finished drink and cookie, C signals* QUESTION YOU DRINK MORE *and reaches for either coffee pot or coke bottle with offer to pour. Follows this with* QUESTION YOU EAT MORE *and offer of cookie plate. If P takes more of either or both, C signals* I DRINK MORE/I EAT MORE *and acts in accordance.*]

[*In this case, C signals* I EAT/DRINK MORE—QUESTION YOU EAT/DRINK MORE *P is expected to signal* YES/NO *appropriately. If P limits signal to* YES/NO, *C signals* EAT/DRINK *and P is expected to clarify by imitating the proper signal, both for self and C behavior. C then signals* QUESTION HOT/COLD DRINK OK, *and P is expected to signal* OK HOT/COLD DRINK. *C signals* EAT OK, *and P responds either* EAT OK *or* EAT NO OK.]

[*C gathers up paper cups and napkins, signals* QUESTION. *P is expected to signal* REJECT. *If so, C responds* YOU REJECT *and P is expected to put them in waste basket. If P does not respond above with* REJECT, *C then signals* QUESTION REJECT *and P is expected to imitate. C proceeds with* YOU REJECT *and P is expected to dispose of rubbish properly.*]

[*C points to clock and signals* TIME YOU WALK—SEE YOU TIME FUTURE— GOODBYE.]

The clinician from this point continues to plan daily sessions to incorporate adequate repetition of previously acquired signals, using greeting procedures, coffee breaks, and repetition of demonstration segments with P demonstrating to C so that P retains use of all acquired signals. Each session should contain stimuli from C that will enable P to move each signal from recognition to imitation, to replication, to retrieval, to actual use in serving the day's activities.

The introduction of other persons into the coffee break may provide opportunity for additional challenges, with the P acting as host. When the clinician decides it would be profitable to do so, P may be taken for a coffee break to another location. Other specialties may be willing to cooperate on this, such as PT and OT. Or other specialties may be invited one at a time to visit and participate at the speech clinic. Some variation may be introduced by having the clinician take the P to the hospital canteen for the coffee break. P would be expected to do the ordering. Such a visit can also introduce the concept and signal for MONEY, as a preparation for other purchasing visits. A family member or friend of P can also be involved in such a trip when it is repeated. Emphasis on having the P act as host quite often strongly reinforces his use of the signals. Canteen personnel with whom P will be dealing should be properly alerted to the signals to be used. If necessary, C can precede in the line and order exact items P will order. C can use both speech and signals. This gives P the model for the correct signals.

Under these new circumstances P may need this. It also provides instruction to the canteen personnel in recognition of the signals of the Ps. Prior to this first canteen visit, clinic sessions must have identified other forms of food and drink as also contained in the signal. Milk and orange juice can vary the drink list, and raisins, nuts, popcorn, toast and jam can vary the food items. It may be helpful, prior to a canteen visit, to use a canteen food item in the clinic to establish the P's preference.

Signal Group C. WATER TEA TIME MORE CHOP.

TASK A
Add WATER to the list of available DRINK choices.

TASK B
Add TEA, HOT/COLD, to the list of DRINK items. Use above new items at all sessions, and alternate the old items, especially those which P has mastered and used well. The only exception to this occurs if P uses signal correctly in effort to obtain a favorite drink which is not offered on the day's menu. P should be given the missisng item that is signaled correctly. If milk and/ or orange juice are used and are popular, the clinician may wish to establish identifying signals for them, such as DRINK—NO COLOR for milk and DRINK COLOR SUN for orange juice. For Ps who cannot progress to these, it is advisable to have these two drinks used alternately as the cold drink, rotating the soda or cola with them. This alternation of drink choices provides variety and at the same time generalizes many of the items.

TASK C
Continue the use of MORE with all drinks and edibles. The latter should be restricted to a variety of finger foods.

TASK D
Continue use of CHOP (ended) in relation to termination of activity segments of each session and also of session.

TASK E
Associate TIME with beginning and end of all activities and also of session.

At this time, the clinician will wish to include with greetings on any occasion the usual quiries about the other person, QUESTION YOU GO, and suitable interchange socially. The ten signals listed as "habituated" should all be part of every session, with the P adding them and moving them up the objective ladder. A constant objective from this point forward, should be to have the P initiate all signals of which he is capable when any appropriate opportunity presents an opening.

Signal Group D. MAN WOMAN HUSBAND/WIFE BABY BIG/LITTLE.

TASK A
Establish meaning of BIG and LITTLE with matching or grouping tasks with objects, form boards, shapes, etc.

TASK **B**

If P is able to match with pictures, continue with pictures as above.

TASK **C**

If Task B is successful, include pictures of men, women, boys and girls. These can then be used to identify same in signals, with girl as WOMAN LITTLE and boy as MAN LITTLE.

TASK **D**

If B and C are not successful with pictures, proceed to have C identify self as MAN or WOMAN appropriately. Same for P. Arrange walking, or wheelchair tour of facility, identifying each person met. C executes proper signal, P imitates. C leads P eventually to initiate the proper identification.

TASK **E**

Even when P does not react to pictures, it is frequently observed that there is recognition of photos of family members. These can be used for the MAN/ WOMAN and girl/boy identities. The same is true for BABY.

TASK **F**

To demonstrate to P the use of MAN/WOMAN in code when in language we would use pronouns, a man and a woman friend might be invited to attend the coffee break. The P if able to do so, might act as host to his friends as well as to C. C can contribute to P's understanding of this use by signaling appropriately on the DRINK requests of the guests, such as: MAN DRINK HOT—WOMAN DRINK COLD—; WOMAN DRINK TEA—STIR—NO POUR; MAN DRINK COLD—POUR NO—STIR NO; MAN DRINK MORE—WOMAN NO DRINK MORE—.

TASK **G**

If the guests in F are husband and wife, this offers opportunity to indicate proper use of MAN RING for husband and WOMAN RING for wife. If P is married, the spouse may be also included in this and similarly identified. A comparison of wedding rings sometimes clarifies this well.

TASK **H**

If P responds to pictures, several group family pictures might be used for identification of MAN, WOMAN, *boy, girl*, BABY, *husband, wife*.

Signal Group E. SEE CRY (*sad*) DANCE (*happy*) HEART PAIN BOSS (*doctor*) PILL (*medicine*).
(C arranges for cooperation of doctor, or for someone to impersonate doctor in white coat and stethoscope, with small bottle of pills in pocket.)
(C meets P at door of clinic.)

P: HELLO

C: HELLO—QUESTION YOU WALK

P: I OK QUESTION YOU WALK

C: I OK THANKS—SEE YOU—HEART ME—DANCE—QUESTION—HEART YOU—DANCE—SEE ME

P: SEE YOU—HEART ME DANCE

[*C facilitates and then elicits repetition, if necessary.*]

C: (to secretary) HELLO—SEE YOU—HEART ME DANCE

SEC: SEE YOU—HEART ME DANCE

C: (to staffer) HELLO—QUESTION YOU WALK—

S: I NO HAPPY—I CRY

C: QUESTION YOU CRY

S: PAIN—HEAD—BIG PAIN

C: COME—SEE DOCTOR

[*Doctor enters from office.*]
HELLO DOCTOR—WOMAN BIG PAIN HEAD—

D: (to Sec) WOMAN DRINK WATER—EAT PILL

[*Secretary brings cup of water, S takes pill with water.*]

S: THANKS DOCTOR—PILL OK—

D: YOU SLEEP—PILL REJECT PAIN—GOODBYE

S: GOODBYE—I SLEEP (S and D leave)

C: HEART ME DANCE—I NO PAIN—QUESTION YOU PAIN YES/NO

P: NO

C: PAIN NO

P: PAIN NO

C: QUESTION YOU HEART CRY

P: NO—HEART NO CRY

C: QUESTION HEART DANCE

P: YES—HEART DANCE

C: QUESTION YOU SLEEP

P: YES/NO

[*If P replies in affirmative, C may offer a nap on clinic sofa, or return to ward, or early ending of session if P is out-patient.*]

This sequence may be repeated for several sessions with a different person having a pain in a different location. Various remedies may be offered; various suggestions made, such as YOU SEE DOCTOR, YOU SLEEP, YOU EAT PILL, YOU PHONE DOCTOR, with appropriate action following.

In following greeting sequences, both DANCE and CRY may be introduced as responses to QUESTION YOU WALK. Staff persons may also introduce DANCE when showing a letter, or a present, or a new outfit, or a special cake for the coffee break. A tooth ache might be indicated by one staffer in response to QUESTION YOU WALK, and suitable advice to SEE TOOTH DOCTOR.

Appropriate questions directed to P will provide opportunity for P to use these signals meaningfully.

Signal Group F. WASH LOCK TALK PHONE BOX WATER CHAIR (*toilet*).

The signal WASH can be introduced in any coffee break session, when plastic rather than paper cups are available. It can be generalized to WASH hands before eating and WASH cups and dishes after eating. It can then be routinely alternated with REJECT, by using paper cups on one day and plastic on another. Paper napkins always provide opportunity for REJECT, which should also be generalized to other uses such as throw away, don't like that, get rid of that, etc.

If the P is taken to a wash room for the hand washing, the concept LOCK can be introduced as usually such wash rooms are locked in hospitals and clinics. Lock can also be generalized by having P's session first in morning when clinic is opening, and occasionally last in day, when clinic is closing up. It can be related to P's own key ring. It can be related to locked materials cupboards in clinic.

Use of wash room can also be occasion for establishing signal for toilet: WATER-CHAIR. This can be demonstrated by placing a straight chair beside toilet and indicating similarity, SIT. Water in toilet can be indicated by WATER signal, and comparing it with water from faucet in sink.

TALK can be demonstrated by C showing both mouth (by pointing to mouth) TALK and hand (pointing to hand) TALK. C signals to P: I MOUTH TALK—YOU NO MOUTH TALK—YOU I HAND TALK—. This can be extrapolated to others, some of whom use only one, some use both systems. P can be expected to indicate which people are mouth TALK and which are HAND TALK people.

BOX is used and easily understood for the TV, which is clarified to SEE HEAR BOX. After the concept is introduced, a portion of later sessions may be profitably employed in showing P certain preprepared materials from video cassettes which can be used as a basis for signal conversation later about the video.

PHONE talk can be introduced through a phone contact with a family member, with C using signals to P and then transposing P's signals to family. P can be encouraged to ask for PHONE call about various needs. PHONE ward to ask when P must return, or to find something left behind, or to receive authorization for P to take walk outside, etc.

Signal Group G. SHELTER WRITE MONEY DRIVE.

SHELTER can be introduced as indicating the building in which clinic is located. If weather permits a walk or wheelchair trip around the hospital grounds can indicate other shelters, other buildings, including garage, roofs over picnic tables, big buildings, small buildings.

A similar interior trip can include visit to:
chapel: SHELTER PRAY
canteen: SHELTER EAT PAY
library: SHELTER BOOK
pharmacy: SHELTER PILL
auditorium: SHELTER PICTURE (*movies*)
speech clinic: SHELTER HAND TALK
garage: SHELTER DRIVE (*car*)
home: SHELTER ME (a photo may help)

DRIVE can be implemented by viewing from clinic window passing cars, taxis and buses. This provides also an opportunity to demonstrate some agglutinations to the patient. Taxi is CAR MONEY. Bus is BIG CAR MONEY.

MONEY can be demonstrated by itself. A trip to hospital canteen or gift shop can also indicate its use. This can be also associated with the check book: WRITE MONEY. Other methods of writing should also be demonstrated, such as the typewriter. Some patients who have indicated no potential for writing with pen or pencil have achieved some limited letters on a typewriter.

Signal Group H. ALL RAIN GET/GIVE HEART.

ALL can be introduced in a group session, using YOU ME ALL to indicate everyone present. Then similarly it can be applied to ALL the liquid refreshments at the coffee break, indicating each by its specific and then grouping them ALL DRINK. The same applies to the various finger foods. After this, every suitable occasion to demonstrate inclusiveness of this circular gesture should be used to enable P to generalize this concept.

RAIN is best introduced on a rainy day, when it is easy to indicate what is happening. After that, it can be applied to the shower in the bathroom, which is BOX RAIN ME. Similarly a snowy day permits the distinction between RAIN and SNOW to be demonstrated easily.

Since the P already has been introduced to the idea that happiness and sadness are located in the HEART, he usually achieves the concept of LIKE as related to the gesture for HEART. With some patient's who had problems in relating to body interior, use of a small, red, paper heart pinned on the chest appeared to help. It was abandonned as soon as P made the gesture without looking for the paper heart. After this P was able to use HEART without this cue.

While GIVE and GET are illustrated in the Signal Repertoire as separate signals, they are really the same thing in different directions. You give and I get; you get when I give. It has proved most effective to introduce this as one concept. The signal should be made in the direction in which the gift passes. For example, to signal the idea that I give you the box, I signal: I GIVE (moving away from myself to you) YOU BOX. If I am asking you to give me the box, I signal: YOU GIVE (moving my hand from you to me) ME BOX. There is no way to signal the concept "want." If the C and P will think in action, it will be clear that when "I want . . ." I mean "You give me. . . ." So the signals GIVE/GET can be used to express the concept that is served in English with the verb want.

SUMMARY

The patterns, tasks and suggestions for both demonstration of meaning in a situational context and leading the patient to use the signals meaningfully in an ascending fashion on the scale of objectives can all be applied to the remaining signals in the repertoire.

It is vital for the success of the P that the C emphasize meaningful use of acquired signals as soon as they have been acquired at the level of imitation, but especially as soon as they are at the level of retrieval. The principal goal of the program is communicative *use* of the signals. This goal is achieved when the P *uses* even a few signals. It is not achieved if he *uses* none, but imitates 250. The quality of the P's use of signals is much more important that the quantity of signals he can execute.

APHASIC PATIENTS TALK BACK

Some false assumptions occur in many treatment situations. Many aspects regarding the patient are misinterpreted. Some of the patient's capacities are overestimated, and some underestimated. They may also be true of feelings, needs, and wishes, all of which should be given adequate consideration and human respect.

In *Aphasic Patients Talk Back* (Skelly, 1975) fifty aphasic patients who had recovered a useful level of speech were interviewed. All had been classified as severely impaired on admission. Structured questions and open-end topics were presented. Free flow of opinion and feeling was encouraged. All the interview content was analyzed. Twelve areas of unanimous, serious concern to aphasic patients were identified.

Ability to Comprehend

All who were interviewed stated emphatically that they understood what was said in their presence much sooner and much more completely than the literature on aphasia would lead one to believe. These persons reported that they were traumatized by much that they heard. They phrased this in various ways: "They talked about me as if I didn't have any brains or feelings"; "They often sounded as though they thought I was as good as dead, and then of course I wanted to be."

There is a common assumption that when a patient cannot or does not respond, he also does not receive. This inference may be unwarranted. Every patient interviewed indicated that his capacity to understand returned very shortly after his trauma and that it consistently increased long before he was able to respond to what he heard. Many stated that in the immediate posttrauma period they experienced fear and anguish. They believed these feelings might have been assuaged had they received reassurance and even some explanation of what had happened to them. But, as they commented, "nobody talked *to* me, only *about* me."

Speed of Input

The aphasic persons who were interviewed all thought that they would have achieved successful communication earlier if the speakers had spoken more slowly. One patient compared the rate of speech he heard to the sound produced when a tape recorder is played at a high speed. One patient said that when conversation was too fast "it was just noise to me." Another was able to say, "I hear all right but, you see, I hear more slowly since my stroke."

Amount of Input

The project participants all agreed that "everyone asks too many questions at one time." The person with aphasia is often unable to formulate a reply under optimal conditions. Any interfering stimulus, such as a question or even a repetition of the first question, can prevent his processing an answer. Yet, under these conditions, the patient's progress is often judged by his response. His chart may read as a result of this input overload, "Patient unable to answer questions." This entry may affect treatment planning and consequently the patient's entire future. Actually, a barrage of questions can disrupt communication flow for a normal speaker. Parents, teachers, police, and lawyers frequently use it as a disruptive approach in certain situations. Our respondents assured us that, even early in their recovery period, they could have answered some questions presented to them if they had been asked one at a time.

Length of Response Time

The respondents said that they needed more time to prepare and produce an answer. Their general impression was that no one waited a sufficient length of time for an answer. Many reported frustration on numerous occasions by the interruption of their thoughts with repetition of questions just as they were about to reply. "When everybody tried to hurry me, all they did was throw sand in my gears" and "I think my wheels go round a great deal slower now, but nobody seems to know this but me."

Perception of Cues

The aphasic patients displayed awareness of and sensitivity to nonverbal communication from the personnel around them. It is of course true that many persons, including hospital personnel and family members, have difficulty tolerating the consequences of the aphasic persons' impairment. Most people control any overt indications of their annoyance at delayed or inappropriate responses. Yet they are frequently unaware that this behavior is inadequate. The participants cited numerous subtle signs of impatience from those around them which were deeply discouraging—audible sighs, tightening of the mouth muscles, shoulder and eye movements, and drumming fingers. The aphasic persons agreed that such behavior affected their morale, motivation, and progress adversely.

Level of Evaluation Tests

The participants considered many of the tasks they were directed to perform during a test or treatment as silly, useless, or insultingly childish. They were particularly emphatic about requests to recite the alphabet; use of childish language, pictures, concepts, and stories; and tests and drills involving nonsense syllables. They objected to the uselessness of counting backwards and repeating numbers in reverse order. They were puzzled by the number of demands for information they thought the questioner already possessed. When several people in the same institution presented the same or almost the same test materials successively, the respondents concluded that the hospital either did not know what it was doing or cared so little that no one knew the test had already been performed.

Participants had been daunted by the testers' manner, which was either bellicose or indifferent. Questions were hurled at the aphasic person in a voice that somewhat frightened him or were presented so blandly as to extinguish motivation for cooperation. One patient said that a questioner "barked at me as if I were a dog. I thought he might hit me if I answered." The reverse effect obtained with another aphasic person: "I felt he couldn't care less and probably wouldn't listen even if I did say something."

In some disciplines, seemingly useless tasks may yield useful information. But if the patient does not understand this, he may fail to respond not because he cannot but because he declines to. He may be rejecting conduct he considers foolish in an adult.

Destructiveness of Noise

Noise pollution and its effects were described in many ways: "I thought I was going noise crazy!" "I always thought a hospital was supposed to be a quiet place. It was worse than the airport."

The participants said that noise hurt them "and not just in the ear." They thought much of the noise was avoidable with a little care and some common-sense rules. All mentioned the prevalence of television sets, their high volume, and their continuous output. They suggested that earphones be required for all hospital sets. They also commented on the loud voices of hospital personnel and suggested that room doors be kept closed to contain noise. They also mentioned door slamming, pan rattling, loud bells, and constant loudspeaker announcements, as well as squealing wheels on hospital equipment.

Any high level of noise generated in a hospital is usually amplified by the hard wall and floors that are installed to facilitate cleaning. Noise studies in hospitals by an audiologist could identify sources of ambient sound that might be reduced.

Influx of Personnel

In the participants' opinions, they were observed too frequently by too many varied groups. These unidentified people, whom the aphasic person did not see as related to his illness, appeared unexpectedly around his bed, in his physical therapy cubicle, or in the examining room. All participants reported that this invasion of their space irritated them seriously. One person said that after this experience he knew how the animals at the zoo felt on holidays.

The size of the groups was disturbing, too. When we explained that these were teaching visits, all the participants voiced their willingness to contribute to health education. They remarked, however, that had someone explained the visits to them before they were made, the visits would have been more tolerable. They suggested less frequent visits, smaller groups, and that lectures about a patient's medical condition be held elsewhere before the bedside visit.

Need for Information

Many decisions affecting patients are made for administrative or medical reasons—frequently, it seems to the patient, without considering his viewpoint. Aphasic persons see this as lack of regard for their feelings and even for their rights. They expressed a need to have explanations as well as directives and orders. The usual assumptions that aphasic patients do not understand and that consequently explanations are superfluous were both contradicted by this study.

Respect for Personhood

Irrelevant questions which violate the aphasic person's privacy and often injure his dignity were mentioned. Those most frequently cited were inquiries about his finances. The manner and imputations rather than the basic inquiry were considered offensive.

The participants regarded their progress as a private matter and resented the frequent requests to "show off" their achievement.

Responsiveness to Needs

The last point the group made is common to every modern organization: "Too much yakketty before any action." The participants thought that responses to their needs and wants were needlessly delayed, a delay that was in some way related to their inability to talk.

The data from these aphasic patients cast additional light on two long-held tenets in aphasiology concerning spontaneous recovery and short duration of treatment.

The spontaneous recovery period is usually described as the six to twelve weeks immediately post-trauma. It has been assumed that the patient will recover language during this time. Yet from the data obtained, this period would be better termed "optimum treatment period," the period when early speech rehabilitation is initiated.

The second insight concerned the duration of treatment. These patients demonstrated that additional improvement, sometimes at a very high level, can and does take place for two or more years following onset.

Consistent exploration of patient feedback in aphasia may provide a basis for further reevaluation of treatment policies and procedures. Such feedback may be important in modifying the behavior of those who care for the patients, to reduce patient frustration and accelerate speech rehabilitation."

DEVELOPMENTALLY IMPAIRED PATIENTS

Many speechless patients of both brain-damaged categories (adventitious and developmental) can profit from alterations of the customary approaches in communication rehabilitation. This is particularly so in the case of the patients with concept deficits. All those classified as severely or profoundly impaired who exhibit lack of language comprehension appear to share some common rehabilitation needs. These include:

1. *Concrete, active demonstration* of the use of reality objects, performed in:
2. *Structured situational* presentation approximating daily-life occurrences, where:
3. *Meaningful action* replaces meaningless (for them) drill, through:
4. *Planned repetitions* accompanied by:
5. *Adequate variety* to promote:
6. *Interest and attention,* as well as:
7. *Generalization of concepts,* by means of:
8. *Selected stimuli,* to which the individual is *able* to respond, and consequently secure:
9. *Approval and reward,* and eventually:
10. *Acceptance*

For both groups of brain-damaged patients, initial programmed sequences based on these premises may provide communication rehabilitation for specific patients.

TREATMENT PROGRAM C

Goal. Communication of basic needs in Amer-Ind with approximately fifty signals acquired over a period of one year.

Subgoal. Acquisition of approximately 30 signals within a six-month period, used for (a) social contacts, (b) recognition of meaning in terms of obeying signaled directives, and (c) execution in imitation, replication and retrieval, and (d) some indication of transitional use with at least five signals.

Objectives. Established in sequence on a five-week pattern, with each sequence repeated five times within the half-year, with each five-week sequence focused on five specific signals. Weekly objectives are as follows:

Week 1. Recognition of signal modeled by clinician; assisted imitation of signals modeled; assisted imitation of actions signaled.

Week 2. Unassisted imitation of signal; unassisted imitation of action signaled.

Week 3. Replication of signal; initiation of appropriate action.

Week 4. Retrieval of signal through clinician question; initiation of appropriate action.

Week 5. Patient initiation of signal, through questions, to control clinician action.

Criteria. (For weekly advance) Patient performs objective on four of the five signals in eight of ten tasks.

Scheduling. The daily schedule should include four daily encounters between clinician and patient. These may at the beginning be as short as ten minutes, and then be extended with increasing tolerance, concentration and progress. Two of these may occur in the morning, two in the afternoon. Each day should include signal sessions with an involvement of other professional staff for reinforcement by inculcating them in Amer-Ind Code so they may use it appropriately for control of patient action and respond to it with appropriate behavior when the patient signals to control the behavior of persons in the environment. Each daily schedule should also include supplementary activities to assist progress in signaling, such as tasks for motoric control improvement and concept development.

The morning session might begin with the signal segment which has been programmed, followed by a sequence of gross motor exercises for imitation with the objective of improved motor coordination and imitation of clinician action. This can lead to adaptation of gross arm movements as preparation for more precise signal execution. Finer hand and finger movements can be added, as appropriate. The programmed signal sequence can then be repeated. This scheduling provides the patient with variety of activity, plus early repetition of the signal program, on one visit to the communication clinic.

An afternoon schedule might include repetition of the programmed signal segment, followed by concept development activities with plaque and form boards, sorting, matching shape, color, size in preparation of application of these concepts to hand shapes and possibly to mouth shapes for future communicative use. These would then be followed again as in the morning by a repetition of the programmed five signal sequence.

The actual length of each activity should suit the attention span and physical tolerance of the specific patient. All effort should be made to increase the length.

Throughout all the above activities, the social signals and the other signals to be habituated should be used frequently and appropriately by the clinician without any demand for use by the patient. Any spontaneous appropriate replication by the patient should of course be immediately rewarded.

Reporting. The Fristoe Tally-Graph provides an efficient method of recording responses daily at each session. Separate blocks used for each task enable the clinician to plan future repetitions for signals less accurately produced as well as those where the objective has not been attained at criterion. Use of the Tally-Graph automatically summates the daily progress. Since these are always in terms of criteria, weekly summations are easily and efficiently produced from the daily data sheet.

At the five week segment intervals, a progress report should review the program for continuation, any needed change in goal, criteria, objectives, tasks, as well as possible termination for the particular patient. Precipitous judgments on termination are inadvisable. Many patients have very slow initial gains but these accelerate later to increases which lead to successful fulfillment of the five-week criteria.

PROGRAMMED SIGNALS FOR PROGRAM MODEL

Segment I	Segment IV
(weeks 1–5)	(weeks 16–20)
WALK (go)	Brush = WASH + POINT (teeth)
WASH	COMB (hair)
SIT	POSSESS (mine, yours)
EAT	SHELTER (house, home)
DRINK	SLEEP (rest, tired)
Segment II	**Segment V**
(weeks 6–10)	(weeks 21–25)
TIME	HOT
REJECT (throw away)	COLD
WATER	SAME
STAND (up)	DIFFERENT
COME	toilet = WATER + SIT (chair)
Segment III	**Habituation Signs**
(weeks 11–15)	
YOU	HELLO STOP
I/ME	GOODBYE QUIET
MAN	OK PLEASE
WOMAN	QUESTION THANKS
TALK	AGREE (yes)
	NO

Segment I

Programmed signals: WALK (go), WASH, SIT, EAT, DRINK.
Habituation: HELLO, GOODBYE, OK.
Furniture: Desk and desk chair, two additional chairs (one beside desk), access to a sink, a small table.
Materials: Two small plastic plates, two small plastic cups, small box of a sugared or fruited cereal which can be a finger food, small pitcher or bottle of juice, milk, or cola. (Food and drink items can be varied each day). Clock with large face on desk or wall.
Clinician communicates with patient *only* in signals. Words in capitals are concept labels, from the Repertoire. They indicate that the person is signaling.

1.* P is brought to door by an escort, who knocks at door, showing P how to knock. P knocks. When sure C is present, escort leaves.
2. C: HELLO (holds signal.) If P does not imitate, C provides tactile and kinetic assistance to shape P's signal.
3.* P. HELLO.
4. C rewards with palm to palm touch and smile.
5. C faces self and P toward sink.
6. C: WALK.
7.* C assists P to signal WALK.
8. C synchronizes leg and finger movement of WALK.
9. C: WASH.
10.* P: WASH.
11.* Both C and P wash hands and dry with paper towel.
12.* C disposes of paper towel in waste basket. P does also.
13. C: WALK.
14.* P: WALK.
15. C and P return to clinic desk.
16. C: SIT
17.* P: Sits.
18.* P: SIT
19. C sits.
20. C takes cereal box and plastic plates from desk bottom drawer, puts some cereal on plates and returns cereal box to drawer.
21. C: EAT
22.* P: EAT
23. C eats a grain of cereal.
24.* P eats a grain of cereal.
25. C: EAT. Continues to eat cereal till gone.
26.* P: EAT. Continues to eat till cereal is gone.
27. C removes bottle and plastic cups from desk drawer or box.
28. C: DRINK.
29.* P: DRINK.
30. C pours small portions for self and P and both drink.
31. C: DRINK.
32.* P: DRINK.
33. C pours again and both drink.

34.   C stands, gathers plates and cups.
35.   C: WASH. Points with index at dirty dishes.
36.**P: WASH. Points at dirty dishes.
37.   C: WALK.
38.* P: WALK.
39.   C and P go to sink.
40.   C: WASH. Points to dirty dishes.
41.**P: WASH. Points to dirty dishes.
42.   C and P wash and dry dishes, throwing paper towels in waste basket.
43.   C: WALK.
44.* P: WALK.
45.   C and P return to clinic desk. C puts plates and cups in desk drawer.
46.   C: I SIT.
47.   C points to clock. YOU WALK.
48.* P: WALK.
49.   C: GOODBYE.
50.* P: GOODBYE. P leaves, or is escorted to door, or C phones for escort if it has not arrived.

   Note: * designates points to be recorded for P scoring.

   C should use OK each time P fulfills criteria on a task. A shoulder pat is suggested if P executes task without assistance during first week.

Segment II

Programmed signals: TIME, REJECT (*throw away*), WATER, STAND, COME.
Habituation: HELLO, GOODBYE, OK, QUESTION, AGREE, NO.
Materials: Same as for Segment I. Add paper plates and paper cups.

1.* P knocks at door. Door is open.
2.   C: COME HELLO.
3.* P: HELLO.
4.   C: SIT.
5.**P: SIT (sits).
6.   C sets out paper plates and food.
7.   C looks at his hands. WASH.
8.* P: WASH.
9.   C: STAND.
10.* P stands.
11.* P: STAND.
12.   C stands.
13.   C: QUESTION WALK WASH AGREE (nods head, thumbs up).
14.* P: AGREE. C and P go to sink. C fills basin, makes waves.
15.   C: WATER (draws water from faucet); WATER
16.* P: WATER (both wash and dry hands with paper towels).
17.**C: REJECT (throws paper towels in waste basket).
18.   P: REJECT (throws paper towel in waste basket).
19.* C goes quickly to door. COME. C and P go to clinic.
20.* C stops P at door. STOP (then goes to desk).
21.   C: COME.

22.* P walks to desk.
23.   C: SIT.
24.* P sits.
25.* P: SIT.
26.   C sits.
27.   C: TIME EAT (points to clock).
28.* P: TIME EAT.
29.   C takes bottle from drawer or box. Points to bottle.
30.   C: QUESTION EAT (shakes head); NO DRINK AGREE.
31.**P: EAT NO DRINK AGREE.
32.   C takes food, paper plates, and paper cups from drawer.
33.   C points to food. EAT AGREE.
34.* P: EAT AGREE (both eat).
35.   C: TIME DRINK (pours drinks).
36.   C: QUESTION EAT (points at drink); EAT NO.
37.* P: EAT NO.
38.   C: DRINK.
39.**P: DRINK. (C and P both drink).
40.   C assembles dirty plates and cups. Points to them. QUESTION WASH
      WATER (gets plastic plate out). WASH WATER AGREE. Point to paper
      plates. WASH WATER NO
41.**P: NO WASH WATER.
42.   C: QUESTION REJECT. If necessary, shows that they can be torn up or
      crumpled like the paper napkin.
43.* P: REJECT.
44.   C gives them to P to throw in waste basket.
45.   C: QUESTION TIME YOU WALK AGREE.
46.* P: AGREE.
47.   C: I DRINK WATER (pours water); QUESTION YOU DRINK WATER.
48.* P: AGREE DRINK WATER or NO DRINK WATER. If affirmative, C pours for
      P and both drink. If negative, C drinks alone.
49.   C: GOODBYE.
50.**P: GOODBYE (departs).

Segment III

Programmed signals: YOU, I/ME, MAN, WOMAN, TALK.

Habituation: HELLO, OK, AGREE, STOP, PLEASE, GOODBYE, QUESTION, NO, QUIET, THANKS.

Materials: Plastic cups, paper cups, container of juice, wastebasket, sink, paper towels, homemade paper badges with pins, five badges with signal for MAN, five with signal for WOMAN.

Situation arrangements: Nearby room with a man and a woman who have agreed to cooperate and who have been trained in the specific signals for the occasion. If C and P are both men, another woman should be available, also. If both are women, another man is needed. The site and the personnel involved can be varied each day after the first three visits have been completed with the first group. The size of the group visited can be also varied, at the discretion of the clinician. If the P has early success in this task, two places can be visited on each occasion, to enlarge the P experience.

1.* P knocks at open door. C is drinking from paper cup.
2. C rises. HELLO. Puts dirty paper cup on desk.
3.* P: HELLO
4. C: COME PLEASE. Crosses to door.
5. C: I SHUT (shuts door).
6. C: YOU SIT PLEASE. (P sits).
7. C: (speak) What are we going to do today?
8. C: (showing surprise) QUIET.
   Points to mouth. TALK YOU HAND TALK.
9. C: YOU HAND TALK ME SIT.
10.* P: YOU SIT.
11. C sits.
12. C: QUESTION YOU DRINK (pours juice in plastic cup).
13.* P: DRINK AGREE or DRINK NO   THANKS.
14. C offers plastic cup if yes, pours juice back in container if no.
15. C: YOU HAND TALK ME DRINK WATER
16.**P: QUESTION YOU DRINK WATER
17. C: NO THANKS
18. C holds up dirty plastic cup. QUESTION REJECT.
19.**P: NO WASH.
20.* C: YOU WASH. P does and uses paper towel to dry.
21. C holds up paper towel and dirty paper cup. QUESTION WASH REJECT.
22.* P: REJECT.
23. C: YOU REJECT.
24.**P: I REJECT.
25.* P throws dirty paper cup and paper towel in waste basket.
26. C: (speaking) You and I are going to see some people.
27. C: I QUIET.
28.* P: YOU QUIET.
29. C: I HAND TALK.
30.* P: YOU HAND TALK.
31. C: AGREE YOU I WALK. (C and P exit from clinic.) YOU SHUT.
32.* P: I SHUT.
33. C: I LOCK.
34.* P: YOU LOCK.
35. C and P visit nearby room.
36. C: HELLO.
37.* P: HELLO.
38. M: (speaking) Hello.
39. W: (speaking) Hello.
40. C: (to P) MAN POINT (mouth) TALK.
41. C: WOMAN POINT (mouth) TALK.
42. C: (to P) QUESTION YOU TALK.
43.* P: I HAND TALK.
44. C: YOU   I HAND TALK   YOU SEE MAN WOMAN HAND TALK.
45. C: (to W) QUESTION YOU MAN.
46. W: (signaling) NO I WOMAN.

47.   C: (to M) QUESTION YOU WOMAN
48.   M: NO I MAN
49.   W: (to P) QUESTION YOU (points to MAN, points to self WOMAN).
50.* P: I (correct signal).
51.   W: (speaking) Women come stand beside me.
52.   C: (to P) WOMAN POINT (mouth) TALK QUESTION YOU TALK.
53.* P: I HAND TALK.
54.   C: (to W) I HAND TALK   WOMAN HAND TALK PLEASE.
55.   W: WOMAN COME ME. If there are no other women present, she signals at door of next room and brings woman from there.
56.   C: (to M) YOU HAND TALK.
57.* M: MEN COME ME. If no other men, bring one from next room.
58.   C: (to P) QUESTION YOU MAN WOMAN.
59.* P: I (correct signal).
60.   M: COME ME.
61.   C places badges in two groups. Points to P. CARDS.
62.* P passes out badges appropriately. If not, C assists. All recipients signal THANKS
63.* C: (to P) QUESTION TIME YOU I WALK.
64.* P: TIME WALK.
65.   C: (to Hosts) GOODBYE.
66.   M W: GOODBYE.
67.   C: OK SEE YOU.
68.   M W: OK SEE YOU.
69.**P: OK SEE YOU   GOODBYE.
70.* P: YOU I WALK.
71.   C and P return to clinic.
72.   C unlocks door. QUESTION TIME YOU WALK
73.* P: TIME I WALK.
74.   C: GOODBYE.
75.**P: GOODBYE   OK SEE YOU.

Segment IV

Programmed signals: COMB, POINT (teeth), POSSESS, SHELTER, (house), SLEEP.

Habituation: HELLO, AGREE, OK, STOP, PLEASE, GOODBYE, NO, QUESTION, QUIET, THANKS.

Materials: Two water glasses, different sizes; two combs, different shapes; two toothbrushes, different colors; two tubes toothpaste, different makes; pitcher with drinking water (or faucet); access to sink and paper towels; mirror; food item (six pieces); two paper plates; access to cot and reclining chair with pillow and blanket; cases for toothbrushes after use; two boxes, different in shape, size, and color to hold belongings of C and of P.

1.* P appears at open door and knocks.
2.* P: HELLO.
3.   C: HELLO   COME   SIT PLEASE.
4.* P: THANKS (sits).

5. C: QUESTION EAT
6.* P: AGREE PLEASE.
7. C: QUESTION WASH HANDS.
8.* P: AGREE WASH HANDS.
9. C and P both go and wash hands.
10. C divides six food items, three to each plate.

POSSESS YOU	POSSESS ME
POSSESS YOU	POSSESS ME
POSSESS YOU	POSSESS ME

Indicates plates. QUESTION POSSESS YOU.
11.* P takes one. POSSESS ME.
12. C takes other. POSSESS ME.
13. C and P eat.
14. C: QUESTION YOU DRINK WATER.
15.* P: AGREE/NO. If affirmative, C gives P cup and P gets water from sink or pitcher.
16. C: TIME WASH POINT (points to teeth).
17. C sets out two toothbrushes, different colors.
18. C points to one. POSSESS YOU. Puts toothbrush near P.
19.* P: POSSESS ME.
20. C points to other brush. QUESTION POSSESS YOU
21.* P: NO POSSESS YOU. Places it near C.
22. C: I WASH POINT (to teeth). Takes toothpaste and brush to sink.
23. C: QUESTION WATER WASH. Points to brush.
24.* P: AGREE WATER WASH
25. C puts brush in case. SHUT.
26. C: QUESTION YOU WASH POINT (to teeth).
27.* P: AGREE WASH POINT (to teeth).
28. C: QUESTION WASH. Points to brush.
29.* P: AGREE WASH.
30. C: QUESTION WATER.
31.* P: AGREE WATER. Washes brush.
32. C: SHUT. P puts brush in case.
33. C: YOU SIT PLEASE.
34.* P: THANKS.
35. C puts out two combs, different shapes, but same color.
36. C takes one. COMB POSSESS ME.
37. C points to other comb. QUESTION POSSESS COMB.
38.* P: COMB POSSESS ME.
39. C: POSSESS YOU AGREE. Gives P comb.
40. C: TIME I COMB. Goes to mirror and combs hair. QUESTION YOU COMB
    Sits, puts comb on desk.
41.* P: TIME I COMB. Goes to mirror, combs, sits, puts comb on desk.
42. C puts box in front of P and self, each box the color of the person's toothbrush.
43. C: POSSESS ME. Puts his toothbrush in his box.
44.* P: POSSESS ME. Puts his brush in his box.
45. C holds up his toothpaste. POSSESS ME. QUESTION POSSESS YOU.
46.* P: POSSESS ME. Holds up his toothpaste.
47. C and P put toothpaste in separate boxes.

48. C holds up both combs. QUESTION POSSESS
49.* P: POSSESS YOU. Gives C his comb.
50.* P: POSSESS ME. Takes his own and each places his comb in his box.
51. C: TIME YOU I WALK. Goes to coat rack, points to P's coat. QUESTION POSSESS.
52.* P: POSSESS ME.
53. C helps P put on coat.
54. C points to his own coat. QUESTION POSSESS.
55.* P: POSSESS YOU. C puts on coat.
56. C: COME WALK. They exit from room.
57. C: YOU SHUT.
58. C: I LOCK   YOU I WALK.
59.* C and P: If P is in residence, C leads shortest way to building where P lives. C points out each building as they pass and makes signal for SHELTER, asking P to imitate it, until they arrive at P's residence building.

    If patient is not in residence but lives at home, arrange in advance for family to provide some snapshots of his home and bedroom. Use these for items 60 to 69. For item 70 go to window and point to nearby buildings.
60. C: QUESTION SHELTER POSSESS YOU.
61.* P: AGREE SHELTER POSSESS ME.
62. C: QUESTION SHELTER YOU SLEEP.
63.* P: AGREE SHELTER I SLEEP.
64. C: YOU I WALK SEE.
65.* C and P both go in building to room or ward where P lives, greeting people they encounter, until they are at P's bedside.
66. C: QUESTION YOU SLEEP
67.* P: I SLEEP. Points to bed.
68. C tries bed, stretches, yawns, stands.
69. C: OK I SLEEP SHELTER POSSESS ME   YOU SLEEP. Points to bed.
70. C: QUESTION YOU I WALK.
71.* P: AGREE WALK.
72.* C and P return to clinic, alternating on way in pointing out buildings and making the signal.
73. C and P arrive at clinic building.
74. C: SHELTER POSSESS ME. They go to room with cot and recliner.
75. C points to cot. YOU SEE SLEEP.
76. C looks at watch. QUESTION TIME I SLEEP.
77.* P: TIME SLEEP NO.
78. C: QUESTION TIME YOU WALK.
79.***P: AGREE TIME WALK   GOODBYE   OK SEE YOU.
80. C: GOODBYE   OK SEE YOU.

Segment V

Programmed signals: HOT, COLD, SAME, DIFFERENT, *toilet* = WATER + SIT (*chair*).

Habituation: HELLO, AGREE, QUESTION, STOP, THANKS, GOODBYE, NO, OK, QUIET PLEASE.

Materials: C's colored box and P's colored box with their toothbrushes, toothpaste, combs, a third box of a neutral color, a hot pot (to boil water), an ice pack (with ice cubes which can be taken out), a bowl to hold ice cubes, a sink available, four forks, four knives, four teaspoons, four more toothbrushes, four combs. Of the latter five groups of objects, in each case there should be two that are identical. The other two should be different and also different from each other. The differences should include examples of color, size and shape.

Situation arrangements: Arrange visit to kitchen, alert personnel on signals and arrange to have small servings of hot soup and cold ice cream for C and P during visit. Place straight chair in bathroom near toilet.

1.* P arrives at clinic open door and knocks.
2.* P: HELLO.
3.   C: HELLO.
4.   C: QUESTION WALK YOU.
5.** P: I OK THANKS QUESTION WALK YOU.
6.   C: I OK THANKS.
7.   C places hand around *warm* hot pot. HOT points. YOU HAND HOT.
8.** P touches pot. HOT.
9.   C puts hand on ice in bowl. COLD YOU HAND.
10.** P puts hand on ice. COLD.
11. C goes to radiator and touches it. HOT COME YOU HAND HOT.
12.** P touches radiator. HOT.
13. C puts hand on window glass. COLD YOU HAND COLD.
14.** P puts hand on window. COLD.
15. C goes back to hot pot, points at it. QUESTION.
16.** P touches it. HOT.
17. C points to ice. QUESTION.
18.** P touches it. COLD.
19. C: YOU I WALK. Takes two paper cups.
20. C and P go to sink in bathroom.
21. C turns on hot water. WATER HOT. Feels it.
22.** P puts hand in hot water. WATER HOT.
23. C: WASH HAND HOT WATER (washes). YOU.
24.** P: WASH HAND HOT WATER (washes).
25. C turns on cold water. COLD. Fills cup, gives empty cup to P. COLD WATER DRINK.
26.** P: COLD WATER DRINK. Fills his cup and drinks.
27. C: OK REJECT. Throws paper cup in wastebasket.
28.** P: OK REJECT.. Throws his cup away.
29. C points to toilet. WATER + SIT (*chair*). Runs water from faucet. WATER. Points to water in toilet. WATER. Points to chair beside toilet. SIT (*chair*). Points to toilet. SIT (*chair*). WATER SIT (chair).
30.* P: WATER SIT (chair).
31. C: QUESTION YOU WATER SIT (chair).
32.* P: AGREE/NO. If affirmative, C leaves and waits for P. If negative, proceeds at once to next item.
33. C: TIME YOU I WALK SHELTER EAT.
34. C and P go to canteen, snack bar, kitchen as prearranged.

35.   C: (to personnel there, K) HELLO   OK SEE YOU.
36.   K: HELLO   OK SEE YOU.
37.**P: HELLO   OK SEE YOU.
38.   C: QUESTION I (points to P) SEE SHELTER POSSESS YOU PLEASE.
39.   K: OK   YOU SEE WALK.
40.   C: THANKS. (to P) COME. Goes to stove, touches it cautiously. QUESTION COLD.
41.* P: HOT.
42.   C goes to refrigerator, opens and touches inside. YOU HAND. P touches it. QUESTION.
43.**P: COLD.
44.   C: (to K) QUESTION TIME EAT PLEASE.
45.   K: TIME EAT. C and P are served small cups of hot soup. C and P signal THANKS.
46.   C: QUESTION COLD.
47.* P: NO COLD   HOT. They eat soup and then are served small ice cream cones.
48.   C: THANKS.
49.* P: THANKS.
50.   C: QUESTION HOT.
51.* P: NO HOT   COLD.
52.   C: QUESTION OK.
53.* P: OK.
54.   C: YOU I WALK EAT. (To K) OK SEE YOU   GOODBYE.
55.   K: OK SEE YOU   GOODBYE.
56.* P: GOODBYE. C and P return to clinic.
57.   C: SIT.
58.   C and P sit at desk or table where the boxes and the objects for sorting are located.
59.   C sets out one of the matching forks as pattern. Then C matches each of the other forks to it, leaving the one like it beside its mate, and pushing all the others away.
60.   C points. SAME. Points. NO SAME   DIFFERENT Repeats at each group.
61.   C allows P to examine both groups.
62.   C then mixes them up and sets pattern.
63.**P sorts to pattern. DIFFERENT   SAME.
64.   C demonstrates knife once.
65.**P sorts knives to pattern. DIFFERENT   SAME.
66.   C demonstrates spoon once.
67.**P sorts spoons. DIFFERENT   SAME.
68.   C demonstrates comb once.
69.**P sorts combs. DIFFERENT   SAME.
70.   C demonstrates toothbrush once.
71.**P sorts toothbrushes. DIFFERENT   SAME.
72.   C: COMB POSSESS ME. Puts his comb in his box.
73.**P: COMB POSSESS ME. Puts his comb in his box.
74.   C points to his own toothbrush.
75.   C: QUESTION POSSESS.
76.**P gives it to C. POSSESS YOU.
77.   C puts his toothbrush in his box.

78.**P: POSSESS ME. Puts his own in his box.
79.   C puts other objects in neutral box, then points to clock.
80.* P: TIME I WALK.
81.   C: OK GOODBYE.
82.* P: GOODBYE.

Segment Modification

The programmed segments are repeated four times a day for five days throughout a five-week span. The same signals, materials, and actions, however, focus each week on a different objective. This, in a few instances, necessitates some minor change in order or some minor alteration.

During the first week the emphasis is on the objective of **imitation** of both signal and related action, with any necessary **assistance.** In the second week, the objective is modified to **unassisted** imitation. This does not require any change in signal or order. During both these weeks, the clinician may repeat the model of each signal as frequently as needed. The clinician may hold the model stance as long as necessary for the patient to achieve the objective.

In the third week, the objective is **replication** of the signal. This means the patient must reproduce the signal after the model has been removed. The clinician may repeat the signal as often as needed, but this repetition should be noted. Criterion is satisfied only when the replication occurs after just one modeling.

In the fourth week, the objective is **retrieval** of the appropriate signals for the situation from the patient's memory. This requires some alteration of the fourth week printed model. The clinician now substitutes QUESTION for his prior signal and does not include the programmed signal as a pattern. It is legitimate, however, to indicate the physical presence of stimulus objects such as food, drink, water, sink, or action to enable the patient to retrieve the signal by association with the object or behavior. In this week the patient is expected to initiate appropriate behavior related to the signal, after he has signaled. If the patient fails to retrieve, the clinician may use QUESTION with the opposite signal. If this does not produce success, the clinician may next offer alternative signals, including the signal at issue, in QUESTION. This latter however reduces the task to the replication level in scoring.

In the fifth week, the objective is patient **initiation** of signals. It includes use of signals in directing the actions of the clinician. Some alteration of the model protocol is needed to allow this. The clinician, instead of initiating the signals, should behave as if puzzled or in doubt about what to do, thus encouraging the patient to take charge by initiating both signals and appropriate action in the situation.

By the fifth week, the patient should be using the HELLO first without difficulty. After the greeting, if the patient does not initiate any signal or action, the clinician may use one or more of the following:

(a) Look at own hands, possibly previously soiled, to induce the patient to suggest WASH and direct clinician to WALK WASH;

(b) Signal QUESTION TIME to induce patient to initiate TIME EAT:

(c) Point to dirty dishes to induce patient to sign WASH or REJECT appropriately;

(d) Point to clock to initiate TIME WALK.

If none of these enable the patient to achieve the objective, the stimuli from week four may be used to obtain success. However, this does not meet criteria so the task must be scored at retrieval level then rather than at initiation level.

ADJUNCTIVE MATERIALS AND ACTIVITIES

Signals

The following materials may be used for structuring program units for the second half of the proposed twelve month plan. Useful segments can be based on the following general areas.

1. Identification by the patient of his or her own body parts by use of index pointing as well as simultaneous association with an appropriately related object or action, including but not limited to: head (associated with hat), hair (comb), ears (noise, hifi, hearing aid), eyes (glasses, TV, pictures, looking out window), mouth (eating), nose (bad smell, good smell, kleenex), hands (gloves, hand talk), arms (hug, coat, shirt, dress, sweater), legs (walk, pants, slacks, skirt), feet (shoes), teeth (toothbrush, toothpaste), fingernails (scissors, nail polish), toenails (scissors);

2. Establishment of the signal for OBJECT so the signaler can distinguish for the viewer between the **action** and the **object** related to the action; for example, the action of eating EAT and the food EAT OBJECT;

3. Inculcation of the generic signals for human being, PERSON as distinguished from both OBJECT and ANIMAL;

4. Presentation of the signals MONEY and EXCHANGE with situational learning in purchasing experiences;

5. Enlargement of TIME to include PAST and FUTURE, yesterday, tomorrow, and clock hour schedules, as well as the use of a calendar.

6. Clarification of the concept of DIRECTION, related to real directional needs, such as turn right to the clinic, turn left at the hospital exit to drive me home, sit on the east terrace for the morning sun, my bed is in the west ward.

Our clinical experience in general indicates that addition of the following signals is most helpful for the patient's basic signal repertoire:

HELP	UP	BIG
MAYBE	DOWN	LITTLE
ALL	IN	DANCE (*happy*)
GIVE	OUT	CRY (*sad*)
GET	ON	PAIN

The following signal groups may be used in several ways:

1. To structure review segments;
2. To establish meaningful relationships more firmly between actions and objects;

3. To move the signal stimulus up the symbolic ladder, in terms of the AKMER/Ind Scale, by gradually substituting higher level pictorial stimuli for the lower level actions and objects, although this should occur *only after* it is quite evident that the patient has firmly established the signal concept in relation to the action and object in reality;
4. To formulate periodic progress check where this is required, although daily use of the Tally-Graph can provide this type of data.

Treatment stimuli by type, adaptable to Base 10.

ACTIONS

come	shave	read
drive	see/look	comb
cut	fly	fight
wash	sit	love/like
hear	drink	hold
stop	write	pour
reject	stand	lock
walk	talk	taste
possess	work	buy
eat	depart	sleep

The signals above can be elicited from the patient as associated with certain objects presented by the clinician, or if the signal is presented by the clinician, the patient can point to associated objects. Eventually, the patient may be able to use pictures representing objects and actions. In addition to objects during the reality stimulation phase, the clinician can perform certain real actions for which the patient is then requested to signal, for example, WASH can be elicited by the actual washing at the sink of the clinician's hands, or by presentation of the cake of soap.

OBJECTS

phone	shoes	knife
chair	pants	book
water	shirt	car
time/watch	key	money
radio	comb	pills
toilet	cup	scissors
glasses	pencil	man
TV	blanket	woman
boy	house	doctor
girl	toothbrush	nurse

Where it is possible to present the actual object and have the patient then produce the appropriate signal, it is probably best to do so. However, some additional steps toward conceptualization may be taken by having a significant object represent a whole, for example the nurse's white cap can represent the nurse and the doctor's stethoscope the doctor, provided these symbols have been associated with the persons involved for this particular patient.

It may be possible at this time to show an additional method of distinguishing certain aspects of concepts, such as DRIVE meaning the action, DRIVE OBJECT meaning the car, and DRIVE PERSON meaning the driver.

It may also be profitable to show that different objects can be associated with the same person; as the nurse is also associated with MEDICINE, so is the doctor.

DESCRIPTORS

fast/slow—you/car
big/little—watch/clock
hot/cold—coffee/coke
good/bad—ice cream/vinegar
hard/soft—pillow/floor
tall/short—question you
sad/happy ⎫
sick/OK ⎪
happy/angry ⎬ PERSON/YOU/ME
hungry/thirsty ⎪
sleepy/no sleepy ⎭

Additional variants of the above can of course be compiled from the total repertoire.

ACTION AND DESCRIPTOR

drive	fast/slow
smells	good/bad
talk	noisy/quiet
eat	fast/slow
talk	big/little
tastes	OK/no OK
drink	big/little
sleep	little/big
drink	hot/cold
buy	big/little

The above list can also be extended with other actions and also with numerous objects.

AGENT AND ACTION

man talk	girl wash
girl walk	boy drink
boy eat	man work
woman sit	woman buy
man sleep	man shave

All the above can be acted, with the patient then providing the signals describing the action and the person acting. Eventually, clear action pictures can enlarge the repertoire. Also, the actor in all the above can be reversed and signaled.

PAIRED ASSOCIATES

yes and ——	up and ——
stop and ——	good and ——
hot and ——	hard and ——
woman and ——	fast and ——
little and ——	left and ——

The above contrasts should be related to the environment at first, with both alternatives offered and also demonstrated, for example the floor is hard and the pillow is soft, the coffee is hot and the fruit juice is cold. Mere drill for retrieval should be avoided.

A useful repertoire for the individual patient in terms of associates and alternatives can evolve from acquisition of a wide variety of replies to the usual social greeting: How are you? These include but are not limited to OK, cold, hot, tired, sick, mad, happy, and even use of the signal MAYBE to mean *so-so*!

MOTORIC COORDINATION

Many patients in the Amer-Ind Code program have problems in execution because of impairments in muscular control and coordination. These may be assisted with exercise, particularly if the exercises are planned with specific synergies in mind. A time segment allotted to this type of exercise can also provide variety for the patient if it is placed between two repetitions of the signal segment on his program.

The motor patterns to be followed should be demonstrated by the clinician with objective first of imitation, then replication, then retrieval. Finally, they are shaped to improve particular signals. It may be rewarding to the patients involved if the clinician plans and carries out the motoric exercise sequences without relating them at first to signal meaning. Some of the patients may discover the signal meaning for themselves, and be very rewarded in so doing. Otherwise of course the clinician leads the patient to this recognition.

If the programmed segments suggested earlier in the text are adopted for use with a patient, the first exercise interval might be devoted to the following exercises. These are usually more enjoyable for the patients if they are performed in a small group situation. In such a context, it may be possible to present the difference between POINT and YOU. The first consists of extending the index finger toward a particular object one wishes to indicate; the second extends index and middle finger at persons.

Exercise for OBJECT:

1. Extend both or one of the arms forward, palms down.
2. Lower the middle, fourth, and little fingers, one by one, if possible, leaving the index extended.
3. Close the thumb over the lowered three fingers.
4. Lower the right arm and relax the hand.
5. Point the extended left index at various objects in the room.

Exercise for YOU:

1. Extend both arms forward, palms down.
2. Lower the fourth and little fingers.
3. Close the thumb over the lowered fingers.
4. Lower the right arm and relax the hand.
5. Point the extended two fingers of the left hand toward each person in the room successively.

Exercise for I/ME:

1. Extend both arms forward, palms down.
2. Drop all four fingers forward, toward the floor.
3. Curl the four fingers until tips touch the palm.
4. Extend the thumbs toward each other.
5. Lower the right hand and relax fingers.
6. Bring left arm toward self until thumb touches chest.

Exercise for differentiation between I/ME and YOU:

1. Have group repeat exercise for YOU.
2. Follow it with exercise for I/ME.
3. Have one individual execute exercise for YOU, pointing at only one other person.
4. This other person responds with signal for I/ME.
5. Go round the group with 3 and 4, until each has executed both sequences.

Exercise for WALK (seated):

1. Place both feet flat on floor, knees touching.
2. Advance left foot its own length and return it to position.
3. Advance right foot and return it to position.
4. Repeat until the two feet have each performed the forward–back movements a total of three times.
5. Stand up and stretch arms above head.
6. Lower arms and sit.
7. Place feet side by side with heels close to chair and knees touching.
8. Place index finger of left hand on right knee.
9. Place second finger on left knee.
10. Fold other fingers under thumb.
11. Repeat 4 above with the index finger and middle finger imitating the leg movements.

Exercise for WASH:

1. Extend both arms forward, palms down.
2. Move hands toward each other until right hand can be placed on top of left hand, crossing it.
3. Bend both elbows bringing hands toward body.
4. Slide right hand toward fingers of left and off them.

5. Move right hand under left hand.
6. Slide left hand toward fingers of right and off them.
7. Move right hand under left hand.
8. Repeat the 3–4–5–6 sequence until it has been performed three times.

Exercise for EAT:

1. Extend both arms forward, palms down.
2. Bend index fingers until they touch thumb tips.
3. Lower one arm and relax it.
4. Move joined index-thumb of other hand to touch table surface in front of patient.
5. Lift joined index thumb to touch lips.
6. Repeat 5 three times in all.

Exercise for DRINK:

1. Have plastic glass in front of patient.
2. Extend both arms forward, palms facing.
3. Bring hands together around glass.
4. Lift hands upward retaining glass shape.
5. Separate hands retaining glass shape.
6. Place one hand on knee and relax.
7. Lower other hand, retaining shape of glass, to table.
8. Lift shaped hand to face until thumb joint touches chin, then lower it to touch table.
9. Repeat number 8 for total of three times.

Exercise for SIT:

1. Sit facing a table.
2. Place both hands on the table about 18 inches apart, with just the fingers on the table, palms down.
3. Bend the hands at the base of the fingers and flex the wrist so that the palmar surfaces of hands form right angles with the fingers.
4. Lift hands from table without losing shape.
5. Bend elbows to elevate hands upward.

Exercise for COLD:

1. Extend both arms laterally.
2. Swing right arm to place right palm on left shoulder.
3. Swing left arm to place left palm on right shoulder.
4. Pat shoulders with palms three times, slowly.
5. Accelerate the rate of the patting until it resembles the shivering of cold hands.

With the above suggestions as illustrative patterns, similar routines may be created for other signals in the program. Physical therapists are usually both interested in and helpful with this activity.

MATCHING AND SORTING

Recognition of shape patterns is a fundamental skill for development of effective hand signaling. It is also highly related to concept formation. Usually, activity concerned with forms and blocks of various colors, sizes and shapes is interesting to the patient as recreation. It can be profitably placed between two repetitions of the formal programmed signal sessions.

Many matching activities will suggest themselves to the clinician from the tasks in the Leiter International Scale, a nonverbal test of problem solving. Of course no clinical task should replicate any of the test tasks exactly, but should rather be designed to build the patient's skill toward mastery of the principle involved.

Simple clinician-made materials will serve. The matching may begin with circles, squares and equilateral triangles cut from colored paper. Simple form boards may be involved with wood or plastic counters to fit the shapes. Two sizes are recommended, and later a sequence of sizes can be added. Colors may help some patients, may confuse others. In any case, when shape or size is the objective, the color cue should be faded.

The ovoid, rectangle and diamond shapes may be added, also in different sizes. All may be presented in the primary and secondary colors. Begin simply with three counters and increase the complexity of the choices as the patient progresses.

Finger tracing of the pattern in the form board appears to assist the patient to visualize and execute the shaped movement. Many can be led to trace the pattern in air with the index with this type of tactile and kinetic stimulus. This type of finger tracing with the index is applicable to the signal BOX, for example, as well as to ROUND, ADD, and MULTIPLY. Watching and sorting activities also formulate the concepts for BIG/LITTLE as well as SAME/DIFFERENT.

The signal for COLOR as well as the methods of signaling different colors can be included in this type of activity, also. Red is the lips, blue is the sky, yellow is the sun, green is the grass. Brown is the earth, white is lack of color, or COLOR NO, while black is COLOR AGREE (yes).

The clinician can design specific tasks for each patient, tailored to his methods of attack on the Leiter tasks, in terms of the following ladder of difficulty, moving each task up the ladder:

1. The clinician indicates a choice and the patient accepts it or rejects it. Demonstrations of the acceptable should precede the presentation of the task. If the patient uses a head nod and head shake these can be associated first with the thumbs up gesture for AGREE and the thumbs down for NO. These can be varied to include the OK for agreement and the REJECT for disagreement.
2. Patient sorts forms progressively through color, size, shape to match a model. These tasks may be extended later to include object function, sound-maker, pitch, etc.
3. Patient compares visually colors, shapes, size and points to one matching a model. This can begin with simple presentation of one red and one

blue to match a red and increase in complexity until he chooses the one counter which is correct color, shape and size.

4. Patient sorts without a model.
5. Matches like with like in pairs.
6. Rejects the one that is different from the group.
7. Arranges a series first with a model and then without.

The above tasks may also be conducted with objects. For example, objects used in the first of the programmed signal sessions may be sorted into categories of functional relationship, as follows:

Eat Objects	Drink Objects	Wash Objects
food	glass	sink
paper plates	cup	soap
plastic plates	bottle	plastic plates
knife	fountain	glass
fork	faucet	water
spoon	juice	hands
paper napkin	cola	I/me

After the preliminary sorting and matching tasks have been mastered, many patients find it rewarding to have shape puzzles used as a recreational activity. Since they focus on proper placement of shape, this is an excellent extension of the clinical task. Since shape is important not only to signaling but also to speaking, the puzzles may serve a multiple purpose.

Both the matching and sorting activities, along with the motoric activities may be conducted by other associated professionals and again serve multiple purposes. The physical therapist, the recreational therapist, the gym instructor, the occupational therapist, and the special education teacher all have extensive skills to offer in these areas. Discussion with them of the applicability of this kind of activity to signaling and communication can be very profitable for all concerned and can lead to a much more intensive program for the patient, and to the patient's eventual rehabilitation in communication.

POSTSCRIPT

The current of our times is scientific. Any profession dedicated to rehabilitation of human beings must be soundly based in scientific knowledge and also in professional skills, both of which must be constantly modified as the total body of knowledge and skill expands and changes. But for the purposes of human rehabilitation, science and skill are not enough.

Modern theory proposes that scientific objectivity rules out emotion. This is sometimes misunderstood by scientist and layperson alike: no human endeavour has ever been or ever will be devoid of emotive factors, but these factors are so variable, capable of such power, that science is unable to formulate the language of emotion, or its logic. The scientist, or, as in our concerns, the clinician, must be wary of disaffecting the patient, of giving the impression that detachment, in the name of objectivity, somehow veils a disinterest in individual human beings.

Objectivity may rule out sympathy as an accountable factor, but, in the human sciences, it need not and cannot exclude empathy, for it is simply too valuable. Understanding of the feelings of human beings and applying this understanding in empathic contacts with the patients are as important to effective treatment as is knowledge of syndromes and their relevant techniques. Intuition, motivation, and dedication on the part of the clinician are vital factors in rehabilitation results. It is not enough for the clinician to have empathy for the patient; the clinician must convey this to the patient. The face, the voice, and the total body action speak this message far more reliably than words.

The human treatment of human beings is as important, or perhaps more important, than the scientific treatment. Where there is any possibility that the latter may not achieve its objectives, the former becomes of overwhelming importance to the patients. It may be well to consider that while science leads us to truth, it does not contribute the whole truth.

Science supplies the truth that lights the way. Human communication provides the truth that warms the heart, and this is the art of therapeutics. Kindness is the universal language that links the science to the art. Impaired human beings are more than the sum of their deficits.

CLINICAL SIGNAL
REPERTOIRE

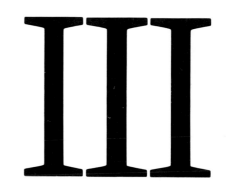

Concept Labels

1. ABOVE	25. BLIND	49. CORN	73. EASY
2. ACCOMPANY	26. BOAT	50. CRAZY	74. EAT
3. ACROSS	27. BORED	51. CRY	75. ENTER
4. ADD	28. BOSS	52. CUP	76. ERASE
5. ADVANCE	29. BOTH	53. CUT	77. ESCAPE
6. AFRAID	30. BOTTLE	54. DANCE	78. EXCHANGE
7. AFTERNOON	31. BOTTOM	55. DAY	79. FAST
8. AGREE	32. BOUNCE	56. DEAF	80. FENCE
9. ALIKE	33. BOWL	57. DEEP	81. FIGHT
10. ALL	34. BOX	58. DEFY	82. FIRE
11. ANGRY	35. BRAIN	59. DEPART	83. FISH
12. ANIMAL	36. BREAK	60. DIE	84. FLAG
13. ARREST	37. BREATHE	61. DIFFER	85. FLAT
14. ARROGANT	38. BRIBE	62. DIG	86. FLY (plane)
15. ASHAMED	39. CAMERA	63. DISTANT	87. FLY (bird)
16. ATTENTION	40. CARDS	64. DIVE	88. FRIEND
17. BABY	41. CARRY	65. DIVIDE	89. FUTURE
18. BEARD	42. CHOP	66. DOMINATE	90. GENTLY
19. BEEF	43. COAX	67. DOOR	91. GET
20. BELOW	44. COLD	68. DOWN	92. GIVE
21. BETWEEN	45. COLOR	69. DRINK	93. GLASSES
22. BIG	46. COMB	70. DRIVE	94. GOODBYE
23. BLAME	47. COME	71. EARTH	95. GRASS
24. BLANKET	48. COMMAND	72. EAST	96. HAND

97. HANG	132. MIRROR	167. PRAY	202. STRAIGHT
98. HARD	133. MOCK	168. PROTECT	203. SUN
99. HEAR	134. MONEY	169. PUSH	204. SURPRISE
100. HEART	135. MONTH	170. PUZZLED	205. SURRENDER
101. HEAVEN	136. MORE	171. QUESTION	206. SWIM
102. HEAVY	137. MORNING	172. QUIET	207. TABLE
103. HELLO	138. MOUNTAIN	173. RAIN	208. TALK
104. HELP	139. MULTIPLY	174. READ	209. TASTE
105. HERE	140. MUSIC	175. REJECT	210. TEA
106. HIDE	141. MUSTACHE	176. RELATION	211. TELEPHONE
107. HIGH	142. NAPKIN	177. RIDE	212. THANKS
108. HOLD	143. NAUGHTY	178. RIGHT	213. THINK
109. HOT	144. NEAR	179. RING	214. THREATEN
110. HUNGRY	145. NO	180. ROUND	215. THROW
111. I	146. NOON	181. SCISSORS	216. TIME
112. IN	147. NORTH	182. SECRET	217. TOOTHBRUSH
113. JUSTICE	148. NOTHING	183. SHAKE	218. TOP
114. KNOW	149. NUMBERS	184. SHAME	219. TOUCH
115. LAUGH	150. OATH	185. SHAVE	220. TOWEL
116. LEFT	151. OBJECT	186. SHELTER	221. TREES
117. LIE	152. OK	187. SHOT	222. TURTLE
118. LIGHTWEIGHT	153. ON	188. SHUT	223. TYPEWRITE
119. LINK	154. OPEN	189. SIT	224. UNDER
120. LITTLE	155. OUT	190. SLEEP	225. UNFOLD
121. LOCK	156. PAIN	191. SMART	226. UP
122. LOOK	157. PAINT	192. SMELL	227. WALK
123. LOUD	158. PAST	193. SMOKE	228. WASH
124. MAN	159. PEEL	194. SMOOTH	229. WATER
125. MANICURE	160. PERSON	195. SNOW	230. WEST
126. MANY	161. PIANO	196. SOFT	231. WINDOW
127. MASK	162. PLEASE	197. SOUTH	232. WOMAN
128. MAYBE	163. POMPOUS	198. SPREAD	233. WORK
129. MEDICINE	164. PORK	199. STAND	234. WRAP
130. MEET	165. POSSESS	200. STIR	235. WRITE
131. MEND	166. POUR	201. STOP	236. YOU

Concept Illustrations

1. **ABOVE**
(kinetic)

higher
superior

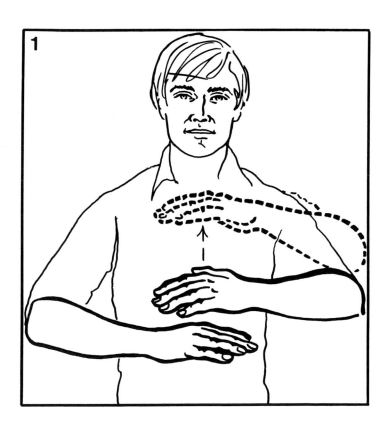

Right hand is placed, palm down, in front of the body at diaphragm level. Then left hand is placed slightly above the right and moved upwards about six inches (or more). The hands do not touch.

2. **ACCOMPANY**
(repetitive)

assist

attend

conduct

escort

follow

lead

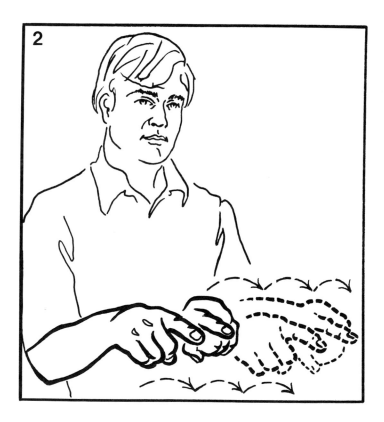

Both hands are extended, palms down, with index extended. Left index is about an inch ahead of the right. Left leads, and the right follows in a brief, forward, jerky movement, which is repeated three times.

3. **ACROSS**
(kinetic)

beyond
bridge
opposite
transverse

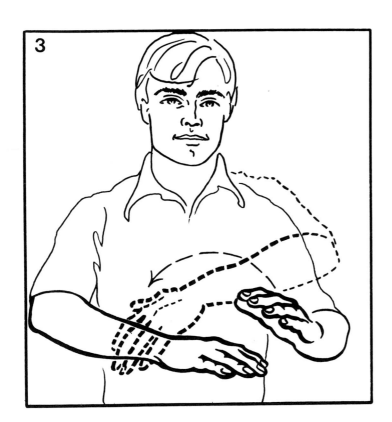

Right hand, palm down, is placed in front of body midline, fingers forward. Left hand is moved toward the right hand, fingers leading, and is elevated to pass over the static right hand.

4. **ADD**
(static)

account
addition
bill
compute
include
plus
sum
supplement
total

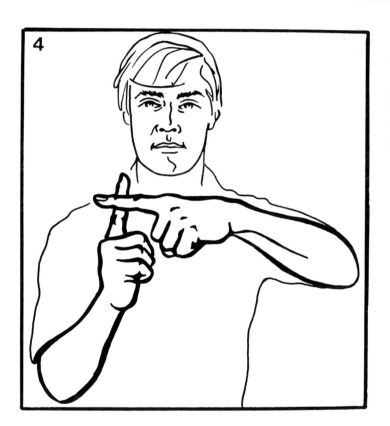

Left index is extended horizontally and the right index intersects vertically.

5. **ADVANCE**
(kinetic)

ahead
beyond
excel
move
progress
promote
surpass

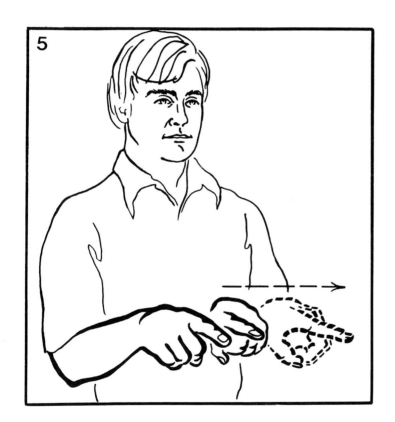

Both hands are extended in front of body, palms down, index fingers pointing forward and touching laterally. Left index moves forward by half its length.

6. **AFRAID**
(static)

alarm

anxious

apprehensive

cowardly

fear

fright

horror

panic

scared

terrified

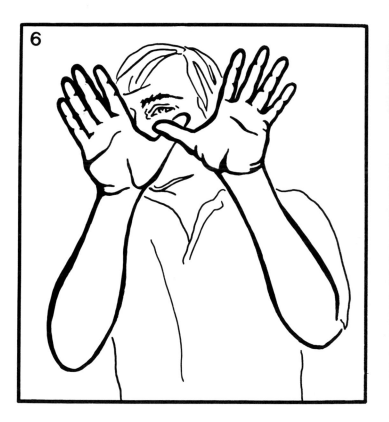

Both hands are elevated, palms forward. Fingers are spread in front of face, thumbs almost touching. Total upper body is leaning backward slightly.

7. **AFTERNOON**
(static)

evening

noon to sunset

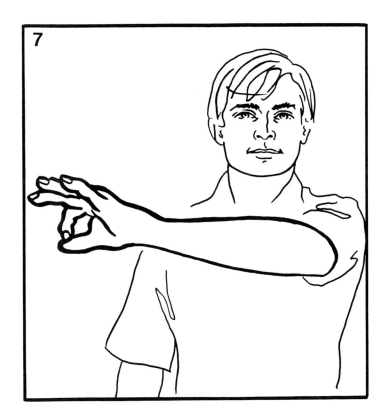

Left arm, bent at elbow, is extended across body toward the right with thumb and index touching and the other three fingers spread and extended. Viewer should be able to see thumb-finger circle, and all three fingers (sun signal). Total means "sun is in the west." (Similar signal is used for WEST: the index points right (west) and the other fingers are folded.) For evening, the index finger is straightened, making the hand flat.

8. **AGREE**

(static)

affirmative

allow

assent

concur

consent

endorse

vote

yes

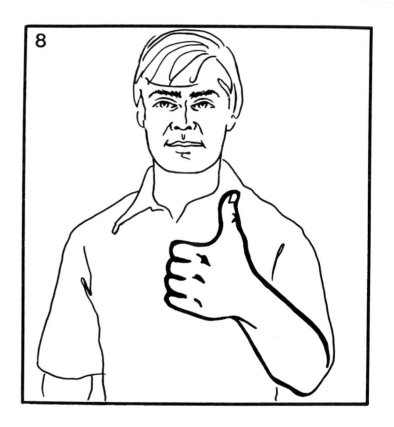

Left fist is extended forward, thumb elevated.

9. **ALIKE**

(static)

comparable
corresponding
equal
equivalent
identical
like
married
matched
parallel
partner
resembling
same
similar
synonomous
together
uniform
unchanged

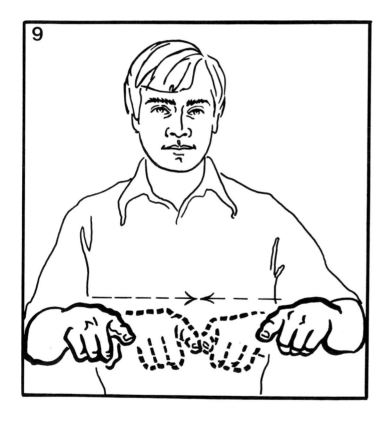

Both hands are extended in front of body, index fingers extended and touching laterally. The other fingers are folded.

10. **ALL**
(kinetic)

complete
entire
every
total
whole

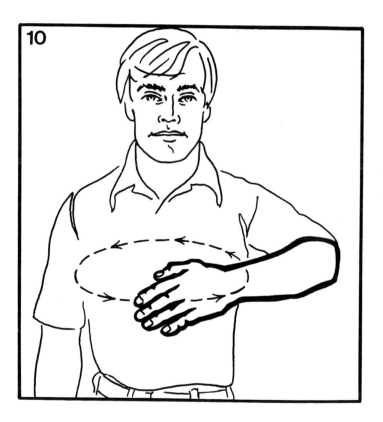

Left hand, back up and fingers extended, moves in horizontal circle in front of body. (Similar to MANY in which fingers flutter to indicate "counting" rather whan "whole.")

11. **ANGRY**
(repetitive)

anger
disturbed
enraged
furious
indignant
irate
turmoil
vexed

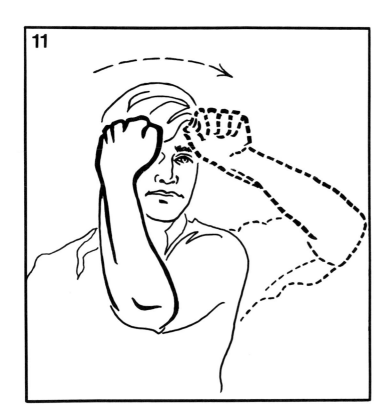

Left fist is placed on left side of forehead with back of hand touching forehead. Fist is rotated to right side of forehead, then back to left side, touching forehead throughout.

12. **ANIMAL**
(static)

alive

beast

creature

organism

quadruped

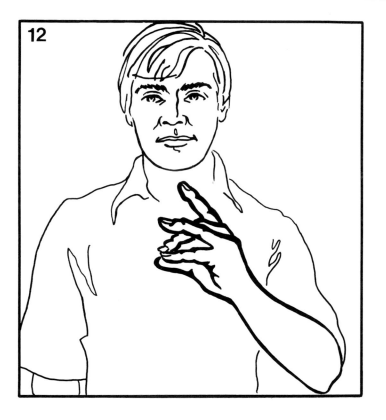

Thumb, middle finger, and little finger of left hand meet to form nose. Index and fourth finger are extended to form erect ears. Shown in profile to viewer. *If patient cannot perform above*, use middle and fourth finger to touch thumb for nose, and erect index and little finger for ears. *Show in profile* so it will not be confused with the deaf sign for "peace." (Indian signal for "peace" is a greeting: HELLO meaning without weapon.)

13. **ARREST**
(static)

capture
custody
handcuffs
prisoner

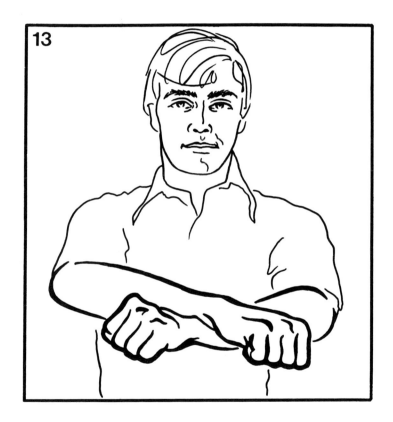

Both arms are extended in front of body and crossed at the wrists, hands limp. (The hemiplegic patient can place the left hand across the inert right hand.)

14. **ARROGANT**
(kinetic)

conceited

contemptuous

haughty

imperious

inconsiderate

supercilious

vain

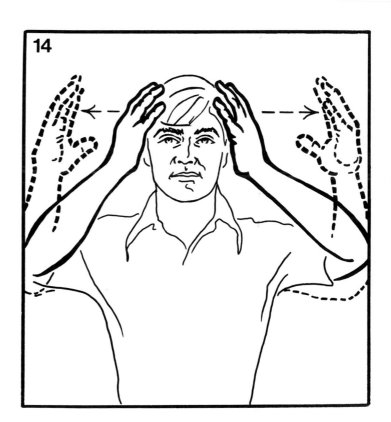

Both hands, fingers spread, are elevated, one to each side of the head. They are moved away from head, laterally, to indicate "swelled-head." Palms are toward head.

15. **ASHAMED**
(static)

embarrassed
humiliated
mortified

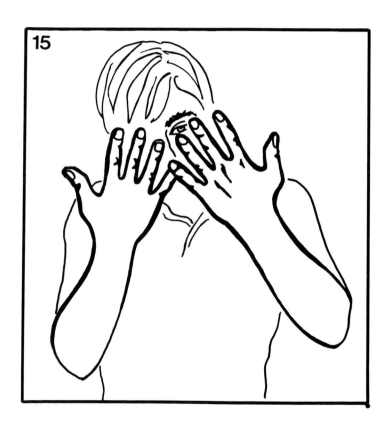

Both hands are placed in front of face, palms to face. All fingers are extended and separated. Signaler hides face and peers through finger apertures. (This signal refers only to signaler. For reference to another person, see SHAME.)

16. **ATTENTION**
(static)

advice

alarm

alert

notice

signal

siren

warning

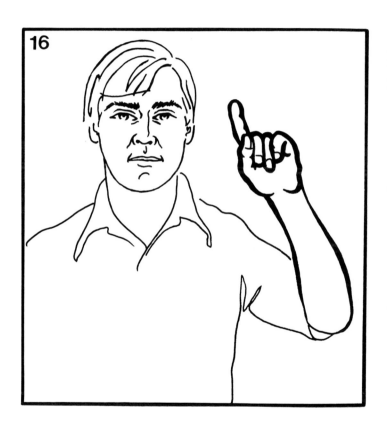

Left hand is elevated at left side of body, index extended upward. Other fingers are folded, palm forward.

17. **BABY**

(repetitive)

babe
child
infant
neonate
pamper
spoil
youngster

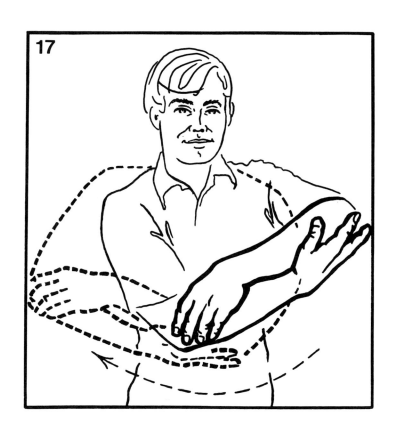

The two arms are crossed with palm of left hand cupping elbow of right and vice versa. The joined arms are then moved as far as possible to the left. Then they are moved to the right and again to the left, creating a rocking or swinging motion (cradling the baby).

18. **BEARD**

(kinetic)

bristles

hairy

hirsute

stubble

unshaven

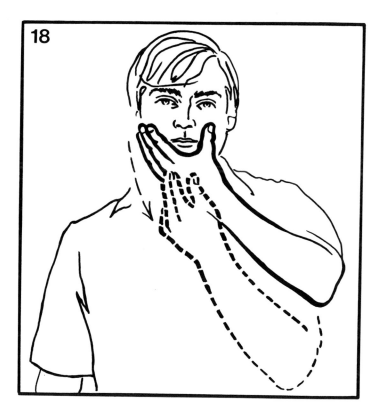

The left hand is raised to chin level, palm toward neck. It is then moved downward, fingers and thumb stroking sides of the chin. Hand continues downward until thumb touches fingers to indicate length of the beard.

19. **BEEF**
(static)

bison
cattle
cow
deer
meat
steer

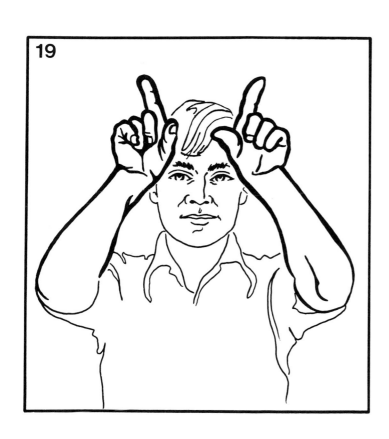

Both hands are elevated to sides of forehead, palms forward, index extended upward at slight outward angle. Other fingers are folded. (Index fingers represent horn of the steer.) Clarifiers: ANIMAL; EAT.

20. **BELOW**

(kinetic)

beneath

lower

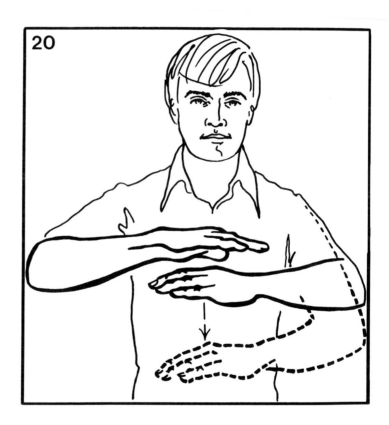

The right hand is elevated in front of body, palm down. The left hand is placed about two inches below it, and then moved downward about six inches.

21. **BETWEEN**
(kinetic)

intermediate

ravine

valley

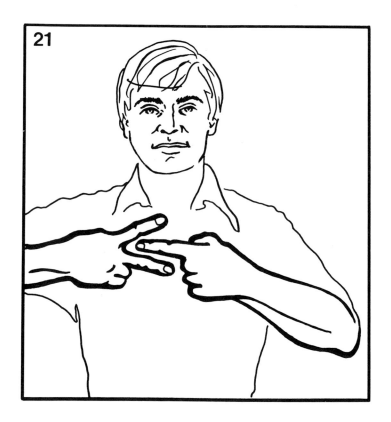

The right hand is placed before the body (slightly above waist height), with back of hand facing out, and index and second finger extended in V shape. Other fingers and thumb are curled. Then the index finger of the left hand points to space created by the V.

22. **BIG**

(static)

bulky

enormous

great

large

massive

much

sizable

vast

(kinetic)

develop

enlarge

grow

increase

stretch

swell

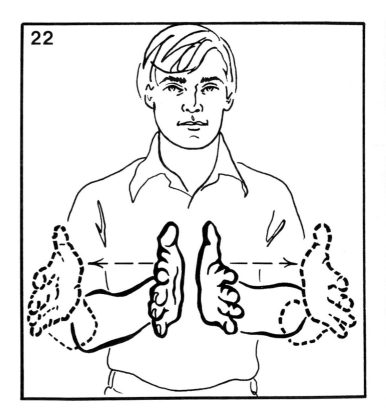

(static) Both arms are elevated at chest height and extended forward, palms facing and about three feet apart.

(kinetic) Both arms are extended at chest height, palms facing and about six inches apart. Then arms are moved laterally until they are about three feet apart, showing the action of growing larger.

23. **BLAME**

(repetitive)

accuse
apologize
confess
criticize
fault
liability
sorry

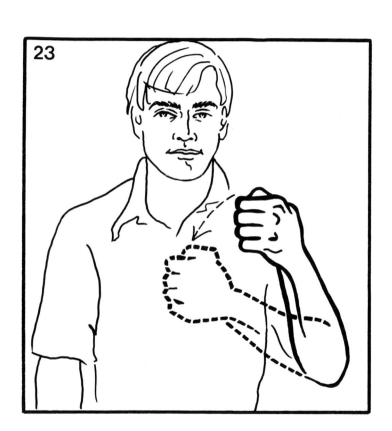

The fisted left hand knocks three times on the breast bone.

24. **BLANKET**
(kinetic)

comfort

cover

quilt

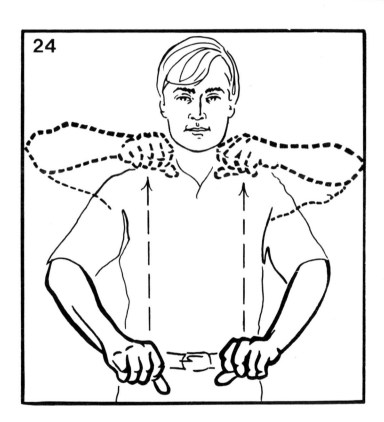

Both hands are fisted at about waist height. Then they move toward the chin, simultaneously, showing the action of drawing a blanket up over the body. (The ancient signal wrapped the blanket around the body, but this is no longer current.)

25. **BLIND**
(static)

sightless
unseeing

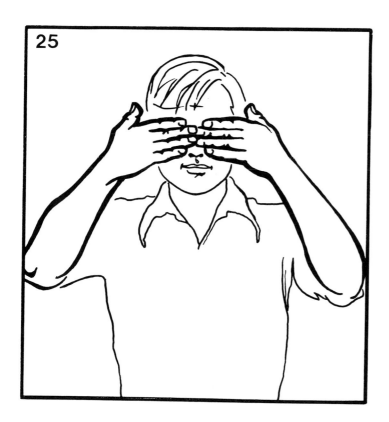

Both hands are raised to the eyes. The joined fingers cover the eyes, palms toward the face, fingers pointing in each case in the direction of the nose.

26. **BOAT**
(kinetic)

canoe
craft
fishing
paddle
sailing
sailor
ship
steamer
transport
travel
vessel
yacht

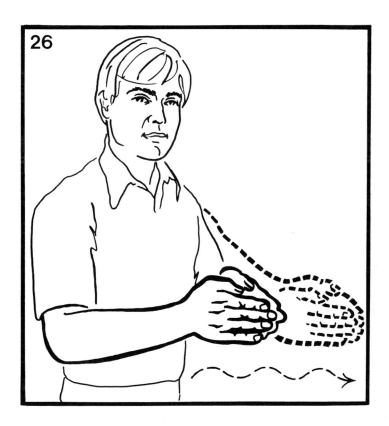

The hands are placed in front of the body, waist height, palms facing. Fingertips are touching to form prow of ship. Then hands are moved foreward as through water, tracing three small wave-like undulations.

27. **BORED**

(repetitive)

indifferent

monotonous

unexcited

uninteresting

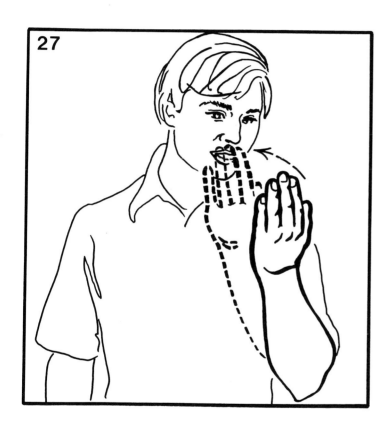

The lips are open and rounded. With palm toward face, the fingers of the left hand gently pat the open lips three times.

28. BOSS
(static)

cardinal [clerical]

chief

commander

doctor [M.D., D.O., D.D.S., Ph.D.]

importance

important

judge–king

leader

physician

professor [Ph.D., Sc.D.]

queen

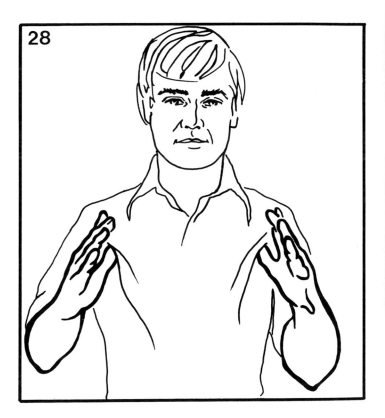

28

Both arms are bent at the elbow. Thumbs are inserted under arms. Fingers are extended upwards and spread. Palms face each other.

29. **BOTH**
(kinetic)

choice
either
other

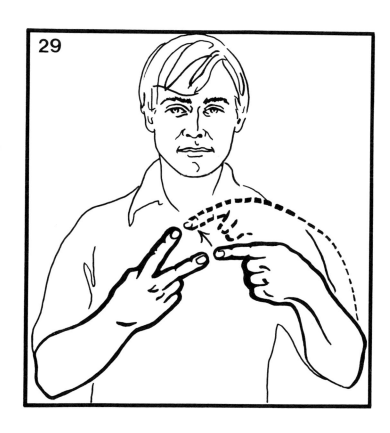

The right hand is held in front of chest, index and second finger extended and spread. Other fingers are curled. The left index points to right second finger, then to right index, and then moves away slightly left. To distinguish BOTH from the other interpretations, add closure of the extended, spread index and second finger.

30. **BOTTLE**
(static)

beer

pop

soda

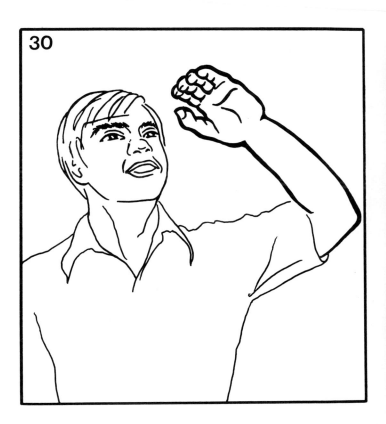

The left-hand fingers are curled as if holding a bottle. The hand is raised above the mouth. The head is tilted back with the lips open.

31. **BOTTOM**
(static)

base
buttocks
foundation
lowest
rump
underpart
underside

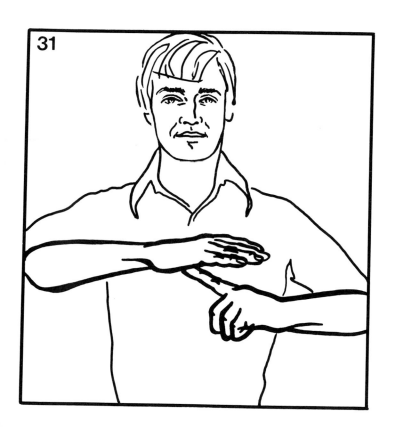

The right hand is held flat, back up, in front of the body. The left index finger points at the palm at a 45 degree angle.

32. **BOUNCE**
(kinetic)

basketball
exercise
game
play
sport

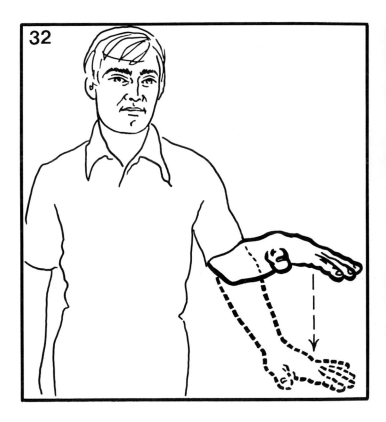

The flat left hand is extended at left side and forward of body, palm down. It is lowered and raised forcefully three times (dribbling). (Contrast: GENTLY, where range of movement is shorter, slower, and more gentle.)

33. **BOWL**
(static)

basin
container
dish
receptacle

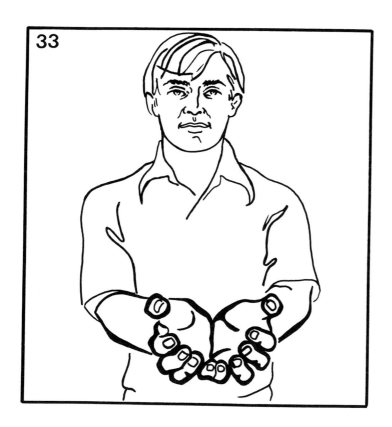

Both hands are held in front of the body, palms up, touching each other from wrist to finger ends. Fingers lie in close contact and are slightly curved. The resulting shape is a bowl or container formed by the hands.

34. BOX

(kinetic)

cabinet
carton
chest
container
crate
receptacle
square
stall
TV
window

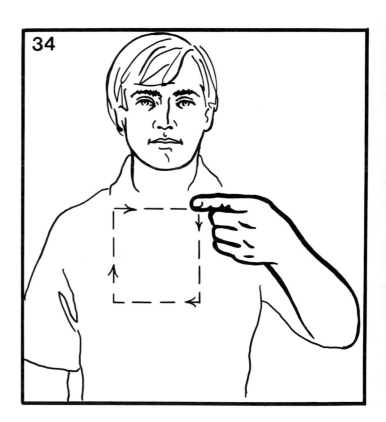

Left index (other fingers curled) draws the outline of a box. The box should be vertically and horizontally consistent with intended meaning.

35. **BRAIN**
(static)

idea
intellect
mind

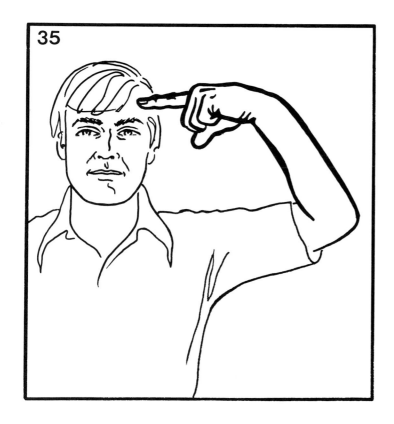

The left index finger touches the left temple. For HEAD, point to top of forehead above hairline. (Compare with THINK, SMART, and KNOW/LEARN).

36. **BREAK**

(kinetic)

burst
demolish
destroy
fracture
shatter
smash
snap
splinter
split

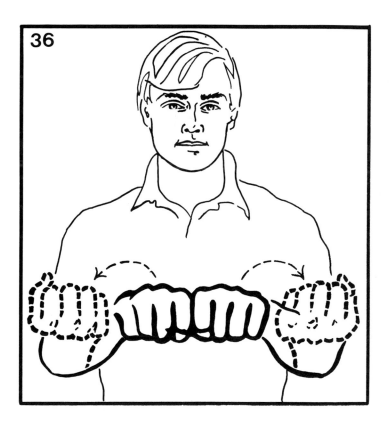

Both fists, touching each other closely, are extended with back up, in front of body. Then they are parted quickly and forcibly by lateral rotation of both wrists as though breaking a stick.

37. **BREATHE**
(repetitive)

breath
breathing
exhalation
inhalation
lungs
respiration
respirator

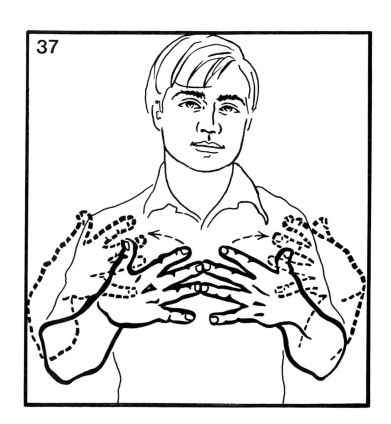

Both hands rest lightly on chest, palms against body, fingers spread. Hands are moved forward and upward away from chest about one inch, then back to chest. Repeat three times.

38. **BRIBE**
(static)

graft

illegal

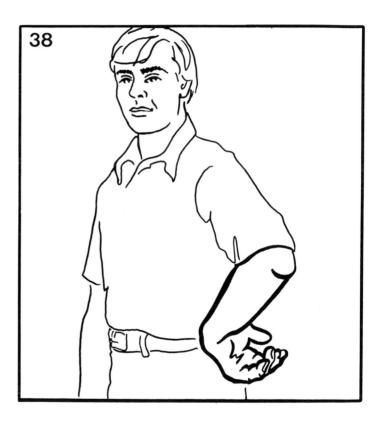

Left hand, palm up and cupped, is held behind the left hip. Total body is turned so viewer may see hand and hip relation.

39. CAMERA
(kinetic)

film
image
photograph
picture

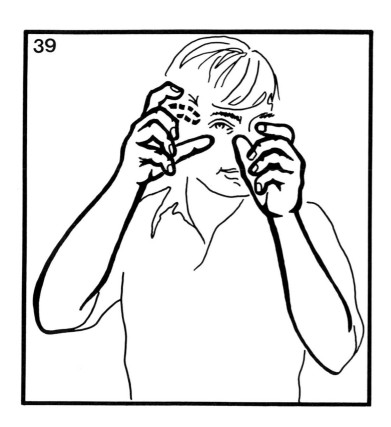

Both hands are raised to face level, before right eye. Left hand supports an imaginary camera; right hand is balancing it. Right index is free to perform quick, light, downward movement as though tripping the shutter.

40. **CARDS**
(repetitive)

deal
dealer
dispense
distribute
game
play

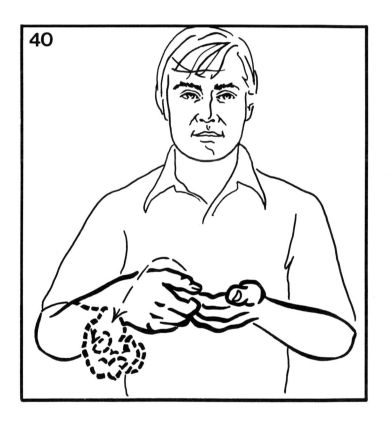

Left hand is extended in front of body, palm up, fingers toward the right. Right hand is slightly above and to the right. Right hand, palm up, moves toward the right, flexing wrist as though taking a card from left hand and laying it on nearby surface.

41. **CARRY**
(static)

deliver
haul
move
shift
transport

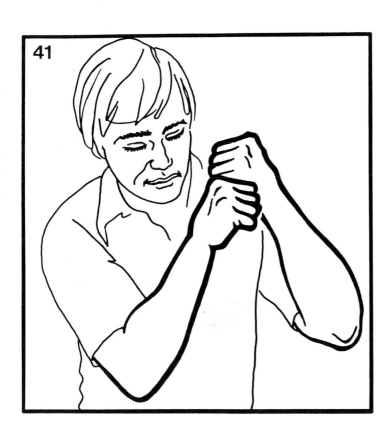

Both fisted hands are placed at left shoulder, left hand slightly higher than shoulder, and right hand slightly lower, as though both were grasping the gathered neck of a sack suspended over the back. (Clarity is enhanced if the torso leans slightly forward.)

42. CHOP

(kinetic)

cleave

cut

end

finished

terminate

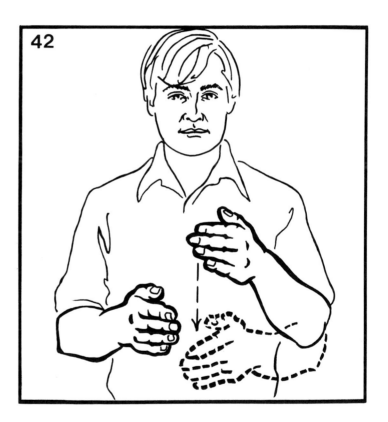

Right arm, elbow bent, is extended forward at 45 degree angle to the body. Right palm is angled toward midline, fingers extended and touching. Left hand, same formation, is elevated about one foot above tip of right middle finger, then is brought down sharply and forcefully, passing as closely as possible to right middle finger tip without hitting it.

43. **COAX**
(repetitive)

incentive
induce
inducement
inveigle
persuade

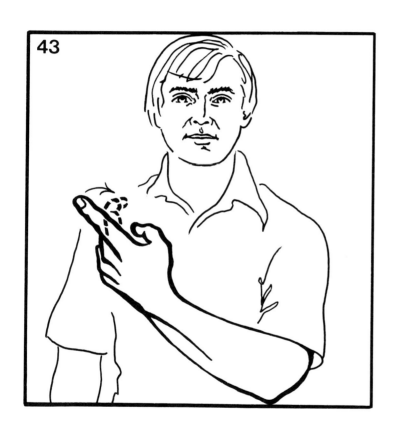

Left hand is raised to chin height, palm toward body, index finger extended upward. Other fingers are folded. Then index is slowly curled toward the body three times. (Meaning is enhanced if signaler smiles.)

44. **COLD**
(kinetic)

chilly

frigid

frozen

icy

shiver

unheated

wintery

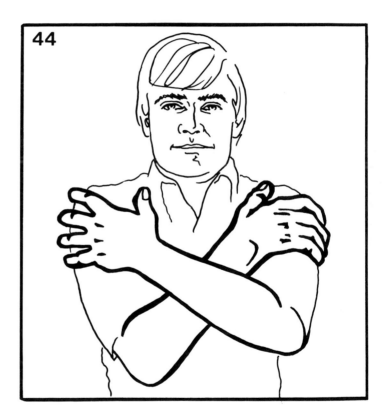

Arms are crossed on chest. Palms of hands are on opposite shoulders. Fingers are spread and slightly gripping. (Signal is enhanced if accompanied by slight shivering movements of hands.)

45. **COLOR**
(kinetic)

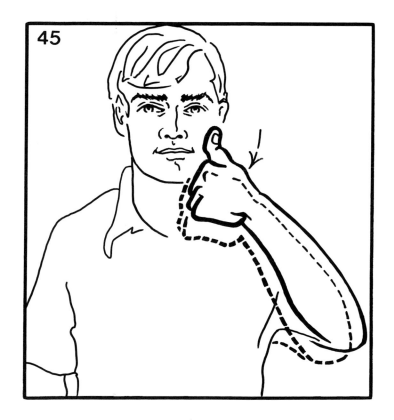

The left thumb is rubbed over the left cheek, back to front, in one stroke. The exact color is then specified by index pointing: blue = sky; green = grass; yellow = sun; red = lips; brown = earth; black = affirmative (much color); white = negative (absence of color).

46. **COMB**
(repetitive)

groom

hair

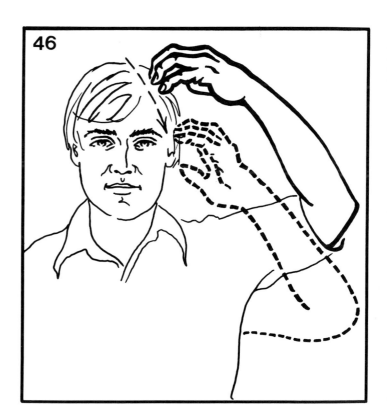

Left hand is elevated to left side of head, fingers spread, palm down. It is then moved downwards, toward the ear, three times. (Fingers represent comb moving through hair.)

47. **COME**
(kinetic)

approach
arrive

(repetitive, executed rapidly)

hurry
pressure
quickly
speed

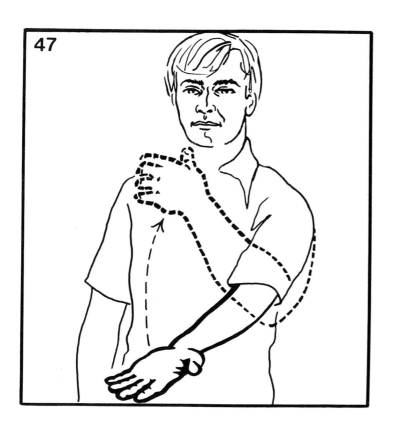

Left hand is extended forward, palm up, fingers toward viewer. Then the arm is elevated, palm toward signaler, moving toward the right shoulder in an arc.

48. **COMMAND**
(repetitive)

order

require

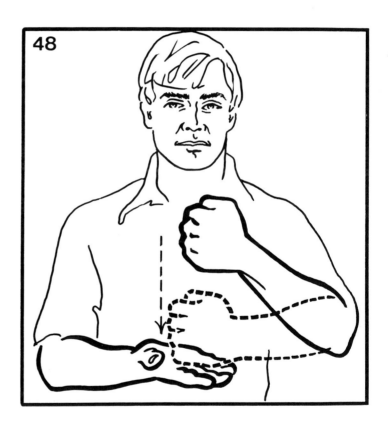

Left hand, fisted, thumb side up, hits right flat palm (or left knee or nearby wooden surface) three times.

49. **CORN**
(repetitive)

grain

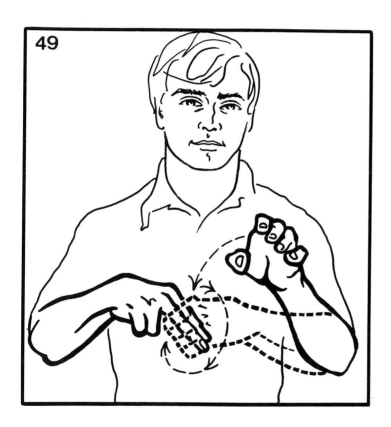

Right index and middle finger are extended to the left, together. Other fingers are folded. Left hand gently grasps right fingers loosely and then rotates three times around the right fingers (as though stripping corn from its cob).

50. **CRAZY**
(kinetic)

dunce

foolish

idiotic

imprudent

irresponsible

nonsense

odd

peculiar

senseless

silly

stupid

unbalanced

weird

witless

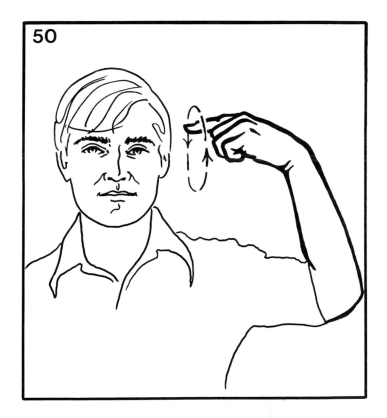

Left hand, index extended, other fingers curled, points to left temple. It then rotates from front to back in a lateral circle. (The brain going backward or in reverse.)

51. **CRY**

(repetitive)

depressed

disconsolate

joyless

lament

melancholy

moan

mourn

sad

sob

tears

tragedy

tragic

unhappy

wail

weep

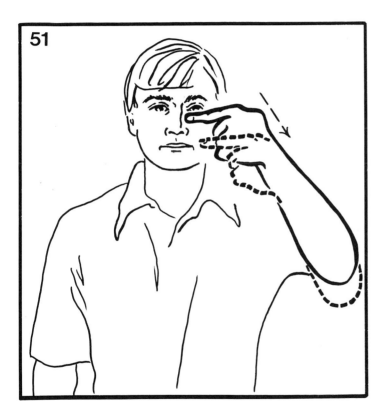

The left index points to nasal side of left eye, then moves down to mouth level, tracing (but not touching) the path of tears on the cheek. Repeat downward movement of index finger three times.

52. **CUP**
(static)

beverage
coffee
drink
liquid

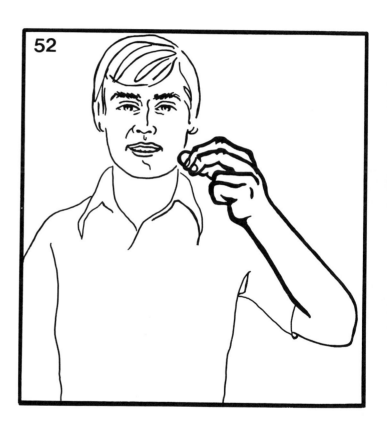

Left hand is positioned at left side of mouth. Thumb tip is touching tips of index and middle finger (as though holding a cup). The lips perform a sipping action.

53. **CUT**

(repetitive)

blade
carve
dagger
dissect
knife
scalpel
sever
slit
split

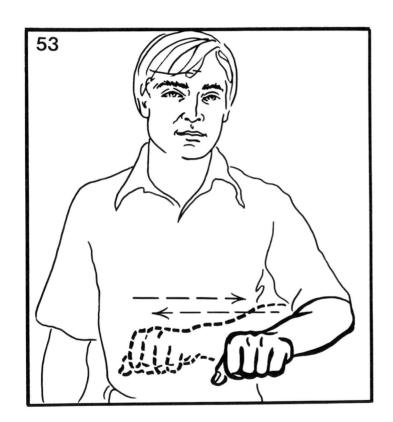

53

Left hand, palm down, fingers bent as though holding a knife, is elevated in front of the body, just above waist level. It is then moved forward and backward in a cutting rhythm three times. (If palm faces right, and movement is larger, the signal can be interpreted as SAWING.)

54. **DANCE**
(kinetic)

celebration

dancer

happiness

happy

party

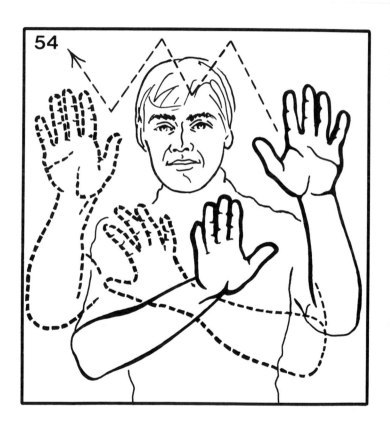

Both hands are elevated. Left hand is at shoulder height; the right hand is beside it and a hand length lower. Then both hands move toward the right in synchrony, exchanging height, with the right hand high and the left hand low. (While changing, the hands move up and down vertically.) The pattern is repeated in reverse, and then a third time, replicating the first.

55. **DAY**
(static)

period of time [24 hr]
dawn to dusk
sunrise to sunset
opposite of night

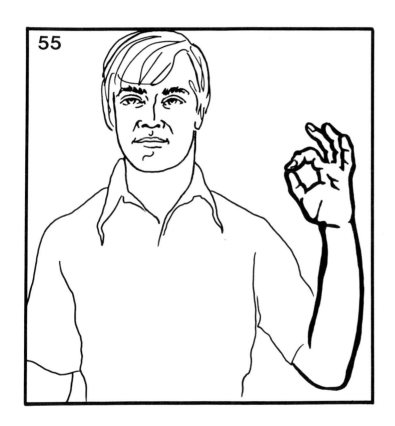

55

The left hand is raised at left side of body, with thumb and index touching. Other fingers are extended, successively bending slightly toward index. (The circle represents the Sun, the three fingers the rays. This is the general SUN signal. When over the head, it specifically means SUN.) When at the left and accompanied by a slight jerky movement, it means OK. (When the arm is at the centerline of body and pointing up, it means NOON.)

56. **DEAF**
(static)

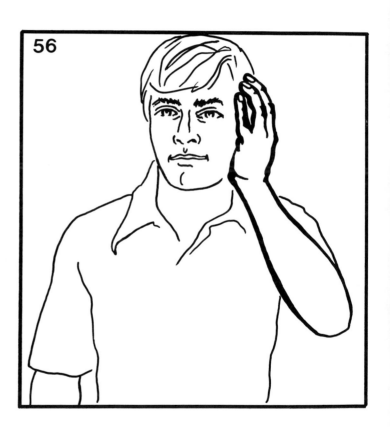

Left hand, slightly cupped, palm toward head, is placed over ear. ("Hard of hearing" is conveyed by DEAF + LITTLE; "won't hear" is conveyed by HEARING + REJECT.)

57. **DEEP**
(static)

below
down
engrossed
involved
profound [thinking]
resonant [sound]
vivid [color]

Left arm is extended downward at left side as far as possible, with some bending of torso. Wrist is flexed, palm up, to show termination of depth. (Compare: DOWN; contrast: HIGH.)

58. **DEFY**

(kinetic)

contrary

defiance

disobedience

insolence

rebel

rebellion

uncooperative

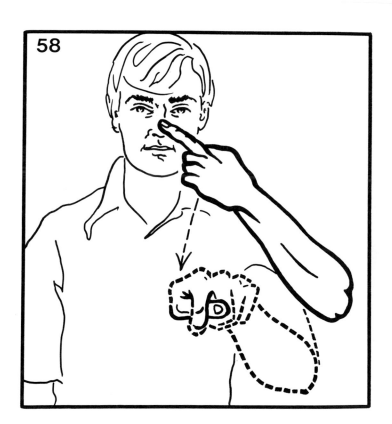

The left index finger touches the nose. Then the left hand is extended forward, palm down and fisted, with thumb inserted between second and third fingers.

59. **DEPART**
(kinetic)

exit

from

go

leave

unwelcome

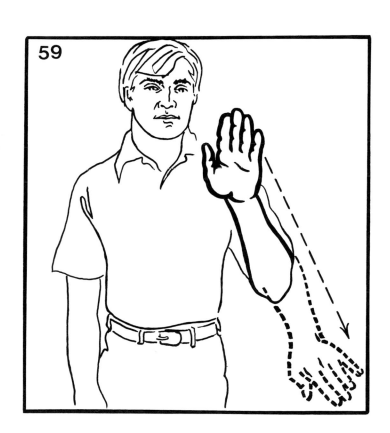

Left arm is raised to shoulder height, elbow bent, palm forward. Then hand is moved downward forcefully until elbow is straight.

60. **DIE**
(kinetic)

burial
buried
bury
dead
death
deceased
dying
funeral

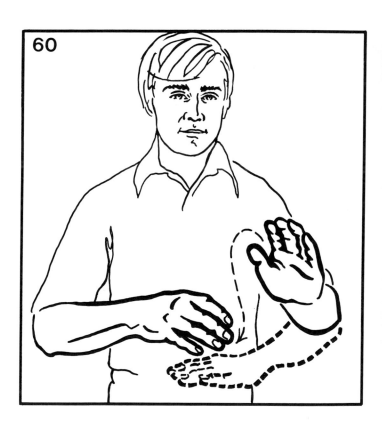

The right hand is held in front of body, palm down, fingers extended forward. The left hand is extended, palm down, but higher than the right hand, and to the left of it. Then, the left hand is moved centrally toward the right hand and suddenly lowered to *go under* it.

61. **DIFFER**
(kinetic)

apart
contrast
demur
different
dispute
deviate
opposed
opposite
separate
unlike

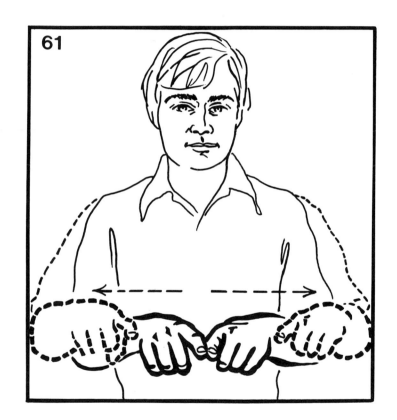

Both hands, palms down, index finger pointed forward, other fingers folded, are brought together at body midline. Index fingers are touching laterally. Then hands are moved apart in synchrony to the width of the body.

62. DIG

(repetitive)

excavate

excavation

farm

farmer

garden

gardener

plant

scoop

shovel

unearth

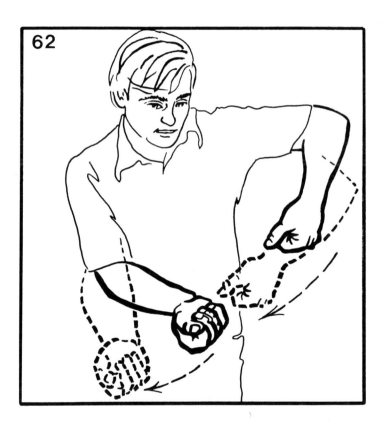

Left arm is raised at left side, elbow bent, with palm toward body. Fingers are curled (as though grasping handle of shovel). Right arm is extended to bring right hand about a foot from and a little lower than left hand. Right hand's fingers are curled, palm up (as though supporting handle of shovel). Both arms move in synchrony from left to right on a descending line. The movement is repeated three times.

63. **DISTANT**
(kinetic)

beyond
distance
far
remote
removed
yonder

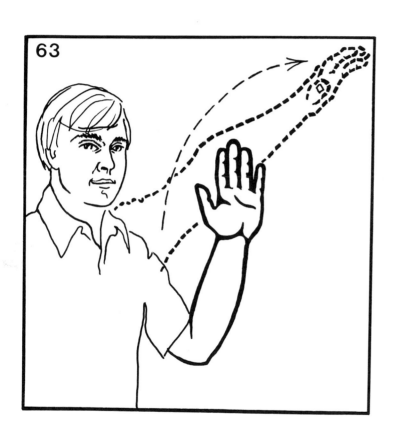

Left arm is extended forward, elbow bent, hand at shoulder height. Palm faces forward, fingers are extended upwards. Then hand is elevated until arm is straight with palm down and fingers pointing forward.

64. DIVE
(kinetic)

diver
diving
lifeguard
plunge
rescue
swim
swimming pool

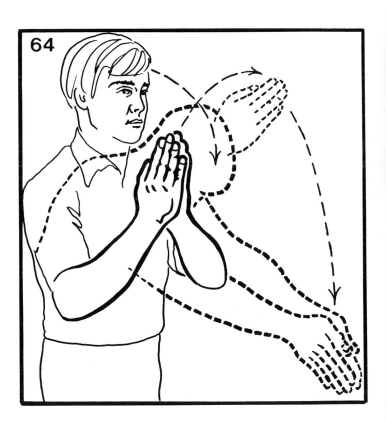

Both hands are joined, palms facing, at chin height. They are then raised to forehead height. Then head and arms are lowered until arms are fully extended downward, fingers pointing downward.

65. **DIVIDE**
(kinetic)

fraction [arithmetic]
half [equal]
part [not equal]
piece
room [of building]
section [microscope]

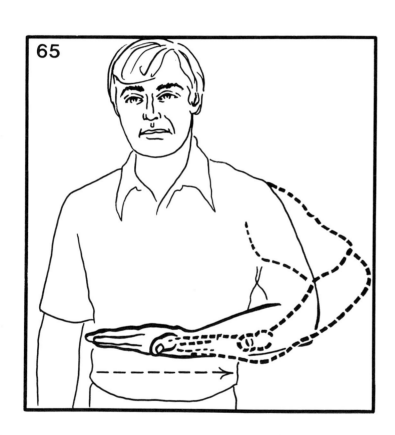

Left arm is extended horizontally across body to the right, touching body. Left hand is palm up. Fingers are extended and touching each other. Left arm is retracted to left, as though dividing the body into two segments. (A wide range of specific meanings within this concept can be accomplished by clarification, additions, or agglutinations.)

66. **DOMINATE**
(static)

control
controller
controlling
dictate
dictator
dictatorial
dominance
dominant
oppress
oppressive
oppressor
ruler
ruling

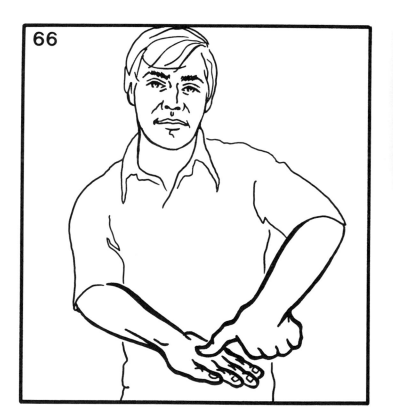

Right hand is extended, palm down, fingers straight at waist height. Left thumb (other fingers curled) is pressed forcefully on back of right hand, meaning "under my thumb."

67. **DOOR**
(kinetic)

entrance
entry
exit
gate
hinge

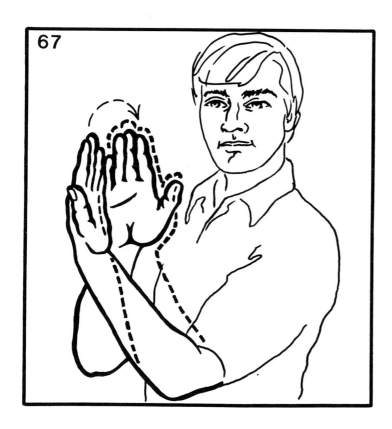

Right hand is elevated at right, palm forward. Elbow is bent. Left arm crosses right at wrist to enable left hand's little-finger edge to form hinge with right hand's little-finger edge. The left hand is rotated at the wrist to show door opening and shutting. "Open" or "closed" can be included in door signal. (See other hinged signals: SHUT; OPEN; READ.)

68. DOWN
(kinetic)

downward [opposite of up]

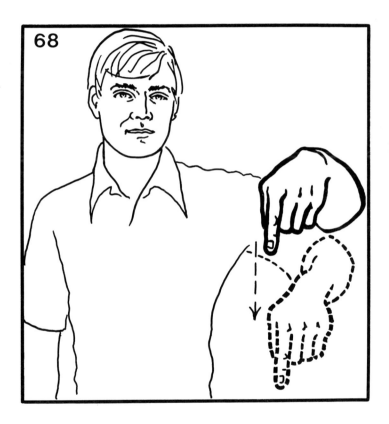

Left arm is extended to left of body, shoulder height, elbow bent at right angle. Forearm is forward, wrist flexed. Index finger is pointing downward; other fingers are curled. Index finger moves downward slowly to waist level.

69. **DRINK**
(static)

imbibe
liquid
partake
refreshment
swallow
thirsty

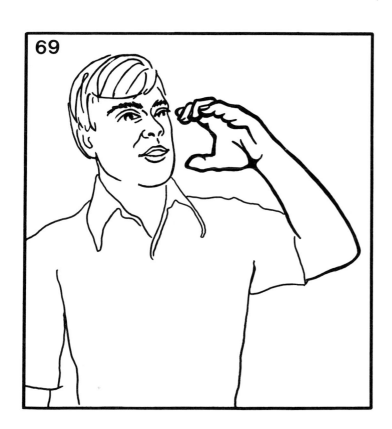

Left hand is raised face high. Thumb is a little below lips, about 1½ inches forward. Fingers are curled toward thumb, leaving space for shape of imaginary glass. Lips are slightly open; head is tilted back slightly.

70. **DRIVE**
(repetitive)

auto

automobile

car

drive

driver

excursion

journey

operate

ride

transportation

travel

trip

vehicle

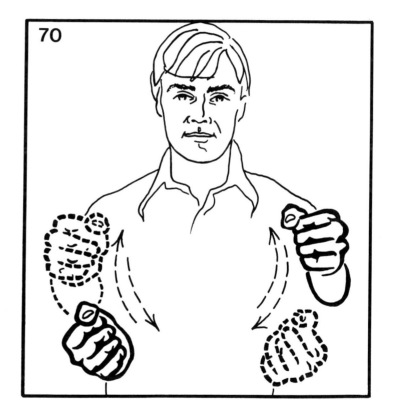

Both hands, palms facing and fingers curled, are extended forward at chest height, about 12 inches apart. They are then moved in opposition through an arc of about two inches, as if steadying the wheel of an automobile.

71. **EARTH**
(static)

country
farm
ground
land

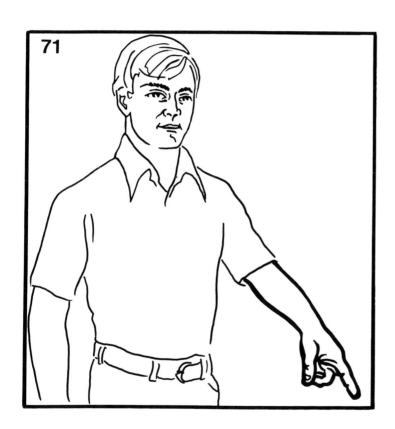

Left arm, index finger extended and other fingers folded, is extended forward and downward at 45 degree angle. Slanting index finger points to earth. (Contrast: DOWN, SOUTH, and HERE regarding angle.)

72. **EAST**
(static)

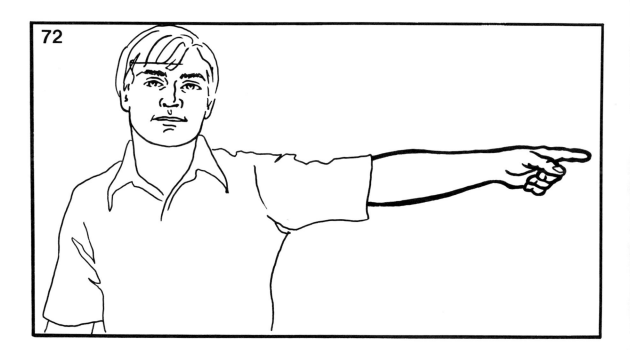

Left arm is extended full length to the left with index finger pointing. Other fingers are curled. (The signaler is like a map: "east" is left and "west" is right.) Compare with signal for MORNING, where left arm is similarly extended, but thumb and index finger meet in the SUN signal circle.

73. **EASY**
(kinetic)

effortless
painless
relaxed
serene
simple
(a) snap
untroubled

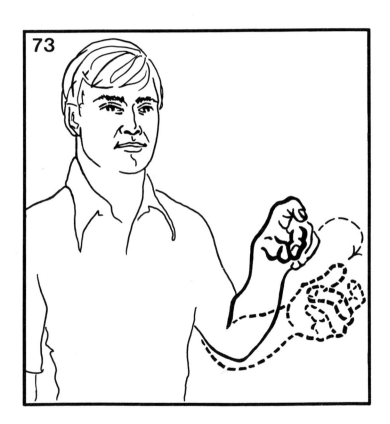

Left hand is extended forward at left, palm down, thumb and middle finger touching. Wrist is rotated to left. Middle finger snaps down thumb, making contact with thumb base (palmar surface) producing characteristic "snap" sound.

74. **EAT**

(repetitive)

feed

food

hungry

meal

nourish

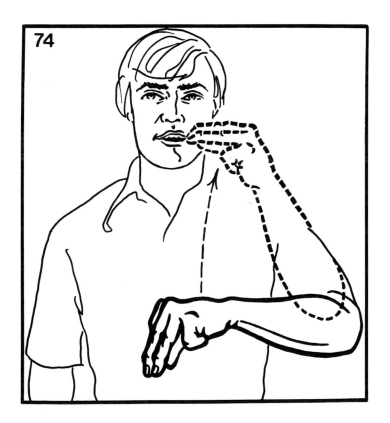

Left hand is extended in front of body, palm down. Thumb, index, and second fingertips are touching (as though holding a morsel of food). Then hand moves to mouth. Repeat three times.

75. **ENTER**
(kinetic)

arrive
begin
commence
embark
enroll
entrance
participate
penetrate
record
register

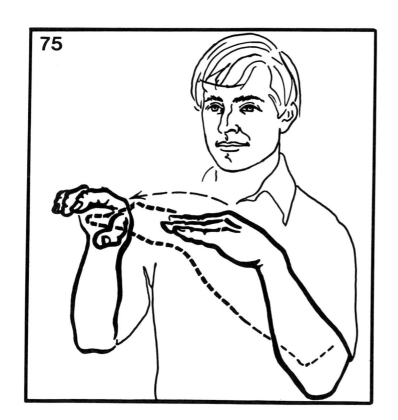

Right hand is elevated at right to shoulder height, palm down. Fingers are extended forward with thumb about one inch below and parallel to the index finger. Left hand is extended, palm down, hand flat, to the level of the opening between left index and thumb. Left hand moves to right hand until left fingers are inserted fully in opening. (May be executed with hands reversed.)

76. **ERASE**
(kinetic)

change

edit

editor

eliminate

eradicate

expunge

forget

re-do

remove

rub

wipe

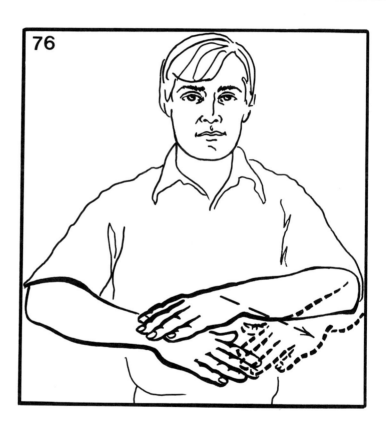

Right hand is extended in front of body, palm down, fingers extended. Left hand is similarly extended above right hand. Left hand moves back and forth along right hand from wrist to fingertips in an erasing motion.

77. **ESCAPE**
(kinetic)

abscond

avert

avoid

breakout

deliverance

elude

exit

flee

flight

getaway

leakage

outburst

seepage

skip

unbound

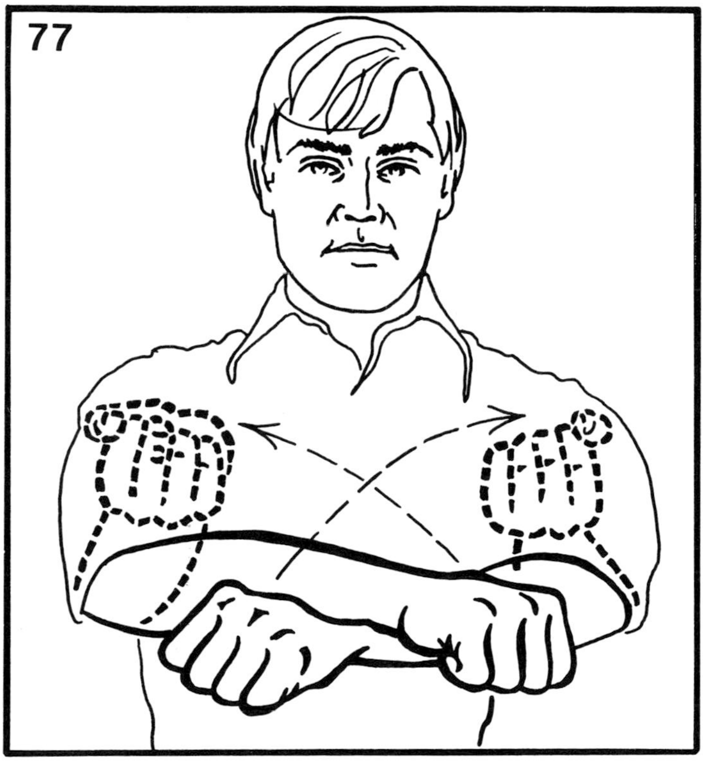

Both hands are fisted and crossed at wrists. The elbows are rotated laterally, bringing palms up. Wrists are a body width apart (breaking the wrist bonds).

78. **EXCHANGE**
(kinetic)

barter

interchange

reciprocate

sell

swap

switch

trade

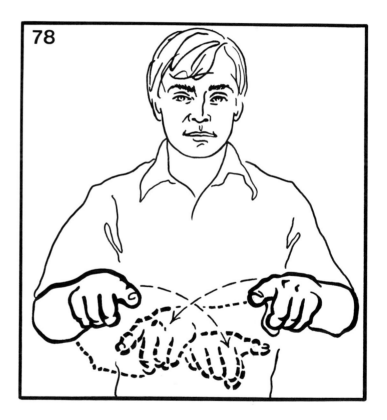

Both hands are extended forward, palms down, index fingers extended. Other fingers are curled. Then wrists are crossed, causing index fingers to EXCHANGE.

79. **FAST**
(kinetic)

brisk
expeditious
quick
rapid
speed
speedy
swift

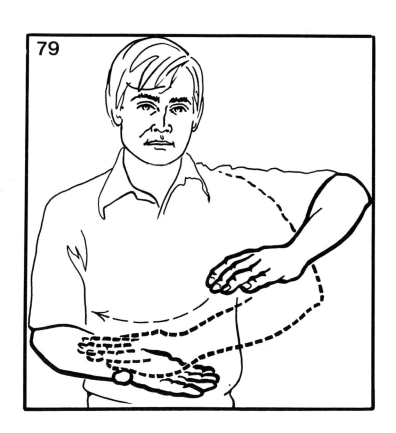

Right hand is extended in front of body center, palm up. Left arm is extended palm down at left, higher than right hand. Left hand is then moved downward and forward to right, contacting and moving quickly over right palm.

80. **FENCE**
(static)

barrier
corral
enclosure
limit
pen (up)
stockade
surround

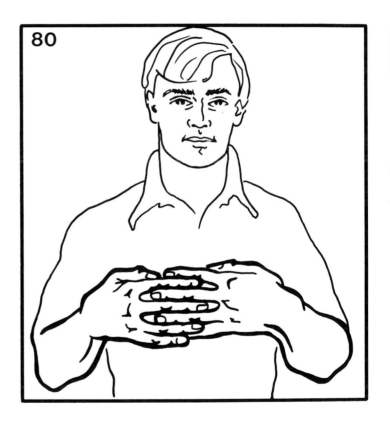

Both forearms are extended forward, elbows touching body sides. Wrists are flexed. Then fingers are interlaced (like rail fence).

81. **FIGHT**

(static)

argue

argument

bout

boxing

combat

dispute

feud

repulse

resist

scuffle

skirmish

spar

struggle

war

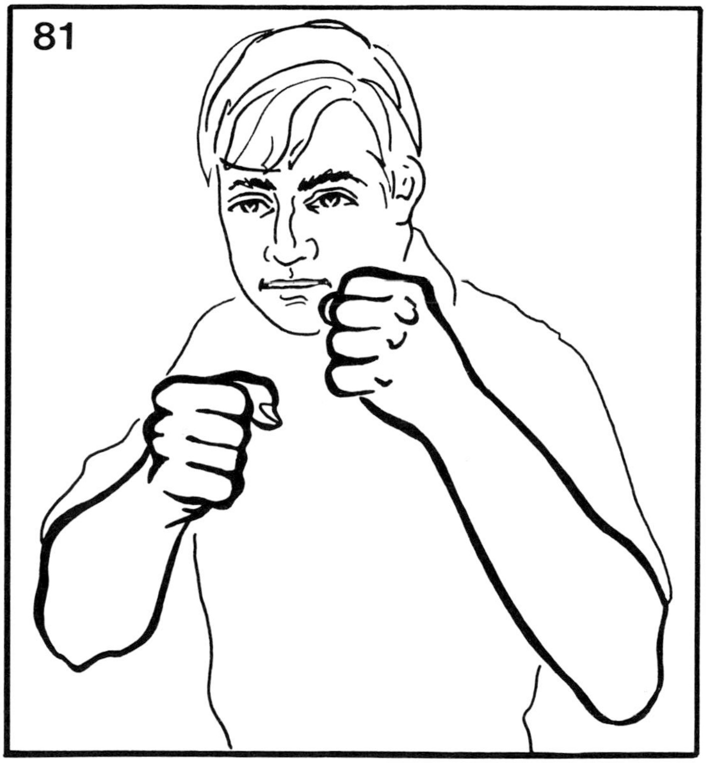

Both hands are fisted and extended forward in front of body. The left is at chin level; the right is slightly lower.

82. **FIRE**
(kinetic)

bake

blaze

brilliant

cook

flame

ignite

kindle

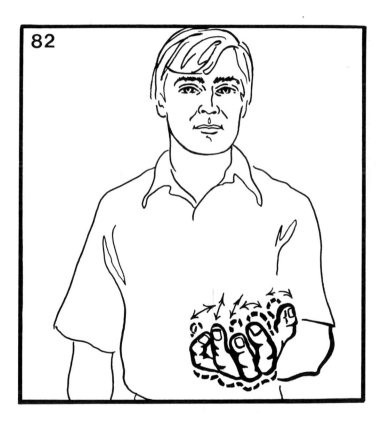

Left hand is extended forward to chest level, palm up, fingers curved upward and separated. Then fingers are randomly moved (to simulate the flickering of flames).

83. **FISH**
(kinetic)

fishing
grope
hook
search

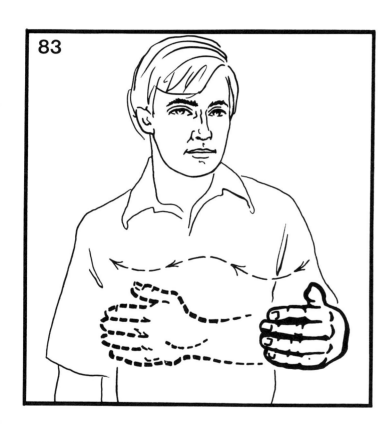

Left hand is extended, elbow bent, at body left. Thumb is up. All fingers are touching and pointing to right. Then the hand moves across body from left to right, alternating forward and backward on a curved trail (simulating the wagging lateral swimming movement of a fish tail).

84. **FLAG**
(repetitive)

banner

emblem

ensign

pennant

standard

streamer

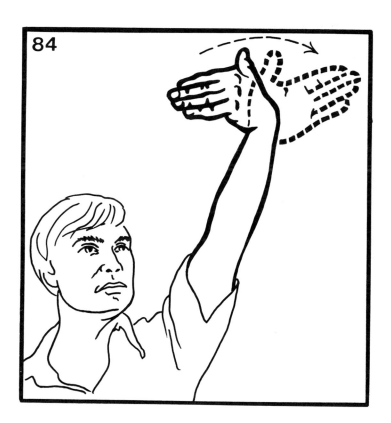

The left arm is elevated at left side of body. Wrist is flexed, fingers touching, palm facing right. Wrist is rotated 180 degrees until fingers point left. They are then rotated again to the right, then back to the left (three "waves" in all) simulating the flag waving on its pole.

85. **FLAT**

(repetitive)

cornbread   flatten   pancake

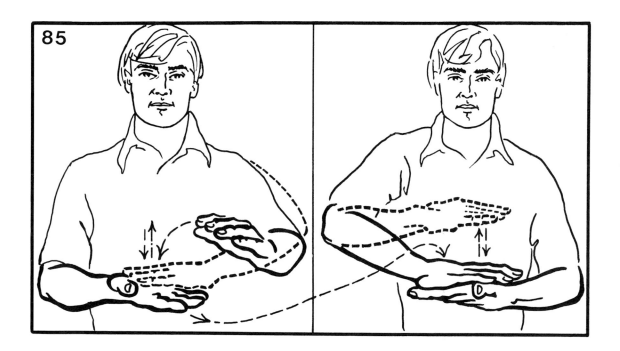

The right hand is held in front of body, palm up. The left hand, palm down, is pressed three times on right palm. Hands are then reversed, right down, left up, and three pressure pats are repeated.

86. **FLY**
(repetitive)

airplane　　　　flight　　　　jet　　　　plane　　　　travel

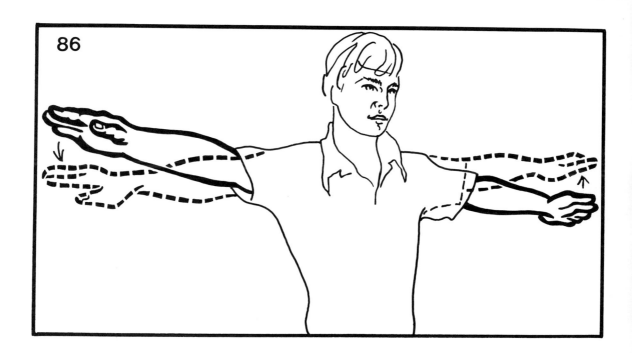

Both arms are entended laterally, elbows and wrists slightly bent. Body leans slightly left, then slightly right. Left arm moves down, right arm moves up; then reverse with left up and right down. Finally, repeat first position for a total of three movements.

87. **FLY**
(repetitive)

bird
chicken
egg
turkey

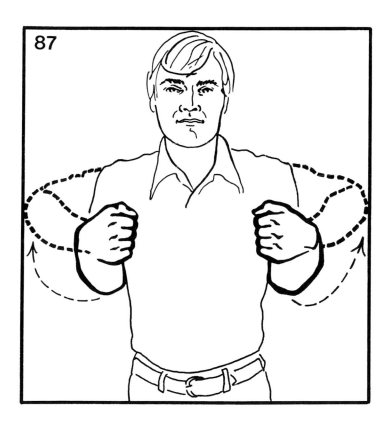

The fisted hands are placed on the chest as far apart as possible with elbows bent. Elbows are raised and lowered simultaneously three times to simulate action of wings in flight.

88. **FRIEND**

(static)

colleague
companion
comrade
confidant
friendship
intimate
pal

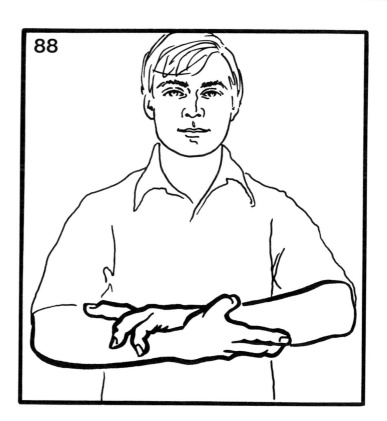

The two hands are joined in front of body, left hand clasping right lower forearm (above). Right hand similarly clasps left lower forearm (below).

89. **FUTURE**
(kinetic)

ahead
anterior
earlier
forward
front
sooner
vanguard

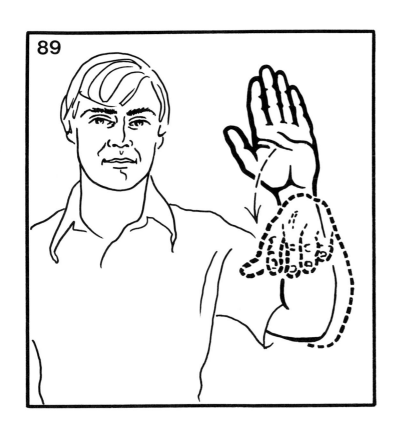

Left arm is elevated with elbow bent and then wrist is flexed, palm down, so that extended fingers point forward.

90. **GENTLY**

(kinetic)

calmly

considerate

kindly

lightly

softly

tenderly

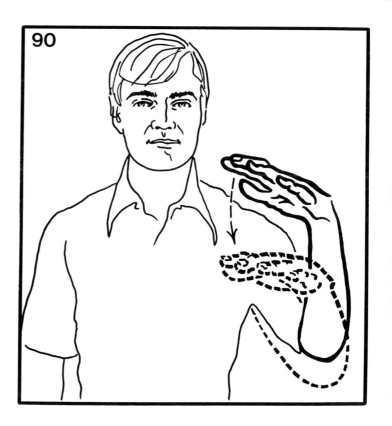

Left arm is extended forward at left, wrist flexed and at about shoulder height, palm forward. Then the arm as a unit moves down, up, and down again. Arm moves slowly and without force. (Contrast with BOUNCE, where arm is lower and movement is fast and forceful.)

91. **GET**
(kinetic)

achieve

acquire

attain

become

gain

obtain

procure

receive

take

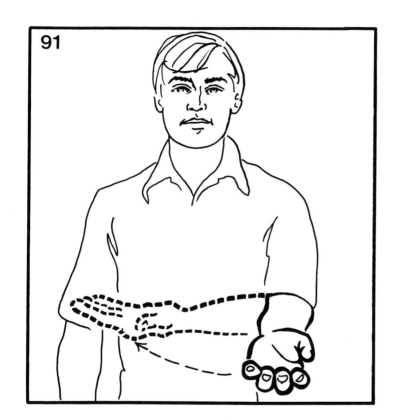

Left arm is extended forward, palm up, at waist level. Hand is cupped slightly. Elbow is rotated in a 90 degree horizontal arc to bring arm across body, touching it. GIVE/GET may be regarded as one concept, with the arc of the arm moving in the appropriate direction for delivery in each specific instance. This signal can also be used to express "want," since this idea really means "you give me."

92. **GIVE**
(kinetic)

award
bequeath
bestow
contribute
dispense
distribute

(repetitive)

donate
endow
offer
present

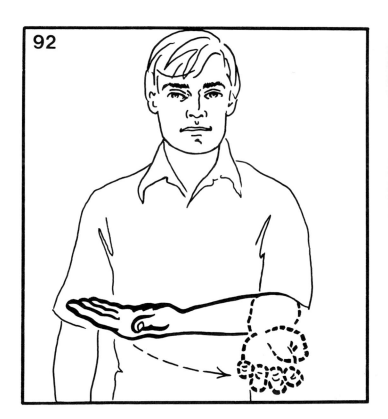

Left arm, palm up, is held across body, touching it. Then elbow is rotated through 90 degree horizontal arc, bringing arm forward toward viewer. (This is the reverse of GET.)

93. **GLASSES**
(static)

glasses [eye glasses]
monocle [circle one eye only]
spectacles

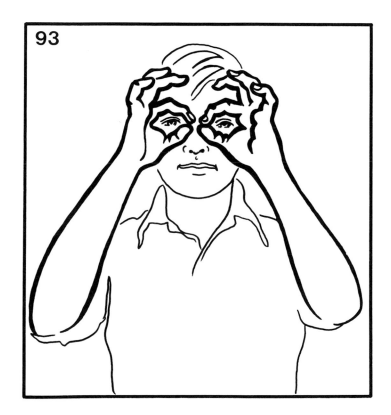

Both hands are elevated to eye level. Thumb and index touch to make a circle around each eye.

94. **GOODBYE**
(kinetic)

bye
farewell
parting
separation

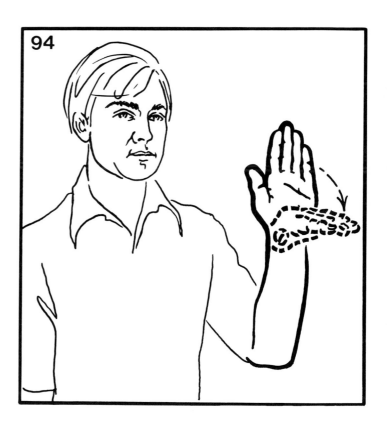

Left hand, palm forward, is elevated at left of body, shoulder height. Wrist is flexed, dropping hand forward, palm down. Repeat three times. (Compare with HELLO, OATH, DEPART, and PAINT for critical differences.)

95. **GRASS**
(kinetic)

grow

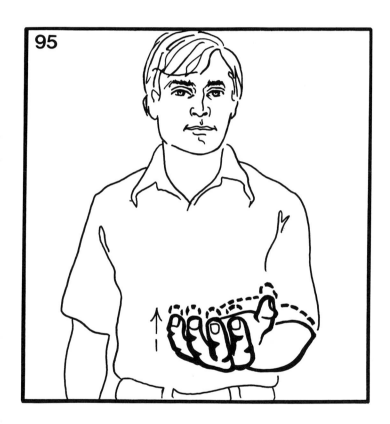

Left hand is extended forward, palm up and fingers up, at left of body. Fingers are then straightened slightly, giving minimal upward movement. (This movement meaning "growing." Compare agglutinations: Flower, Green, Pasture, and Vegetable.)

96. **HAND**
(static)

manually

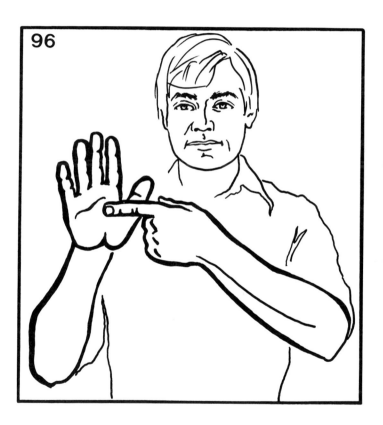

Right hand is elevated at right, palm forward, at shoulder height. Left index finger (others folded) points to right hand. (All body parts are indicated by index pointing; all visible objects can be indicated by index pointing with two exceptions: (1) two fingers (index plus second) are always used for human beings, and (2) the thumb is always used for self.)

97. **HANG**
(static)

affix
append
attach
dangle
suspend

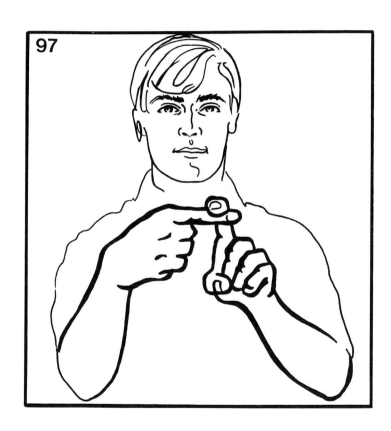

Right hand is elevated to chest level, palm toward body. Index finger is extended toward left; other fingers are folded. Left index finger is hooked over right index; other left fingers are folded.

98. HARD
(kinetic)

metal

rock

stone

unyielding

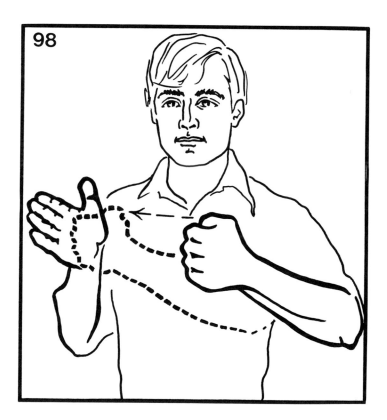

Right hand is extended at right, palm facing left. Thumb is up; fingers are touching. Left hand is fisted, then driven forcefully against the *unyielding* right palm. (This should be done silently. If a smacking noise is produced, the viewer is misled and interprets the signal as "hit." Clarify by contrasting with SOFT.)

99. **HEAR**
(static)

attend

heed

listen

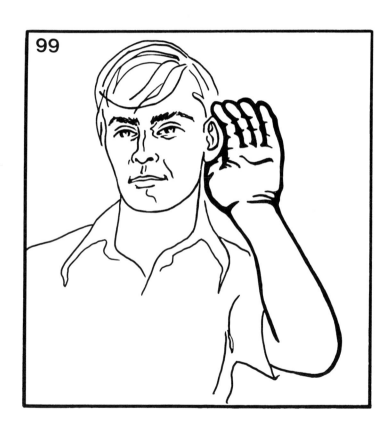

Left hand, palm forward, is cupped behind left ear. Compare with DEAF (ear covered); "can't hear you" (hand cupped in front of ear); "won't hear" (HEAR + REJECT); compare LOUD (hand slapping ear three times).

100. **HEART**
(static)

emotion
feel
feeling
love

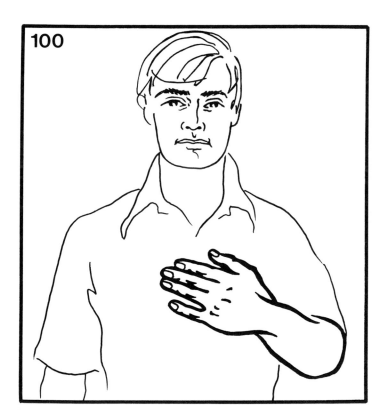

Palm of either hand is laid on chest at heart.

101. **HEAVEN**
(kinetic)

afterlife
ceremonial
ceremony
god
minister
paradise
religion
religious
spiritual

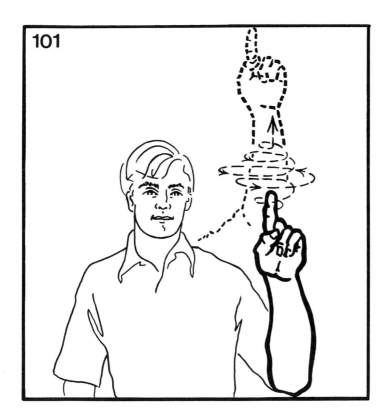

Left hand is elevated at left side of body, shoulder high. Index finger is extended, other fingers are folded, palm faces forward. Left index traces an upward spiral until arm is fully extended. (This signal was misinterpreted by early white settlers in America as "medicine," but it actually means "spiritual." Illustration 129 best conveys the contemporary concept of medicine. The administration of herbs by the wise-woman was always accompanied by spiritual ceremonial by the shaman, who was a combination minister-priest and psychiatrist.)

102. **HEAVY**
(kinetic)

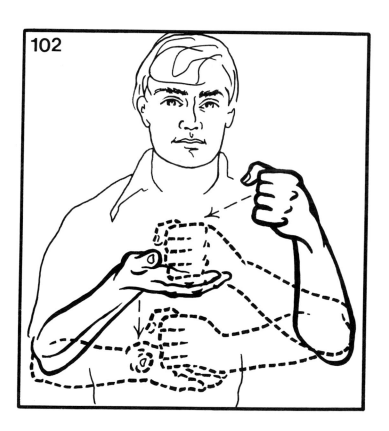

Right hand, palm up, is extended forward. Left fist is placed (like a weight) on left palm, which quickly moves downward. Compare LIGHTWEIGHT. (Each may be used to clarify the other.)

103. **HELLO**
(static)

greeting
Hi
peace

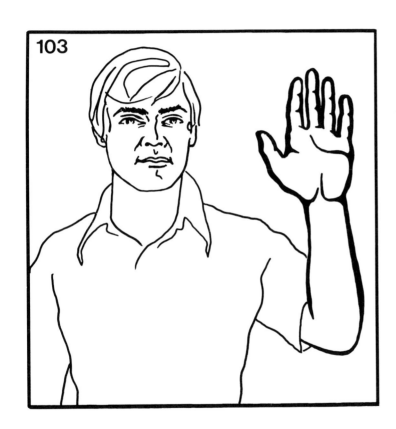

The left hand is elevated at left, head high, palm forward. (The signal says "I have no weapon"; consequently, it means "I come in peace.")

104. HELP
(static)

aid

alleviate

assist

assistance

remedy

rescue

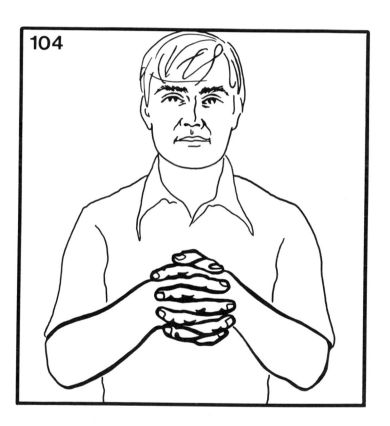

Hands are extended forward in front of body, fingers tightly laced and tensed. Laced hands are directed toward person from whom help is sought. Facial expression of distress can enhance transmission.

105. **HERE**
(kinetic)

location

place

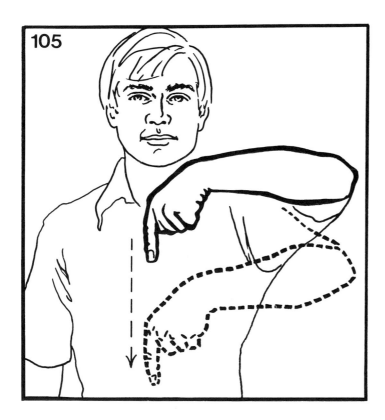

Left arm is raised, shoulder high, elbow bent, hand *centered* on body. Index finger is extended; other fingers are curled. Left index moves downward about three inches. (Compare with EARTH, where finger is slanted and lower; DOWN, which is executed at right side with lengthier movement; SOUTH, which is like HERE, but lower with no movement; NOW, which is an agglutination of HERE + TIME.)

106. **HIDE**
(static)

conceal
defend
disguise
refuge
sanctuary
seclude

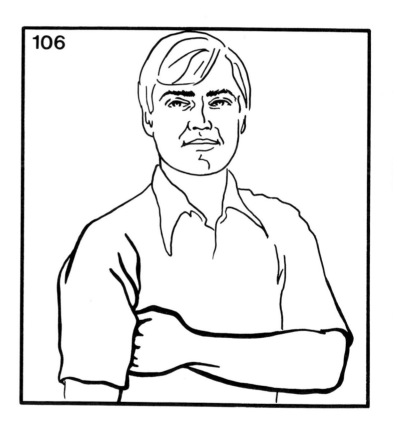

The left hand, palm to body and fingers extended, is placed in right armpit.

107. **HIGH**

(static)

lofty
superior
tall

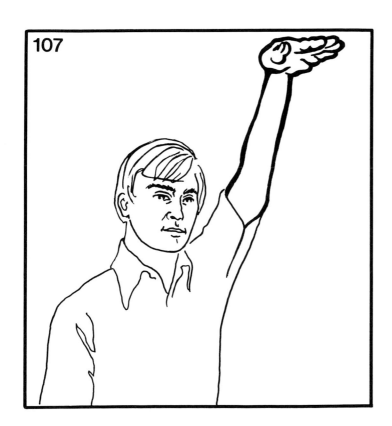

Left arm is elevated at left side as high as possible. Wrist is flexed so downward palm indicates height. (Contrast with UP; compare with DEEP.)

108. **HOLD**
(static)

bag
control
grip
keep

(kinetic)

catch
clasp
clutch
grab
grasp
hinder
nab
seize
snatch

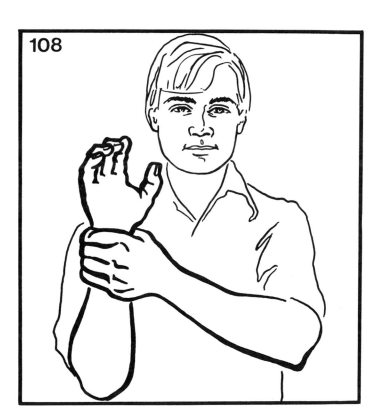

108

Right hand is elevated at right side, shoulder high; elbow is flexed, palm forward. Left hand grasps right wrist. (Speed and force of execution can convey subtle differences in meaning.)

109. **HOT**
(kinetic)

heat
heated
sweat

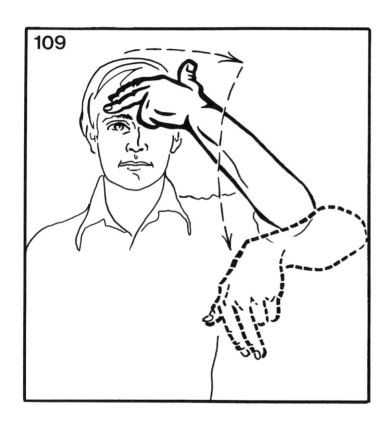

Left hand is raised to forehead, palm toward head. The index and second finger are extended; the others are folded. Paired fingers are moved across forehead from right to left. Then they are lowered to left side with a slight shake as though wiping moisture from forehead and then shaking moisture from fingers.

110. **HUNGRY**
(kinetic)

appetite
hunger
ravenous
starved
starving

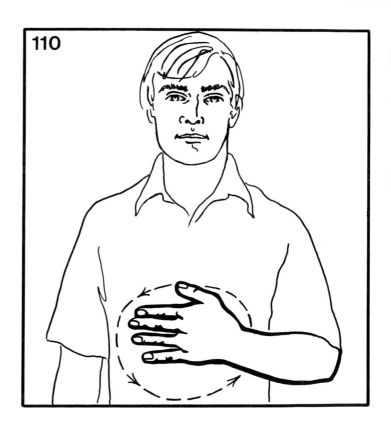

The flat left hand, palm to body, rubs the abdomen in a circular motion.

111. **I**
(static)

me
myself

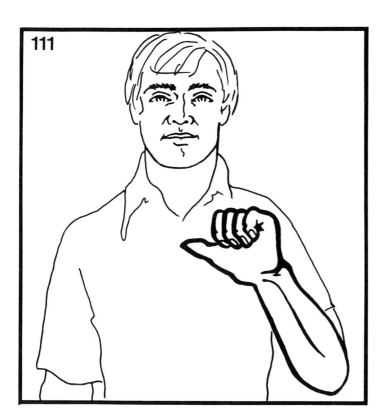

Left thumb points at signaler's chest, touching it. Other fingers are folded.

112. **IN**
(kinetic)

inside

into

inward

within

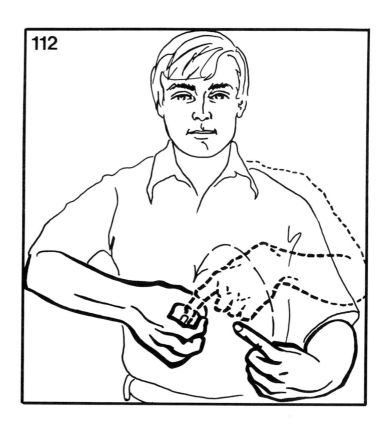

The right hand is centered on body, just above waist height. Index and thumb are up and touching in circle. Other fingers echo circle. Left hand is extended toward right hand but slightly lower. Index finger is pointing; other fingers are folded. Left hand then is brought up and to the right-hand circle, and left index is pointed downward while entering right circle. (Compare reverse actions in signal for OUT.)

113. **JUSTICE**
(kinetic)

balanced
equitable
fair
honest
impartial
law
legal
trial [in court]

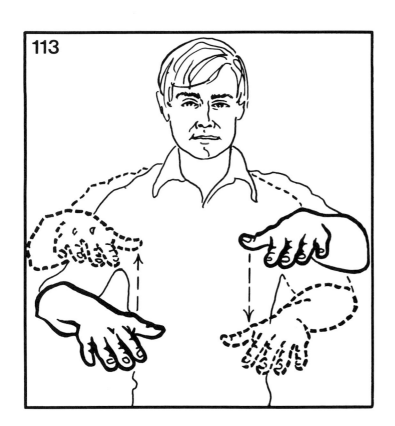

Arms are extended forward, palms down, with fingers spread. Left hand is at chest level and right hand is at waist level. Then they move in synchrony, left down, right up, and reverse, gradually reducing difference in height until they are of equal height. (They are showing the scales of justice.)

114. **KNOW**
(kinetic)

ascertain

discover

learn

notice

perceive

recognize

scholarly

student

teacher

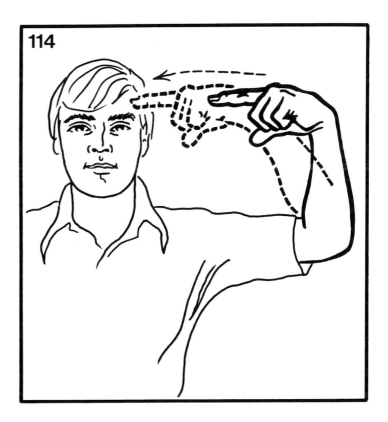

Left hand is elevated to head height and about six inches to the left of head. Index finger is pointing to left temple (other fingers folded). Hand moves toward head until index is touching temple. (Action means: "go into brain.")

115. **LAUGH**
(repetitive)

amuse
funny
joke
jolly
mirth
pleasant

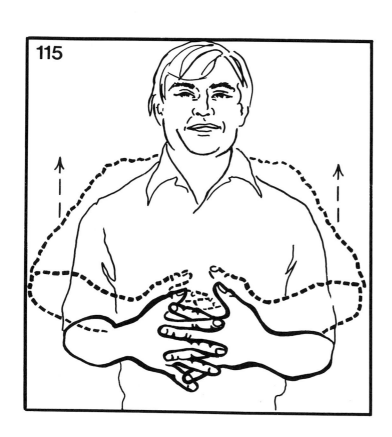

Fingers of both hands are interlaced on abdomen, palms to body. Then arms and shoulders move up and down three times in laughing action.

116. LEFT
(static)

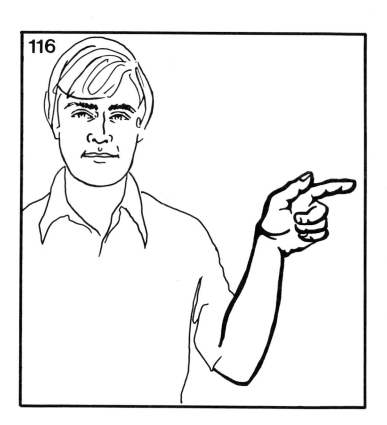

Left index finger points to left. (Contrast EAST, where left arm is fully extended; MORNING, where left arm is fully extended and thumb and index touch to make SUN.)

117. **LIE**

(static)

deceit

deceive

deception

dishonorable

dishonest

false

liar

perjury

untrustworthy

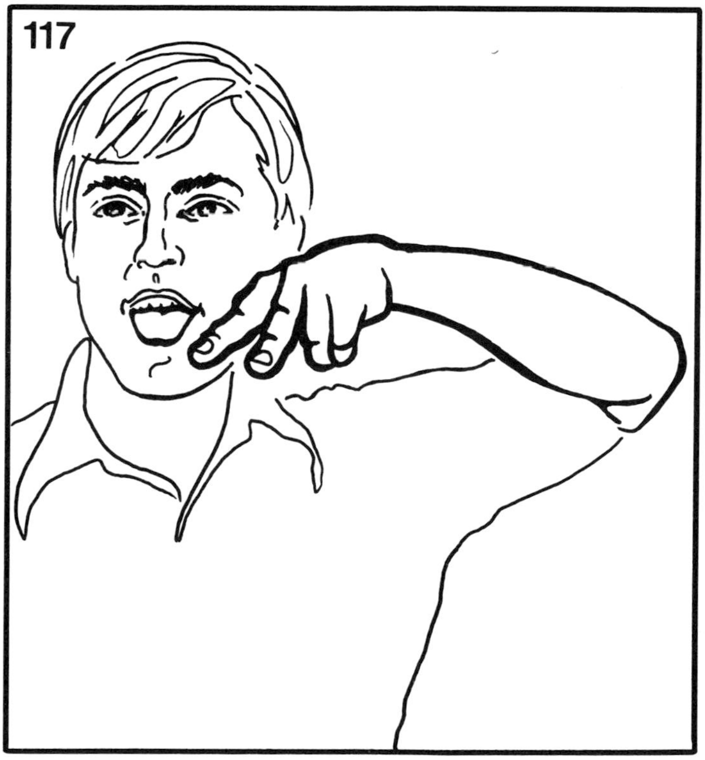

Mouth is slightly open, showing tip of slightly protruding tongue. Left hand is placed beside mouth, palm down. Index and second finger point forward and are separated; other fingers are folded. (The gesture means "two-tongued" or "speaks with a forked tongue.")

118. **LIGHTWEIGHT**
(kinetic)

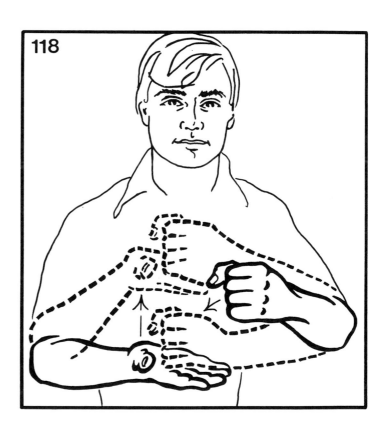

Right hand, palm up, is extended forward. Left fist is placed on left palm, which quickly moves upward. (Compare HEAVY. Each may be used as a clarifier of the other: HEAVY = LIGHTWEIGHT + NO or HEAVY + AGREE; LIGHTWEIGHT = HEAVY + NO or LIGHTWEIGHT + AGREE.)

119. **LINK**

(static)

alliance
association
coalition
compact
confederation
function
join
linked
loop
pact
partner
splice
treaty
union

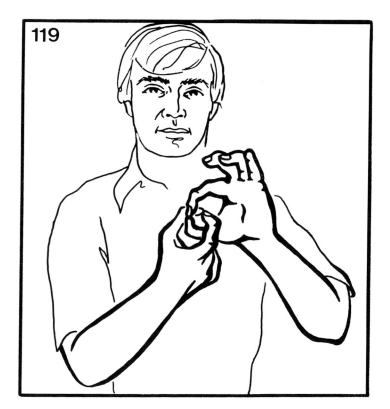

Index finger and thumb of right hand touch in circle. Index and thumb of left hand are brought together inside right circle (making two linked circles).

120. **LITTLE**
(kinetic)

diminutive

meager

short

small

trifle

trivial

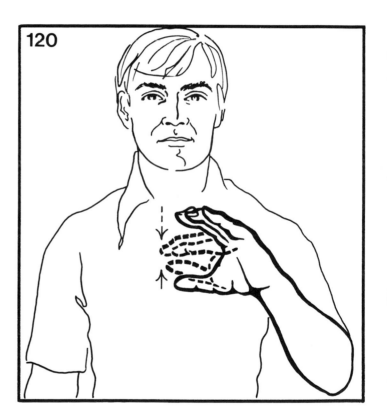

Left hand is held chest high, palm down, fingers all touching. Thumb is lowered as far as possible. Then thumb and finger-group slowly approach each other but without quite touching.

121. **LOCK**
(kinetic)

bolt
fasten
fastening
key
latch
locked
safe
secure

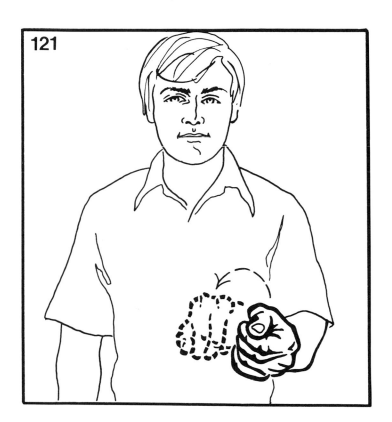

Left hand is extended, fingers curled. Thumb is against index finger (as though holding a key). Then wrist is rotated in action of turning key.

122. **LOOK**
(static)

contemplate
examine
eye
glance
notice
observe
regard
see
view
watch

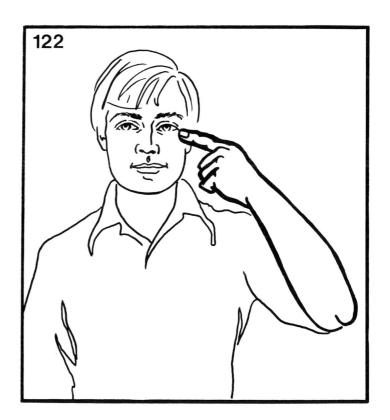

Left index finger points to outer corner of left eye (other fingers folded).

123. **LOUD**

(repetitive)

blaring
boisterous
deafening
noisy

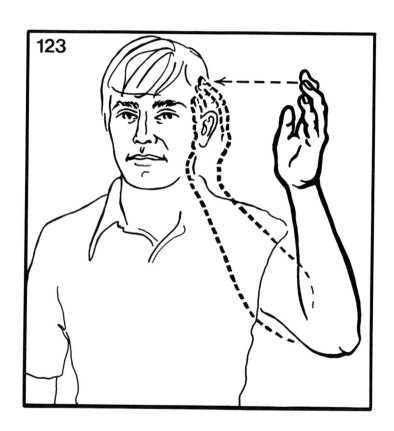

Left hand is elevated at left of body, head high. Palm faces head, then moves to cover ear. Repeat three times. ("Noise" is hitting ear.)

124. **MAN**
(static)

male

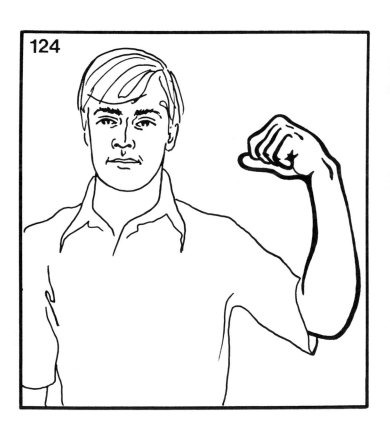

Left arm is elevated at left, elbow flexed. Wrist is flexed, hand fisted, all tensed (to increase bicep). (Compare "strong" (agglutination) where right index finger points to bicep.)

125. **MANICURE**
(repetitive)

file

nails

nail file

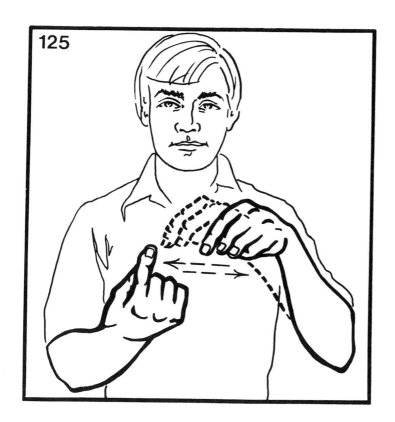

Right index finger is elevated vertically with other fingers folded. Left hand, palm down, is placed to the left and above right hand with thumb against finger pads (as though holding the nail file). The left hand is then moved right, left, right, as though stroking right index nail with file.

126. **MANY**
(kinetic)

abundance

numerous

several

variety

various

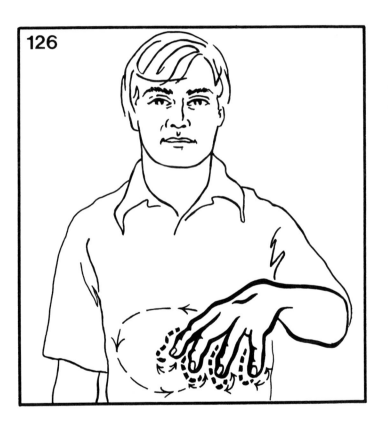

Left hand is placed in front of body, palm down. Fingers are flexed downward and spread. Hand moves in horizontal circle, with fingers fluttering.

127. **MASK**
(static)

camouflage
disguise
obscure
screen
shield

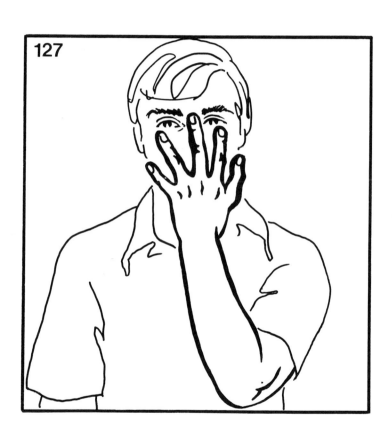

Left hand, fingers spread, is placed over face, palm to face, so that middle finger is over nose. Index finger is at left corner of left eye. Fourth finger is at right corner of right eye. Thumb is on left side of jaw. Little finger is on right side of jaw. (Hand forms a mask over face.)

128. **MAYBE**

(repetitive)

debatable
erratic
fluctuating
hesitant
indefinite
uncertain
undecided
unpredictable
unsure

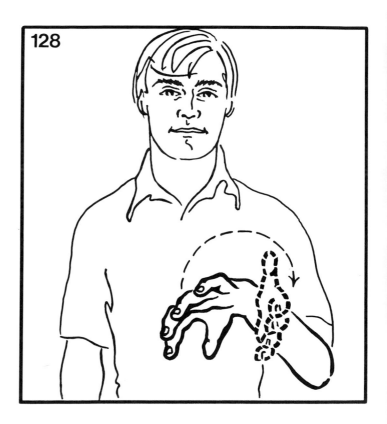

Left hand is extended vertically, thumb up. Fingers are parted. Wrist is rotated until thumb points down and little finger is up; then action is reversed until little finger is up and thumb is down (three rotations).

129. **MEDICINE**
(kinetic)

drug
medication
pill
remedy
salve
shot
tonic

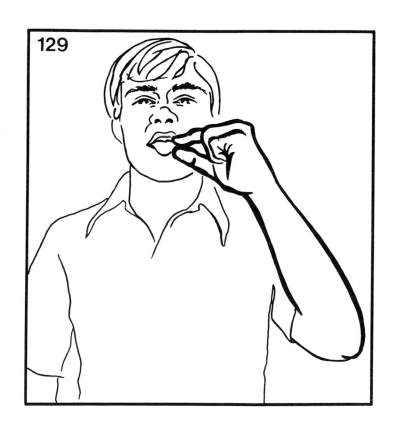

The left index finger and thumb touch and are brought to the open mouth, where the tongue is slightly protruded (to receive the pill). (If necessary, the signal can be clarified by adding the signal for DRINK.)

130. **MEET**
(kinetic)

about

adjoin

confront

encounter

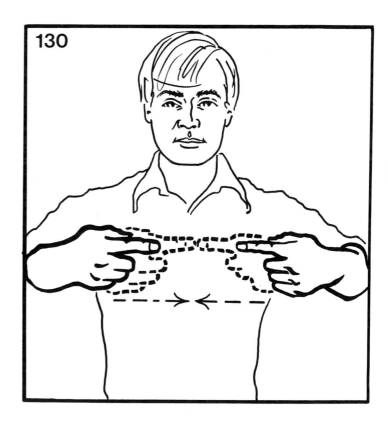

Both hands are elevated chest high, palms facing body. Index fingers are extended toward each other; other fingers are folded. The hands are brought in synchrony toward each other until index fingertips meet at centerline.

131. **MEND**
(kinetic)

correct
cure
heal
improve
restore

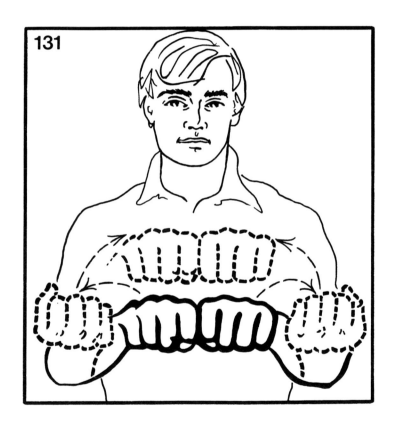

Both fists, back up, are placed in front of body. Thumbs and index fingers are touching. Wrists are rotated to separate fists with a jerk, showing BREAK. Then wrists are rotated slowly in reverse until the hands touch again (put back together).

132. **MIRROR**
(kinetic)

handsome

image

looking glass

pretty

reflected

vain
(repetitive)

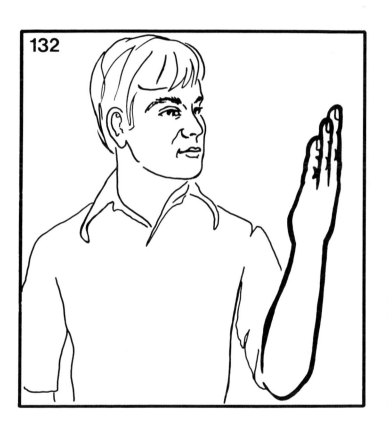

The left hand is held at left side of body. Elbow is flexed, palm toward body. Face is directed toward palm (as to a mirror). The head is turned from side to side (for complete view).

133. **MOCK**

(static)

deride

ridicule

scorn

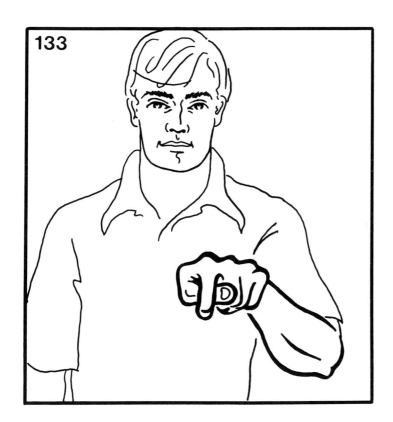

Left hand is extended forward, palm down and fisted, with thumb protruding between index and middle finger.

134. **MONEY**
(repetitive)

assets

cash

cost

currency

funds

pay

precious

revenue

riches

specie

value

valuable

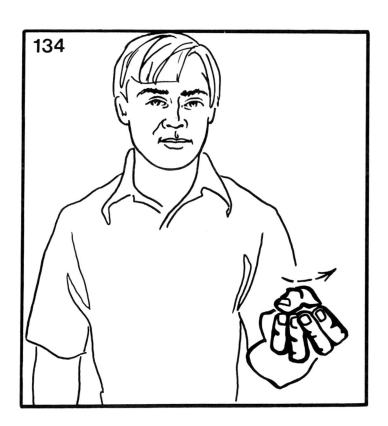

The left hand is extended at left side, palm up. The thumb pad contacts finger pads successively, starting with little finger. Contact of four pads is repeated three times.

135. **MONTH**
(static)

moon

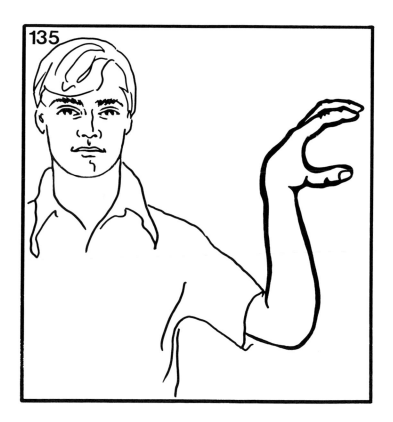

Left hand is elevated at head height at left of body, palm facing left, all fingers curved. Thumb is extended so that line from index finger tip to thumb tip forms the sickle shape of the new moon. (TIME clarifies MONTH if necessary).

136. **MORE**
(kinetic)

additional
extra
further
reserved
supplementary

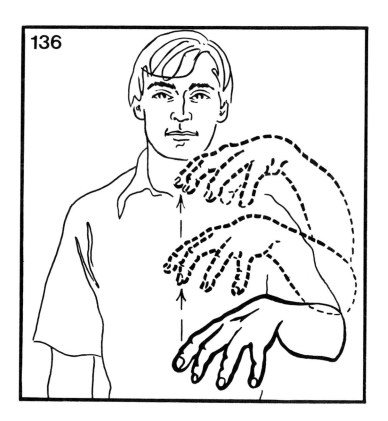

Left hand is placed in front of body, palm down, fingers flexed downward and separated. Hand then moves upward in three stages, halting at each and giving small downward thrust (piling something up).

137. **MORNING**
(static)

dawn daylight forenoon
daybreak early sunrise

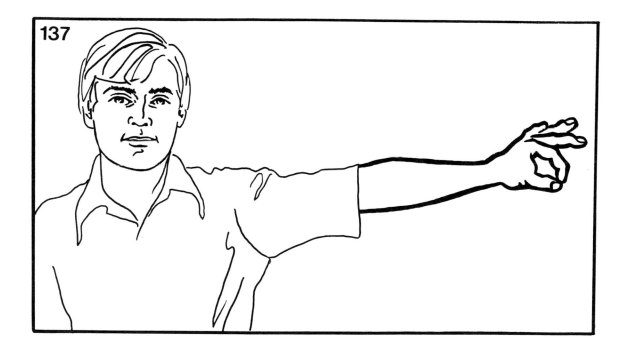

Left arm is fully extended to the left. Palm is down, thumb and index finger are joined at tips. Other fingers are folded. (Compare with WEST, DAY, SUN, OK.)

138. **MOUNTAIN**
(kinetic)

elevation

hill

peak

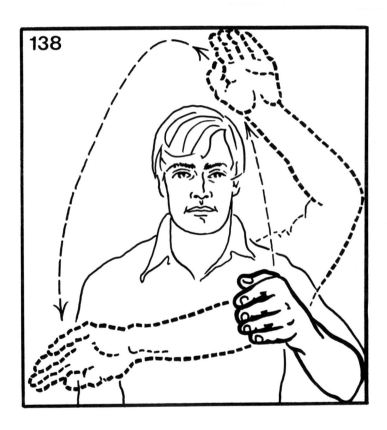

The left hand is extended forward at left of body, palm facing right. Fingers are extended and touching, thumb folded to palm. Hand is raised to arm length tracing a slanted line upward to centerline. It then descends on slant to the right. (The resulting pattern represents the mountain slope rising to a peak.) Where appropriate, agglutination HIGH + EARTH may be used.

139. **MULTIPLY**
(static)

extend

increase

times [arithmetic]

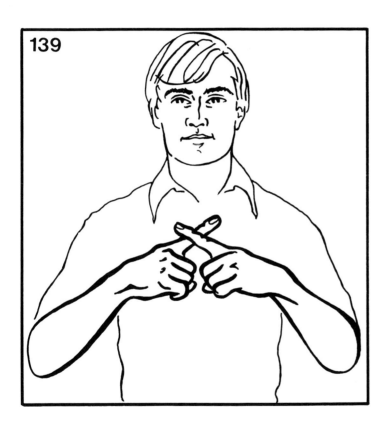

Index fingers are crossed at 45 degree angle in front of body. Other fingers are folded.

140. **MUSIC**

beat [time]
conduct [orchestra]
harmony
melody
play [musical instrument]
rhythm
score [music]
tempo
tune

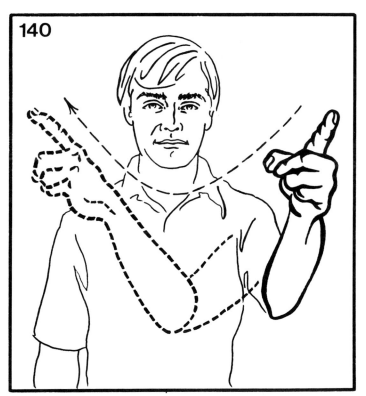

Left arm is extended forward at left side of body, shoulder height. Index finger is pointing forward; other fingers are folded. Left hand is swung through downward arc to the right. Repeat arc to the left, then to the right. (This signal is used in many agglutinations to identify various actions related to music. For example, singing is MUSIC + TALK.)

141. **MUSTACHE**
(kinetic)

whiskers

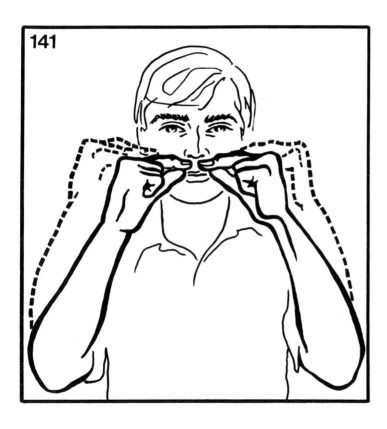

Right hand, index finger and thumb touching (other fingers folded), is placed with tips under right nostril. Left hand is similarly at left nostril. Then both hands move outward synchronously, tracing the mustache along the upper lip.

142. **NAPKIN**
(kinetic)

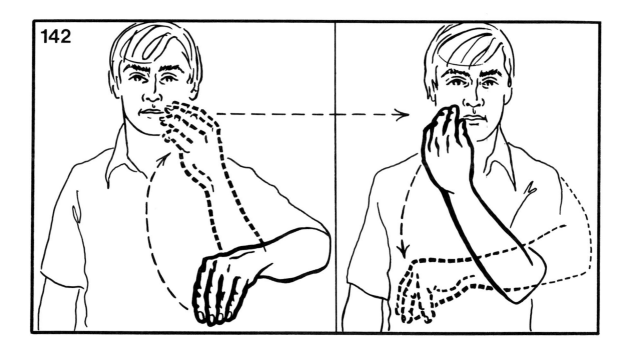

Left hand, palm down, is extended. Thumb pad meets pads of other fingers at lap level. Then fingers are raised to mouth with wrist rotation. The five finger pads pat the right corner of the mouth, then the left corner. Hand is then lowered.

143. **NAUGHTY**
(kinetic)

disobedient
disrespectful
misbehaving

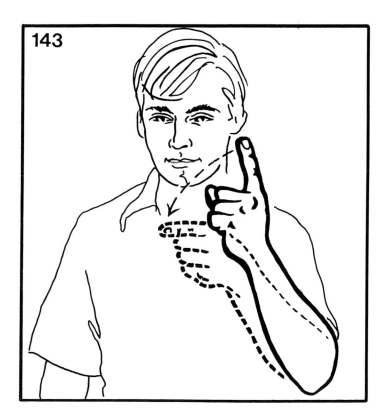

Left arm is elevated to face level, palm toward body. Index finger is extended with other fingers folded. Wrist is rotated to lower index in a short arc three times.

144. **NEAR**

(kinetic)

almost

alongside

close

hereabout

imminent

impending

nearby

proximate

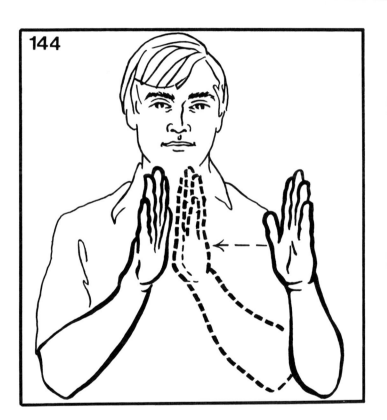

Flat right hand is placed in front of body at chest height, palm toward left. Left hand is elevated at left in same fashion, palm facing right. Left hand is then moved slowly toward right until palms are about an inch apart.

145. **NO**
(static)

denial
disagree
negative
refusal
refuse

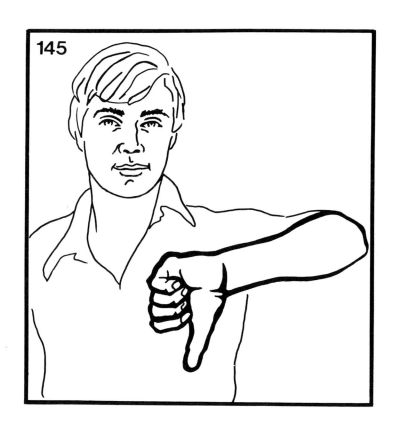

Left arm is extended at left side. The four fingers are folded, but the thumb is extended strongly downward.

146. **NOON**
(static)

meridian

midday

zenith

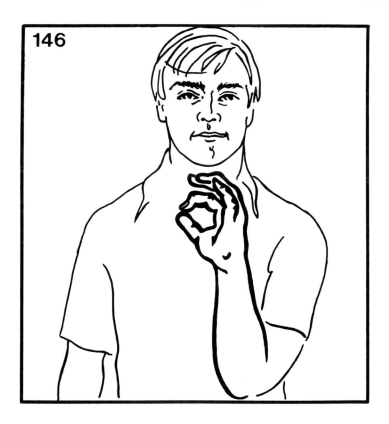

Left forearm is placed vertically at body midline, palm facing right, thumb meeting index finger in a circle. Other fingers are extended as for SUN.

147. **NORTH**
(static)

arctic
northern
polar

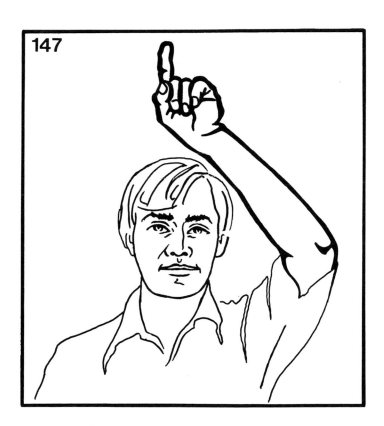

Left arm is elevated, hand over head, palm forward. Index is vertical, pointing up. Other fingers are folded.

148. **NOTHING**
(static)

zero

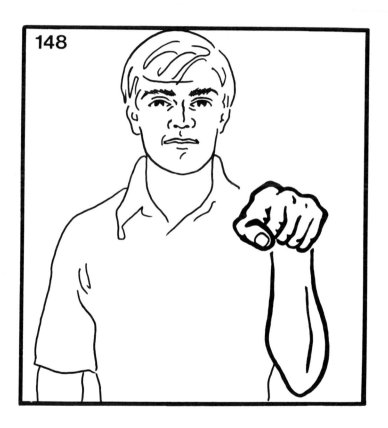

Left fist is held forward at shoulder height, palm down. (This is the arithmetical signal for ZERO, consequently used also as NOTHING.)

149. **NUMBERS**

(kinetic)

accounting   calculate   computer   numerals

accounts   calculator   counting

arithmetic   compute   digits

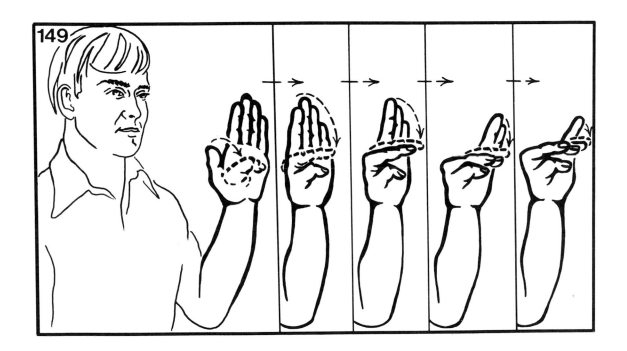

Flat left hand is elevated at left of body, palm forward. Thumb is folded and returned. Next, index is folded and returned. Then each finger is successively folded and returned. Total effect is rapid ripple of motion across fingers of hand.

150. **OATH**

(static)

affirm
agree
attest
avow
covenant
guarantee
pledge
promise
swear
vow

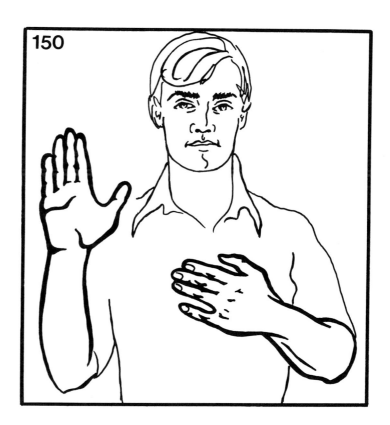

Flat left hand is elevated at left of body, palm front. Right hand is placed on chest over heart.

151. **OBJECT**
(static)

show

thing

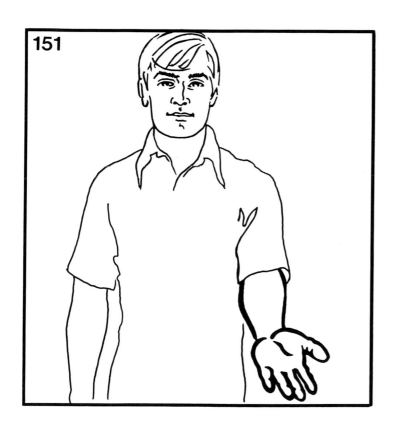

The open, flat left hand is extended forward, palm up (as though holding or showing object).

152. **OK**

(kinetic)

admire

approve

concede

correct

fine

good

healthy

right

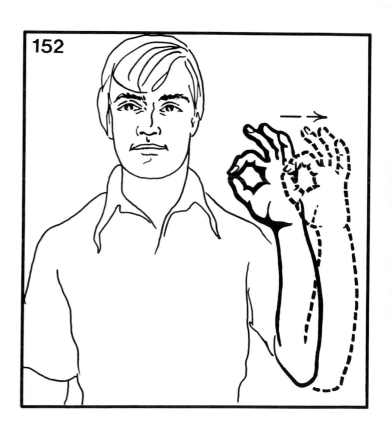

Left arm is elevated vertically at left of body, palm forward, at shoulder height. Thumb and index fingertips touch in circle; other fingers are fanned. Hand is given a slight forward jerk. (Compare SUN, DAY, and NOON for differences.)

153. **ON**
(kinetic)

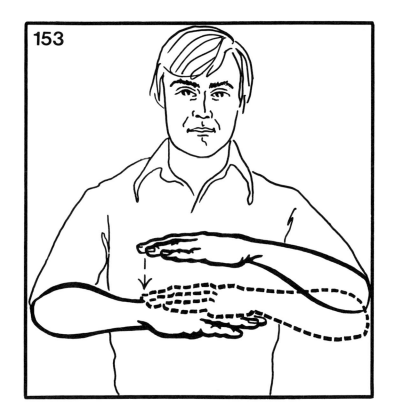

Right arm is extended in front of body, palm down. Fingers are extended toward left. Left hand is placed, palm down, above right hand. It is then lowered until left hand rests on right hand. (Compare UNDER.)

154. **OPEN**

(kinetic)

accessible
coverless
exposed
uncovered

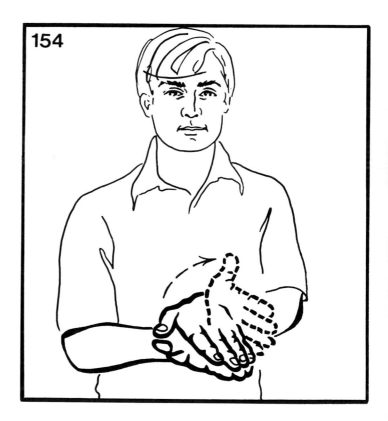

154

Right hand is extended forward, palm up. Left hand, palm down, is placed on top of right palm. Left hand is then lifted and rotated to the left while little fingers remain in contact (as a hinge). (Compare other hinged signals: SHUT, READ, DOOR. Both READ and DOOR can be "opened" and "closed" as part of their own signals.)

155. **OUT**
(kinetic)

exterior
external
outdoors
outer
outside
outward

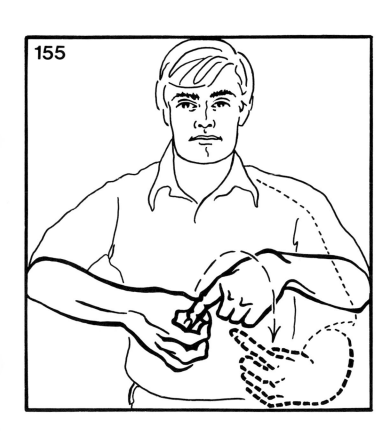

Right arm is extended to center of body, palm toward body. Thumb and index meet; other fingers repeat curve of index. Left arm is extended to center, palm down, index extended; other fingers are folded and index is placed into circle formed by right thumb and index. Then with left wrist rotation, left index is moved out. (Compare IN.)

156. **PAIN**
(static)

ache

agony

distress

hurt

ill

nauseated

sick

sore

suffer

throb

unhealthy

unwell

upset

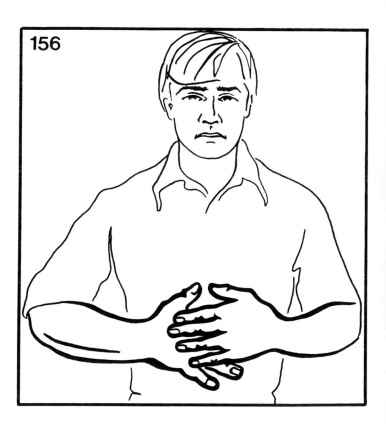

Right palm is pressed to abdomen. Left palm covers fingers of right and presses inward. (Signal is clarified if torso leans forward.)

157. **PAINT**
(kinetic)

coating
decorate
renew

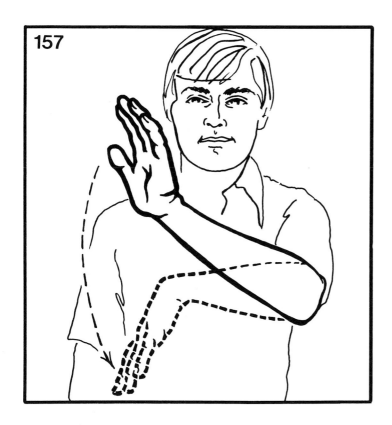

Left arm is extended across body to right, palm down, fingers pointing right. Wrist is flexed and hand moves downward. Repeat flection three times. Hand simulates paint brush. (Compare with GOODBYE, FLAG, and SPREAD.)

158. **PAST**
(static)

after

ago

back

behind

bygone

dorsum

elapsed

later

posterior

rear

retreat

reverse

spine

withdraw

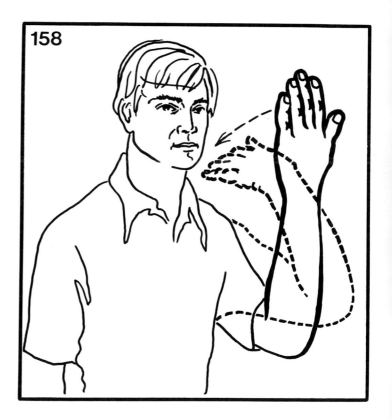

The left arm is elevated, elbow bent and wrist flexed, so that fingers of flat left hand (back of hand up) are pointing over the shoulder to space behind the signaler.

159. **PEEL**

(repetitive)

banana
skin
strip

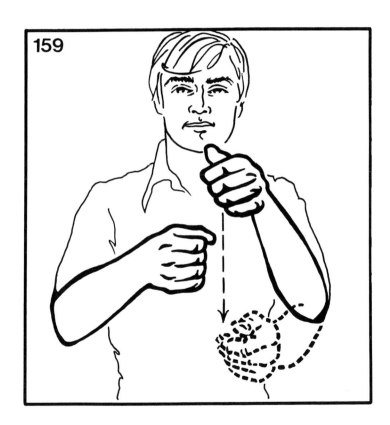

Right hand is extended in front of chest, palm toward body. Thumb and fingers are curled (as around a banana). Left hand, palm toward body, is placed above and to the left of right hand with index and thumb touching. Left hand moves downward past right hand (peeling). Repeat peeling movement three times.

160. **PERSON**
(static)

being

human

people

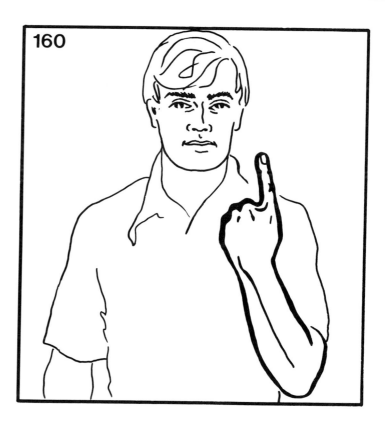

Left forearm is extended upward at body side with elbow touching body and palm toward shoulder. Index finger is erect; other fingers are folded. (Originally, the signal for ANIMAL was executed by putting right hand beneath PERSON signal, meaning "the upright animal." The signal can be clarified this way, or by signaling ANIMAL + WALK + 2 + LEGS.)

161. **PIANO**
(repetitive)

composer
concert
musician

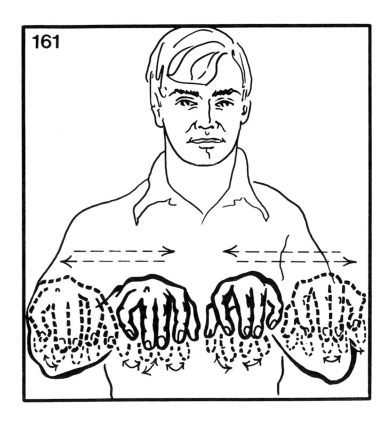

Both hands are positioned before body about one foot apart, palms down, fingers flexed. Then hands move to left and right with fingers moving randomly and the wrist flexed randomly. (Compare with TYPEWRITE, where movement is very limited.)

162. **PLEASE**
(static)

appeal

ask

beg

implore

plead

request

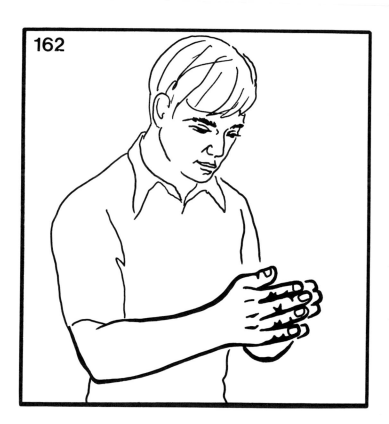

162

Both hands are placed in front of body, palms touching, fingers pointing forward. Head is bowed forward slightly. (Compare PRAY, where fingers point up.)

163. **POMPOUS**
(kinetic)

blustering
egotistic
ostentatious
overbearing
pretentious
snobbish
strut
swaggering

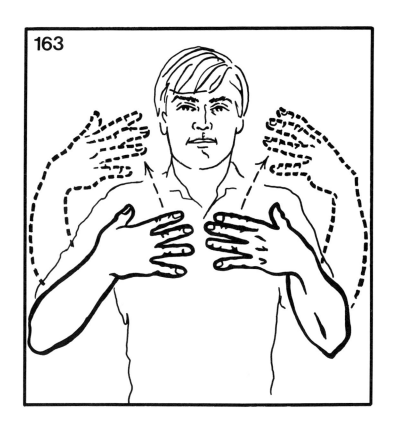

Hands are placed palms on chest, fingers spread. Hands are moved synchronously out and upwards (as if one "sticks his chest out."). (Compare with BREATHE.)

164. **PORK**
(static)

bacon

ham

meat

pig

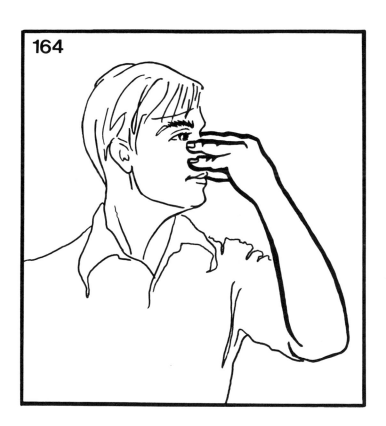

Left hand is placed over nose, with fingers flexed and tips touching face, surrounding and enlarging nose. (Clarifiers: ANIMAL; EAT.)

165. **POSSESS**
(kinetic)

mine
owner
ownership
possession
possessor

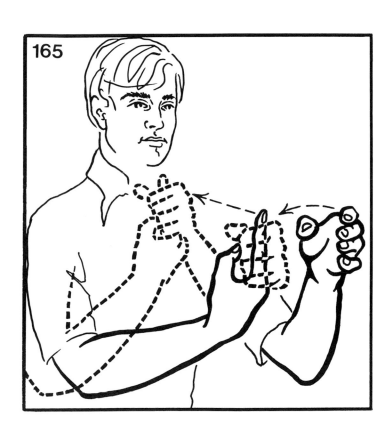

Right index finger is held upright in front of body, palm toward body. Left hand is advanced toward finger and grasps it, pulling finger toward body.

166. **POUR**
(kinetic)

decant
decanter
drain
flow
pitcher

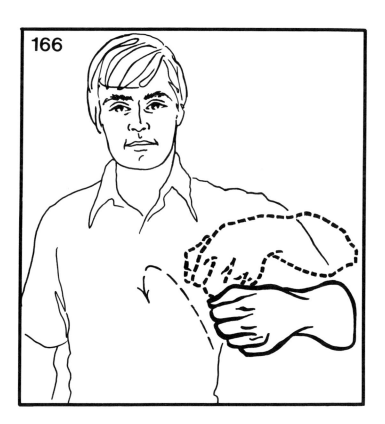

Left arm is extended at right, elbow flexed and elevated. Fingers and thumb are folded (gripping handle of pitcher). Forearm is lifted a little and wrist rotated to right (as though pouring from pitcher).

167. **PRAY**
(static)

implore
petition
plead
request

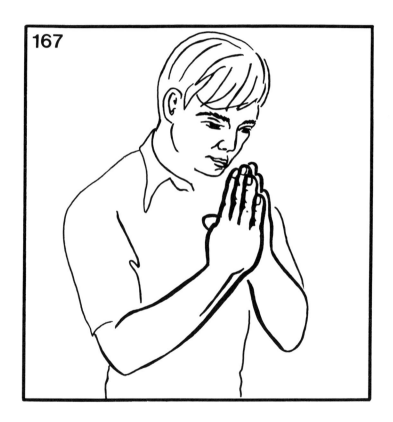

Both hands are placed in front of body, palms touching, fingers pointing up. (Compare PLEASE, where fingers point forward.)

168. **PROTECT**

(static)

cover

guard

insurance

insure

protector

safe

secure

shield

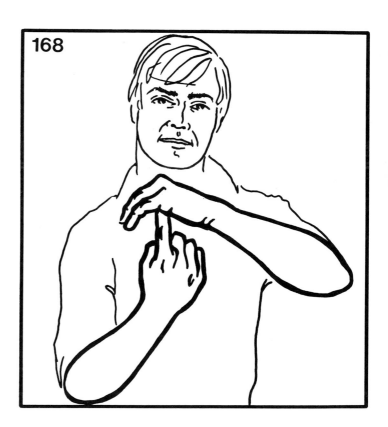

Right hand is elevated forward, elbow bent, wrist flexed, palm toward signaler. Index finger is extended upward and other fingers are folded. Left hand is placed on tip of right index, palm down, fingers pointing right; hand is slightly cupped.

169 **PUSH**
(kinetic)

bump
drive
force
jostle
motivate
move
nudge
press
prod
propel
shove
thrust
urge

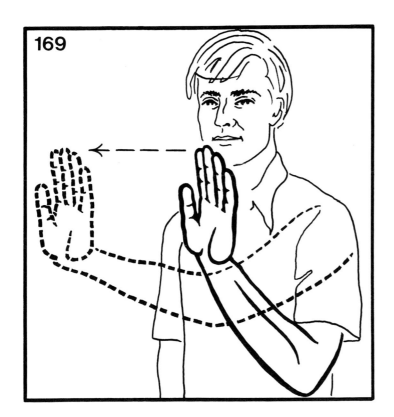

Left forearm is elevated at left of body, palm forward, hand flat. Entire forearm and hand are moved forcefully forward about one foot.

170. **PUZZLED**

(repetitive)

baffled

bewildered

confused

dilemma

doubt

mystified

perplexed

unclear

unintelligible

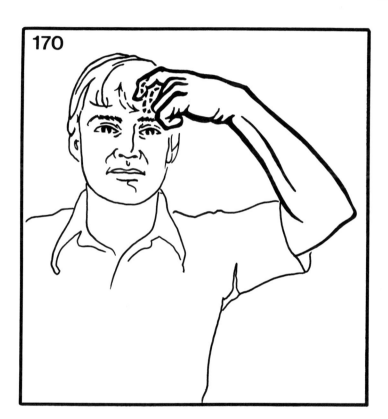

Left hand is elevated to forehead. Index finger is slightly curled; other fingers are folded. The index at hairline moves downward in slant line on forehead (making a scratching motion) three times. (The signal says "hunting in brain" for lost item.)

171. **QUESTION**
(repetitive)

ask
challenge
dispute
doubt
interrogate
issue
moot
query
quiz

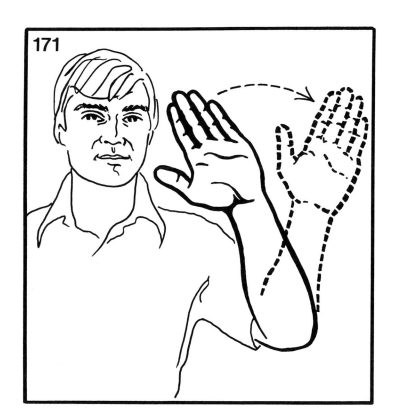

Flat left hand is elevated, palm forward, above shoulder. Forearm moves left, right, then left in sequence with small additional wrist movement.

172. **QUIET**
(static)

calm

dormant

hush

low [noise]

mute

noiseless

serene

silence

silent

still

tranquil

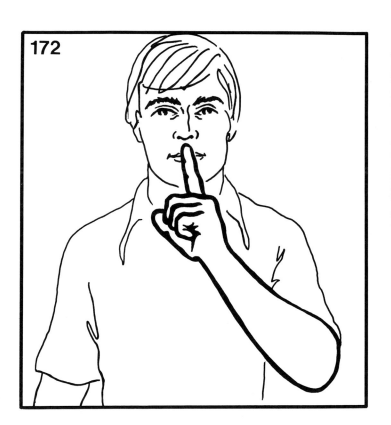

Left hand, index elevated, other fingers folded, is raised towards mouth, with index touching lips.

173. **RAIN**
(kinetic)

deluge
downpour
drizzle
precipitation
shower
sprinkle
torrent
wet

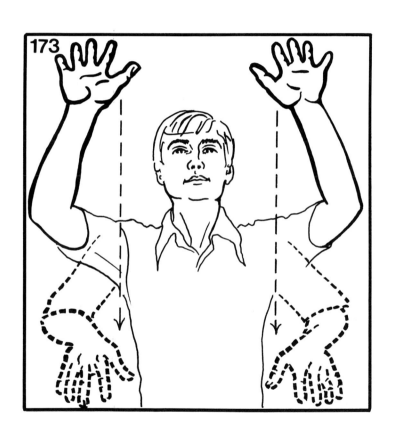

Arms are elevated at sides, hands above head. Palms are forward, fingers spread. Hands are slowly lowered to waist level; movement is accompanied by slight finger flutterings. (Compare SNOW.)

174. **READ**
(static)

album

book

print

publication

scan

study

volume

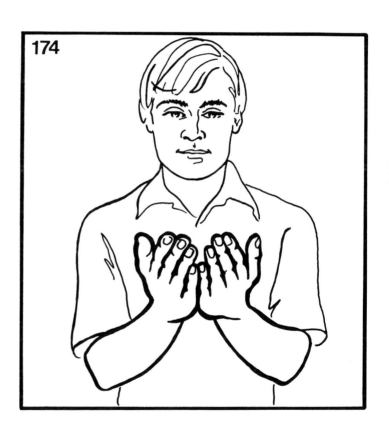

Hands are placed in front of body midline at chest height with edges of little fingers touching (hinged), palm up at 45 degree slant. The eyes should be directed toward the palms.

175. **REJECT**
(kinetic)

abandon
discharge
divorce
forsake
relinquish
subtract
undesirable
worthless

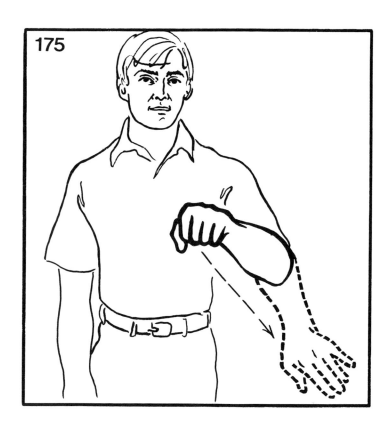

175

The closed left fist is extended at elbow level, then moves forward and slightly to the left as the fingers open with a downward thrust (throwing away the abandoned or rejected object or idea).

176. **RELATION**
(kinetic)

brother
cousin
kin
kinship
relation [by blood]
relative [by blood]
sister

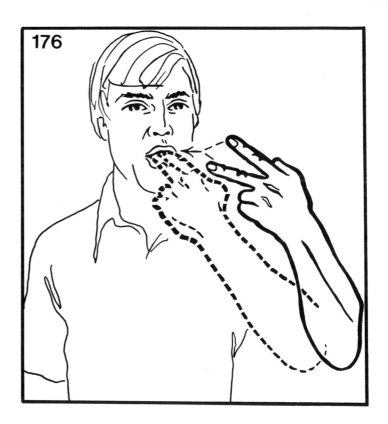

Left hand, index and second finger extended (others folded) is brought to mouth; the two fingers touch and enter lips together. (Signal says "two sucked same place.")

177. **RIDE**

(repetitive)

horse
horseback
rider
riding

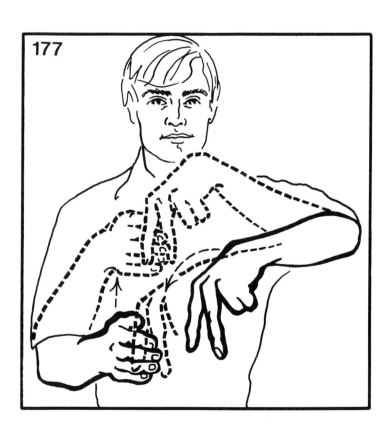

The right hand is extended before body at centerline. Fingers are extended forward and touching, palm facing left. Left hand has index and second finger extended and parted (other fingers are folded). Then fork of parted fingers of left hand is placed over the upper edge of right index finger (rider mounting horse). Then joined hands are moved up and down three times.

178. **RIGHT**
(static)

right [opposite of left]

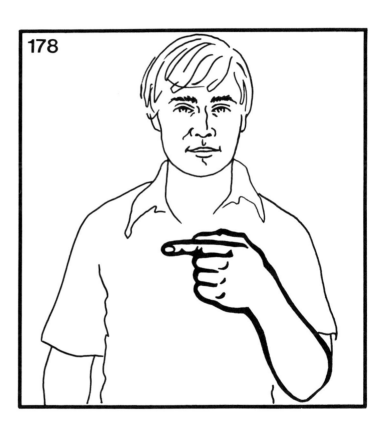

Left arm is extended to right across body. Index is pointing right; other fingers are folded. (Compare AFTERNOON; WEST.)

179. **RING**
(static)

husband [man]
married
marry
wife [woman]

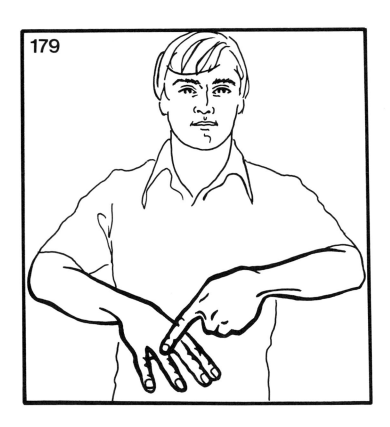

Either index finger points to ring position on other hand's fourth finger.

180. **ROUND**

(kinetic)

    a) circular

    b) globular

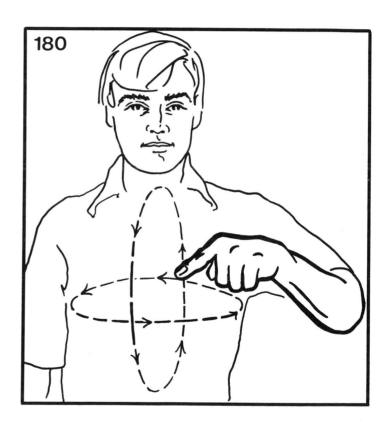

a) For circular, left index finger traces flat horizontal circle in front of body.

b) For globular, add intersecting vertical circle.

181. **SCISSORS**
(kinetic)

clip

cut

shears

snip

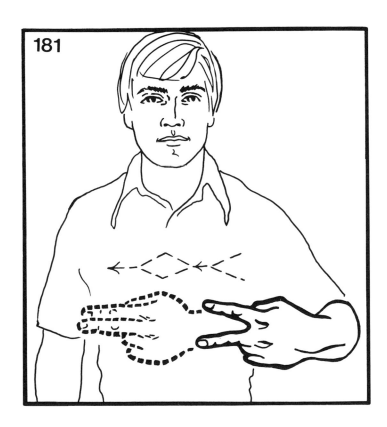

Left hand has index and second finger extended toward right, palm toward body; other fingers are folded. Two extended fingers touch and part (scissors' blade action) as hand slowly advances from left to right across body.

182. **SECRET**
(kinetic)

connivance

conspiracy

conspirator

conspiracy

plot

secretive

spy

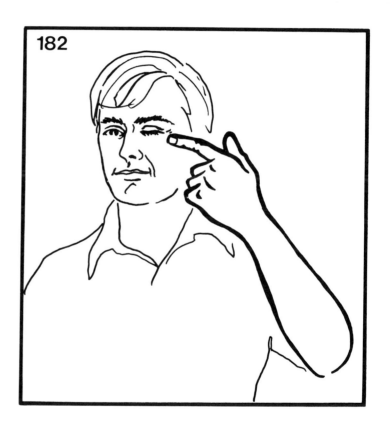

Left hand is raised, index pointing and other fingers curled, to corner of left eye. Then left eye is slowly winked.

183. **SHAKE**

(kinetic)

agitate
jiggle
quake
rattle
vibrate

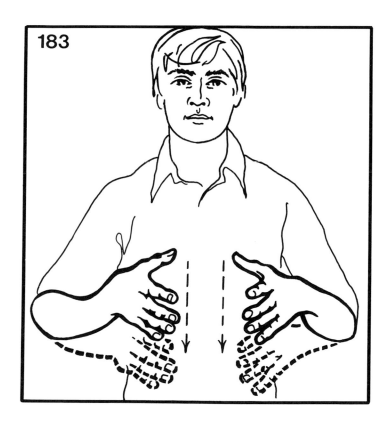

Hands are extended in front of body about one foot apart, palms facing. Fingers and thumbs are spread and curved slightly in a grasping gesture. They are then moved up and down synchronously three times. They may be moved to and from body if appropriate to shaking situation. (This signal is not used to mean that the signaler himself is shaking. The hand tremble of COLD is appropriate then.)

184. **SHAME**
(repetitive)

deride

disgrace

embarrass

ridicule

scorn

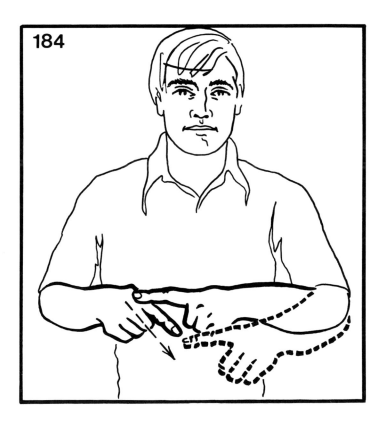

Right hand, placed in front of body, has index finger extended; others are folded. Left hand with index extended is placed at right index knuckle and then moved along index to tip and then off. Repeat three times. (This signal refers to another person's shame. For self, see ASHAMED.)

185. **SHAVE**
(kinetic)

barber

razor

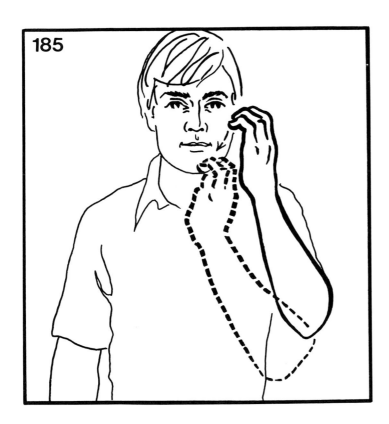

Left hand is placed on left cheek bone, palm facing face, fingers flexed forward. Hand is moved down face to chin, with nails lightly scraping face.

186. **SHELTER**
(static)

build

building

dwell

home

house

residence

roof

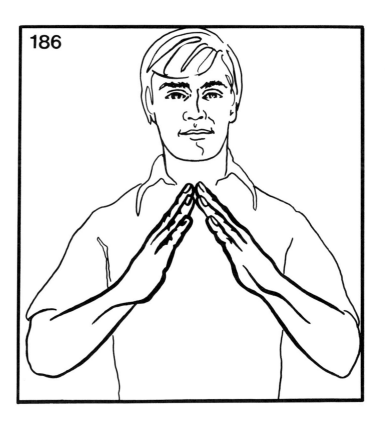

Hands are brought together, chest high, palms facing, tips of middle fingers touching. Wrists are about five inches apart, forming a gable roof line. (The signal can be executed with one hand by forming the gable at the finger-base knuckles or at the wrist. It can be clarified, if necessary, by placing it over the head.)

187. **SHOT**
(kinetic)

drug
injection
medicine

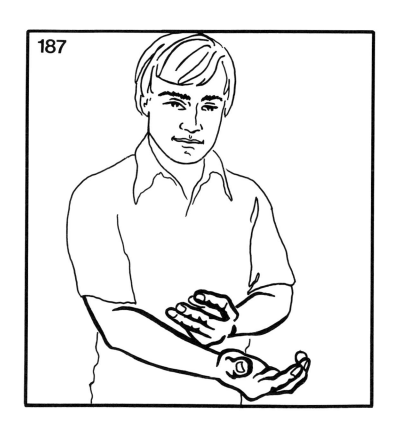

187

Right hand is extended forward, palm up. Left hand is placed near right elbow bend and makes short movement toward skin (as though inserting needle).

188. **SHUT**
(kinetic)

close

enclose

fasten

latch

secure

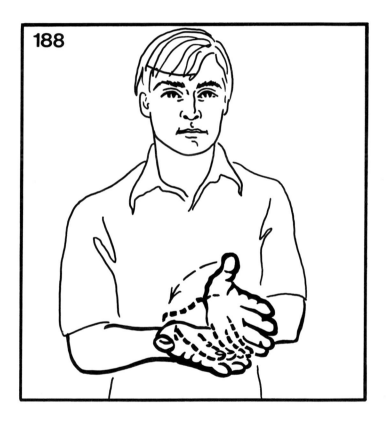

188

Right hand is extended in front of body, palm up. Left hand is placed against right with little fingers touching and left hand vertical (90 degree angle) hinged to right. Then left hand is lowered to meet right, palm to palm. (Compare other hinged signals: OPEN; READ; DOOR.)

189. **SIT**
(static)

chair
furniture
seat

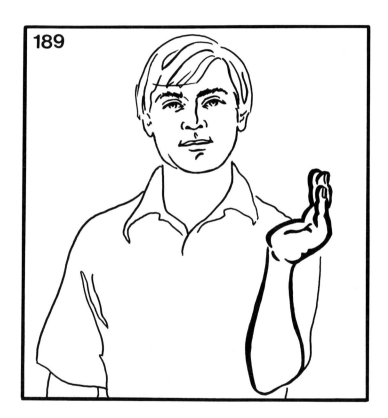

Left hand is elevated, elbow bent and wrist flexed, to put palm upward. Fingers are touching laterally and point upward. The hand forms a chair shape in profile to the viewer.

190. **SLEEP**

(static)

bed

doze

nap

repose

rest

sleepy

slumber

snooze

tired

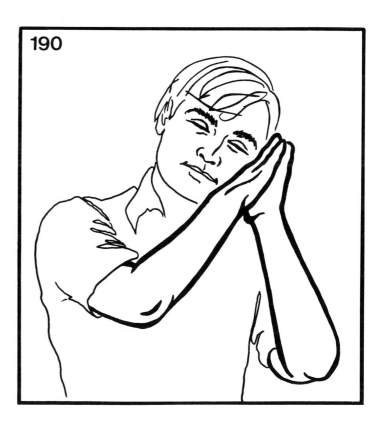

190

Hands are placed palm to palm at left of head, which is tilted left to rest on them. (Can also be executed with left hand only.)

191. **SMART**
(repetitive)

brainy
capable
clever
competent
intelligent
keen
knowledgeable
shrewd
witty

Left index finger is extended upward at left of head; other fingers are folded. Index taps left temple three times (3 brains). (Compare KNOW and BRAIN.)

192. **SMELL**
(static)

aroma

bouquet [smell]

fragrance

odor

perfume

reek

scent

sense

sniff

stench

stink

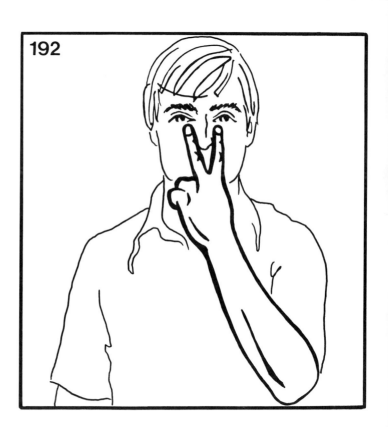

Left index and middle fingers are extended upward and separated; other fingers are folded. Hand is at chin level, palm toward face. Extended fingers lie on either side of nose.

193. **SMOKE**
(kinetic)

chimney
cigarette
fire
fire alarm
fire engine
fire department
fireman
fireplace
pipe
signal
tobacco

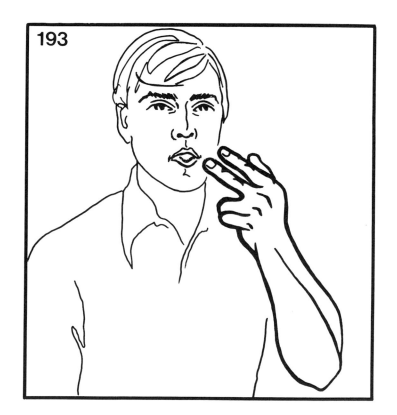

Left hand is raised toward left corner of mouth. Index and middle fingers are slightly parted. Lips make puffing movement for SMOKE (three times).

194. **SMOOTH**
(repetitive)

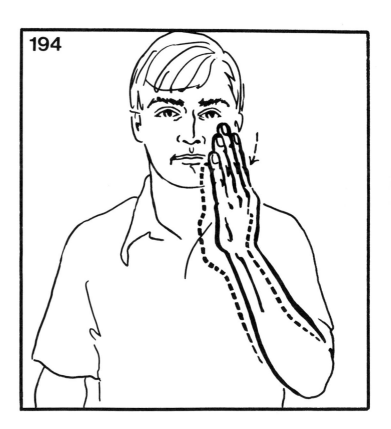

Left fingers stroke left cheek three times. (For clarification add BABY.)

195. **SNOW**
(kinetic)

winter
year

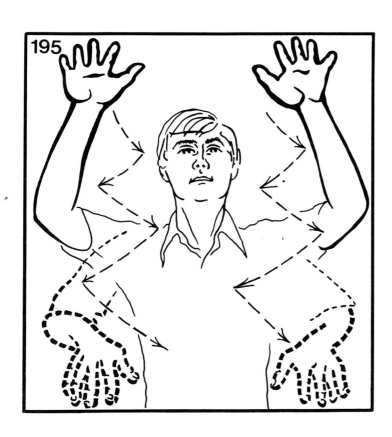

Hands are elevated above head height at left and right, palms forward, fingers spread. Hands are then moved downward synchronously in zig-zag pattern (right and left) with fingers fluttering.

196. **SOFT**
(repetitive)

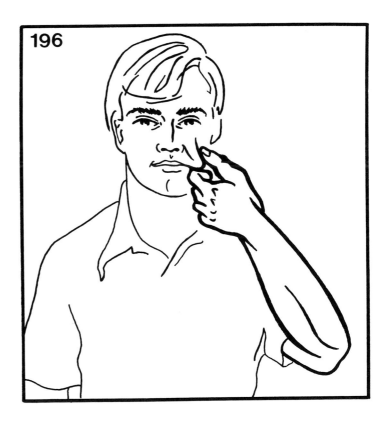

The left cheek is gently pinched between left thumb and index (three times). If clarification is needed, add SMOOTH. If second clarification is needed, contrast with HARD.

197. **SOUTH**

(static)

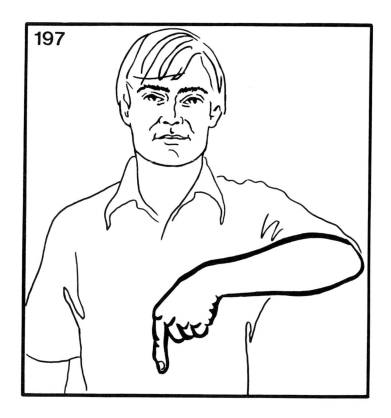

Left hand is placed at body vertical midline in front of chest, palm toward body, index finger pointing down; other fingers are folded. (Compare DOWN; HERE.)

198. **SPREAD**
(repetitive)

bread

butter

smear

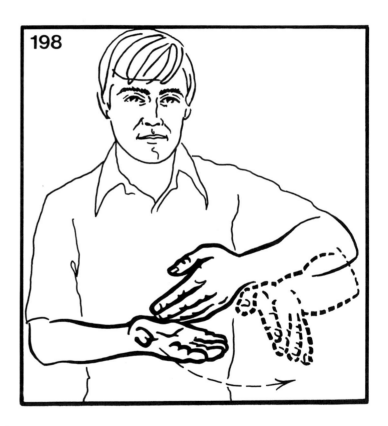

Flat right hand is extended, palm up, to center of body at about waist height. Left hand is placed above it, palm toward body. Left fingers stroke right palm from wrist to fingertips and reverse, then back to right fingertips (three in all).

199. **STAND**

(kinetic)

arise
awake
rise (out of bed)
stand up
wake

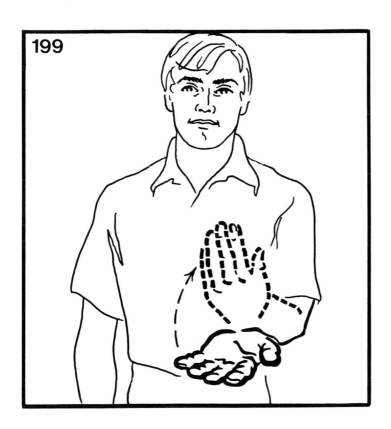

Flat left hand is extended forward, palm up, elbow bent. Wrist is flexed until fingers point upward. (May be used repetitively for emphasis or speed.) For clarification use SIT and then flatten hand upward and erect.

200. **STIR**

(kinetic)

blend

commotion

mix

spoon

sugar

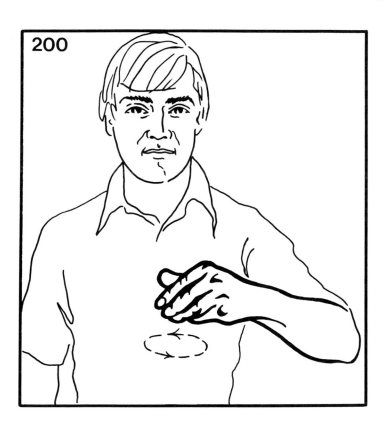

Left hand, palm down, is positioned in front of body. Finger knuckle-joints are flexed, thumb touching index; other fingers are all slightly flexed and touching (as though holding a spoon). Then hand is moved through a small horizontal circle (about three-inch diameter) three times.

201. **STOP**
(static)

block
brake
deter
determine
halt
policeman
prevent
prohibit
restrain
stall
stay

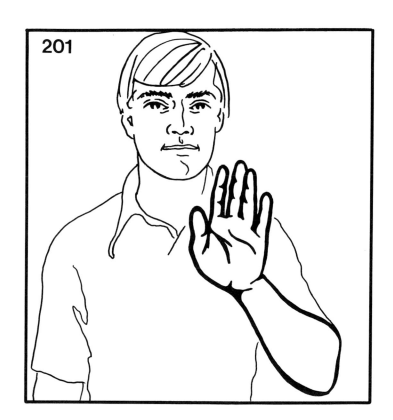

Left hand, palm forward, is extended forward at shoulder height. (Compare for differences HELLO, where the hand is held higher and closer to body.)

202. **STRAIGHT**
(kinetic)

accurate

direct

level

unbent

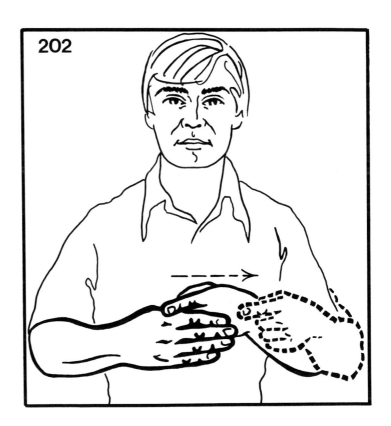

Right hand is placed in front of body, palm facing body. Fingers are straight, touching, and tips point left. Thumb is folded into palm (upper edge of index is now a straight line). Left index points to right index knuckle and then moves left along right index tracing the straight line, which is continued a little beyond the right index fingertip.

203. **SUN**
(static)

light
sunny
sunshine

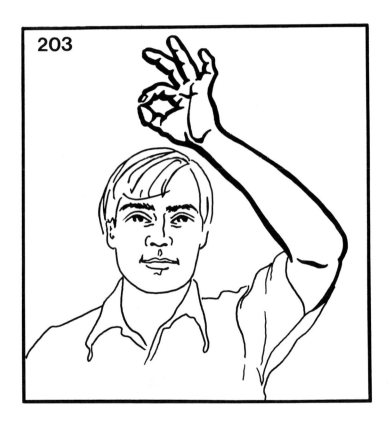

Left hand is held above head, index finger touching thumb to form circle (sun); other fingers are extended (rays). This signal (overhead) almost always means SUN, and occasionally "light." Compare DAY—different position; NOON—different position; OK—different position and kinetic rather than static.

204. **SURPRISE**
(kinetic)

amaze

astonish

astound

daze

dumfound

shock

startle

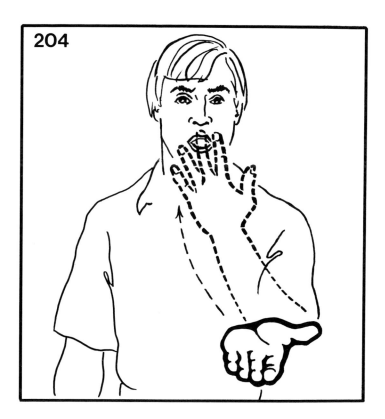

The mouth is rounded and open, then covered by left hand. Fingers are spread, palm toward signaler. Viewer must be able to see open mouth.

205. **SURRENDER**
(static)

capitulate

cede

relinquish

renounce

submit

vacate

yield

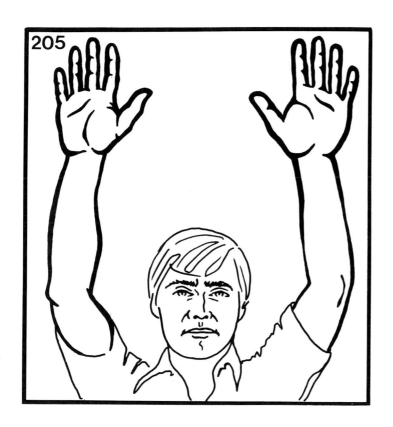

Both arms are elevated above head, at either side, palms forward. (Compare TEN—hands are lower and closer to each other.)

206. **SWIM**
(kinetic)

swimming

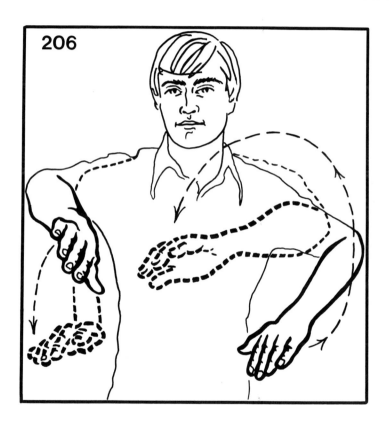

Left arm is elevated at left side of body, elbow at shoulder height, hand palm down. Right arm is extended forward at right, palm down. Left arm moves forward, right arm back, in a thrice-repeated alternation (replicating hand-arm movement of simple swimming stroke).

207. **TABLE**

(kinetic)

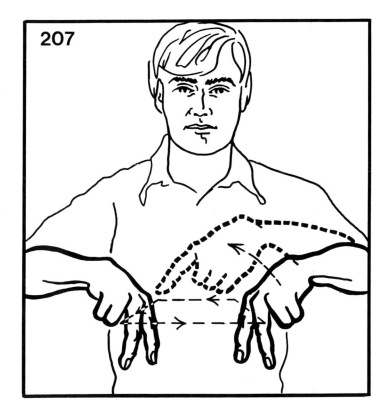

Right hand is extended before body. Right index and second finger (other fingers are folded) are pointed downward and separated (forming two legs). Index is closest to body. Left hand repeats above pattern to complete the four legs. Then left hand is withdrawn and left index traces square table top above the legs.

208. **TALK**
(kinetic)

communicate

conversation

discuss

lecture

say

sermon

speak

speech

tell

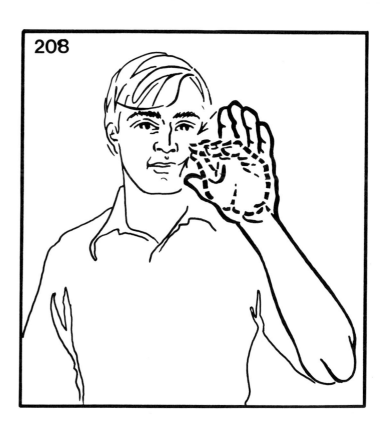

Left hand is placed at left corner of mouth, palm forward. Thumb is lowered (to represent lower lip). Fingers are flexed forward and joined (to represent upper lip). Thumb and joined finger unit are moved toward each other three times.

209. **TASTE**
(kinetic)

flavor
palate
sample

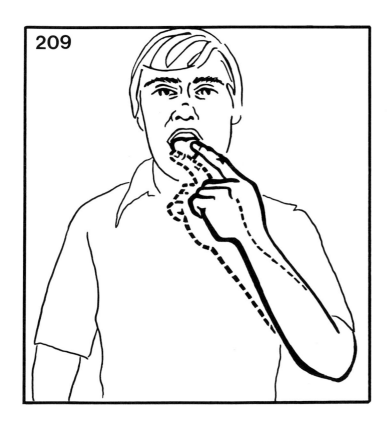

Mouth is slightly open, tongue tip forward. Left index touches tongue at left and moves across tip toward right.

210. **TEA**
(kinetic)

beverage
hospitality
social

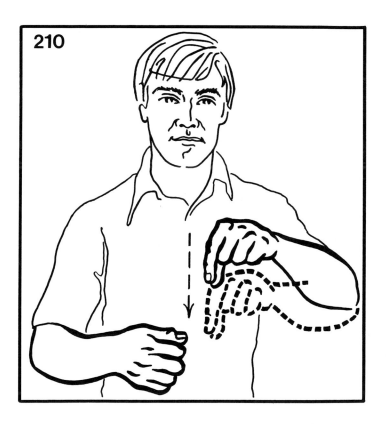

Right hand is held in front of body, palm toward body (holding cup). Left palm is down with index and thumb touching (other fingers are folded). Left hand moves in down-up sequence three times (dipping the tea bag). (Compare coffee—DRINK + HOT.)

211. **TELEPHONE**
(static)

call (phone)
communicate
message
phone

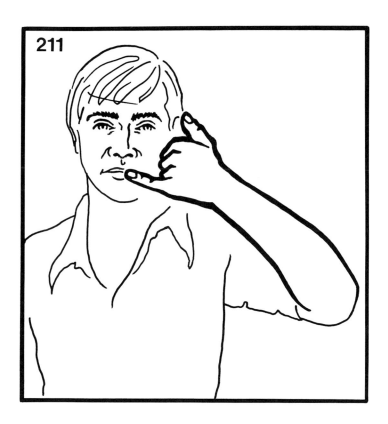

Right hand, loosely fisted, is held in front of mouth. Left hand, loosely fisted, is held at left ear. (Signal can be executed by one hand: Extend thumb and little finger, fold others. Place thumb near ear and little finger near mouth. This can be clarified, if necessary, by index finger dialing circle.)

212. THANKS
(kinetic)

appreciate
bless
grateful
gratitude
thank

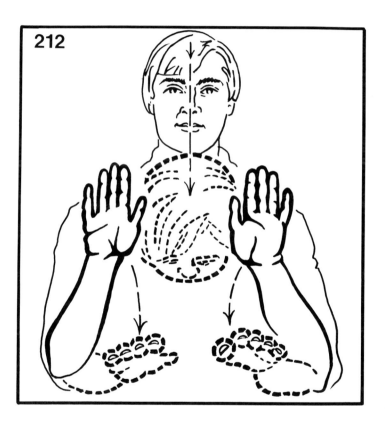

Forearms are elevated at sides of body, palms forward, fingers spread. They are then lowered forward to the horizontal plane, with head bowing simultaneously.

213. **THINK**
(static)

believe
choose
decide
deliberate
imagine
ponder
recall
recollect
reflect
remember
speculate

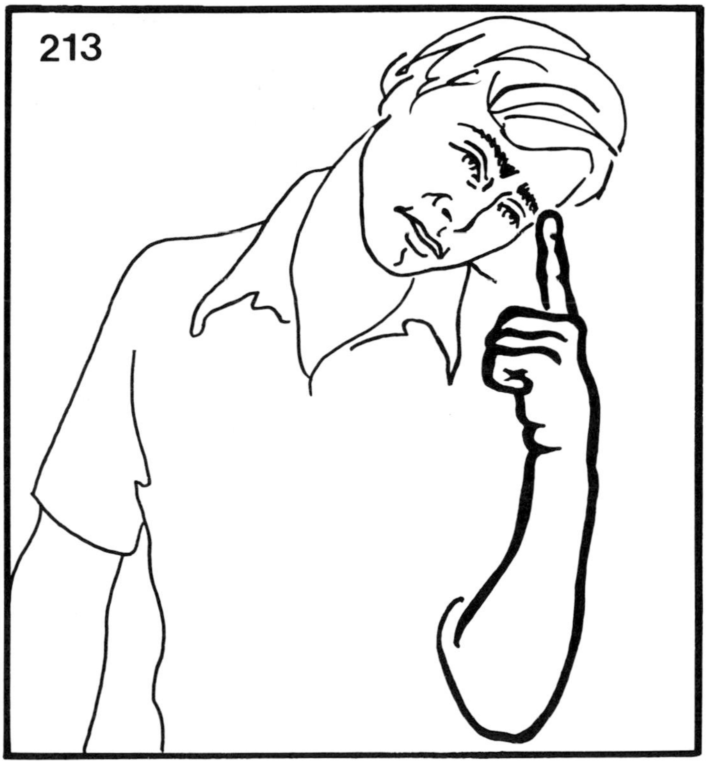

213

Left index finger touches left temple, with head tilted left, resting on finger. ("Brain is heavy with work of thinking." Compare BRAIN, KNOW, and SMART.)

214. **THREATEN**
(static)

alarm

forewarn

imperil

intimidate

menace

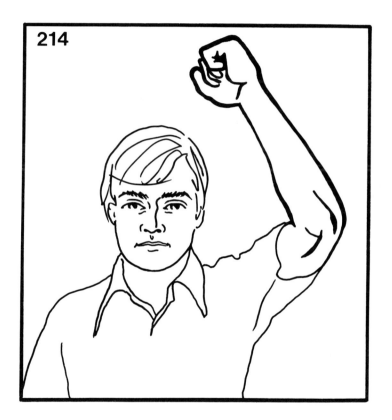

Left fist is elevated over left side of head.

215. **THROW**
(kinetic)

ball
baseball
game
play
projectile

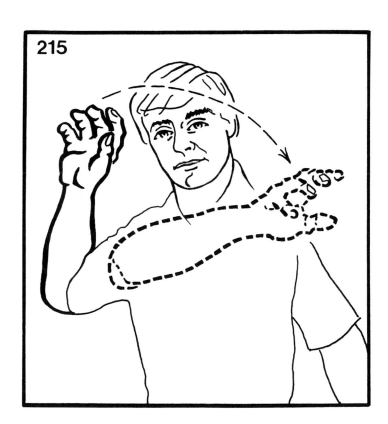

215

The active hand is cupped, as though holding a ball. Then the arm is elevated vertically, palm forward, to shoulder height. Arm is then moved forward with energetic thrust as though pitching a ball.

216. **TIME**
(static)

clock

hour

interval

period

watch

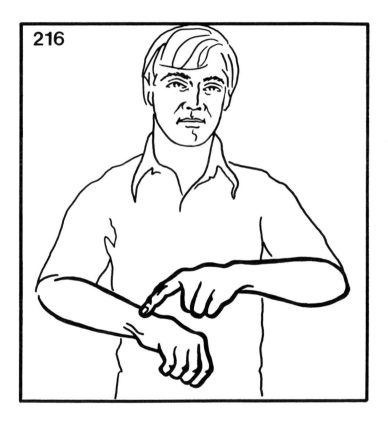

Right index points to left wrist; hands may be reversed. (The signal does not require a watch on the wrist.) The ancient signal was the angle of the arm as it moved from morning to evening, east to west. Now everyone wears the sun-time on the wrist.

217. **TOOTHBRUSH**

(repetitive)

toothpaste

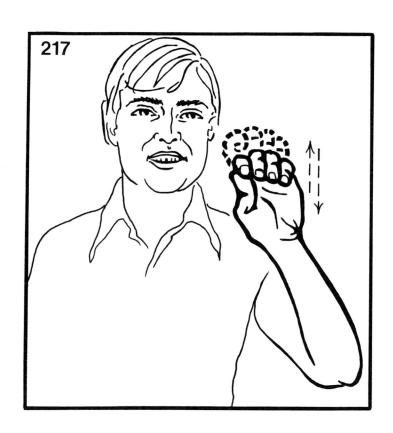

Left hand is raised mouth high at left side of mouth. Palm is forward, fingers curled (holding brush handle). Hand is moved briskly up and down three times. Teeth must be showing through retracted lips.

218. **TOP**
(static)

apex

crest

crown

lid

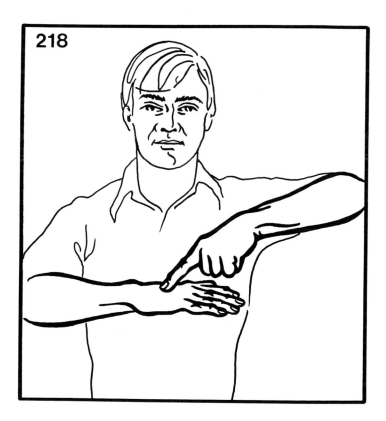

Flat right hand, palm down, is placed in front of body, with fingertips at left. Left index finger points to back (TOP) of right hand with index at 45 degree angle. (Note: The difference in angle is critical to specific meaning.)

219. **TOUCH**
(kinetic)

adjoin   contact   deftness   skill   style

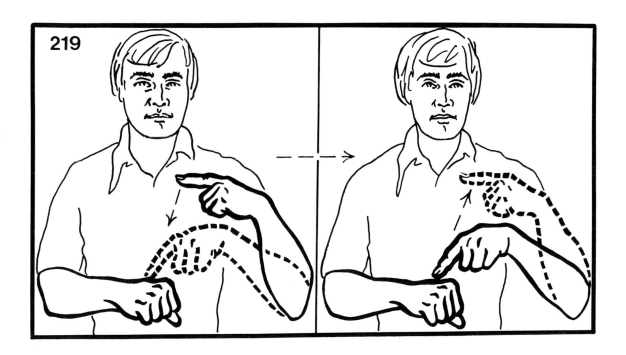

Right fist is extended in front of body, palm down. Left index is extended; other fingers are folded and are about six inches higher and to the left of right fist. Then left index finger lightly contacts surface of right fist and quickly withdraws upward.

220. **TOWEL**
(kinetic)

cloth   dry   wipe

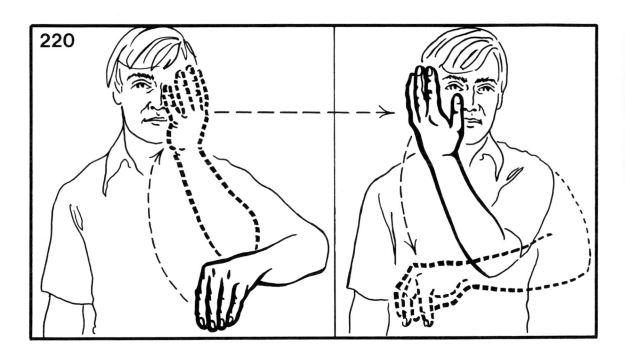

Left hand is extended forward, palm down. Fingertips and thumb tip are touching (as though picking up object). Then hand is lifted to left side of face and open palm pats three times. Hand then moves to right side of face and pats three times. Hand returns to original position where fingers are then opened to release object (towel).

221. **TREES**
(kinetic)

forest
grow
plant
woods

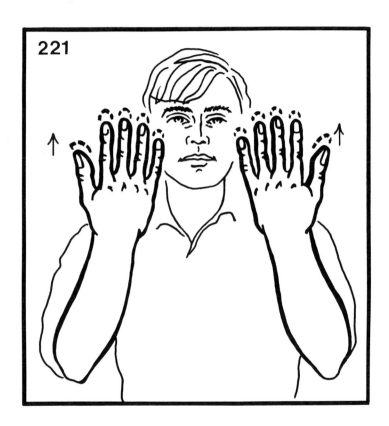

Hands are elevated beside face, palms toward signaler. Fingers are erect and spread. Hands are then slowly moved upward about half an inch (barely perceptible movement) to indicate growth.

222. **TURTLE**
(kinetic)

dependable

patient

persistent

reptile

shell

slow

sure

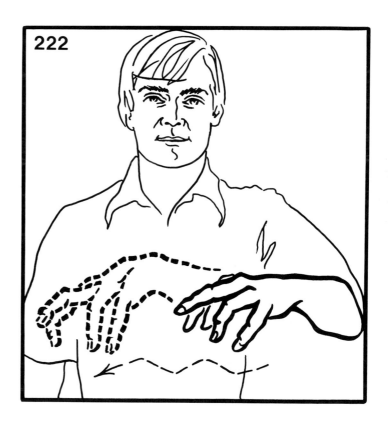

Left hand is placed in front of body, palm down. Fingers point right with middle finger extended. Thumb and other fingers are flexed. Hand is moved forward with a slight rocking movement. (The extended middle finger represents the head; the other four represent the legs.)

223. **TYPEWRITE**

(repetitive)

letter
machine
message
secretary
type
typewriter
typewritten

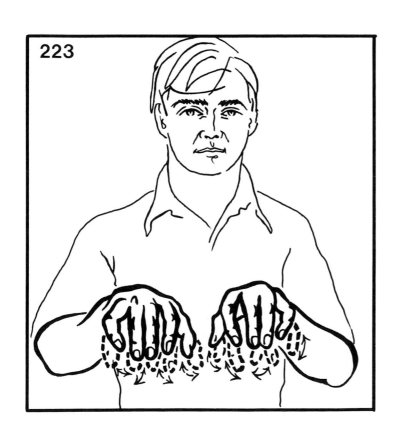

Both hands are extended before body and are about one inch apart. Palms are down and fingers flexed (positioned at typewriter). Then fingers move randomly. (Compare with PIANO, where arm movement is much broader.)

224. **UNDER**
(kinetic)

less

subordinate

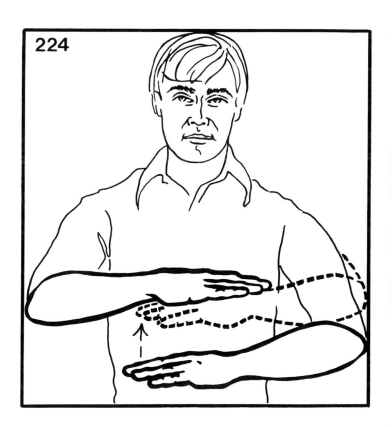

Right arm is extended in front of body, palm down, fingers extended toward left. Left hand, with palm down and fingers extended to right, is placed under right hand. Then left hand is raised until it contacts right palm. (Compare ON.)

225. **UNFOLD**
(kinetic)

disclose
explain
flower
reveal
unfurl

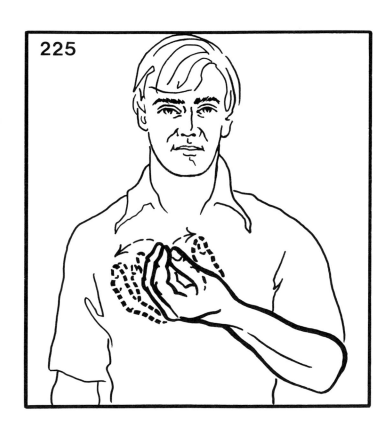

225

Left hand is extended at left side of body. Elbow is bent at right angle and close to body. Wrist is flexed downward; palm is facing upwards; fingertips are tightly bunched over thumb tip. Then very slowly fingers are unfolded until the hand forms a small bowl-like shape.

226. **UP**
(kinetic)

ascent

higher

upper

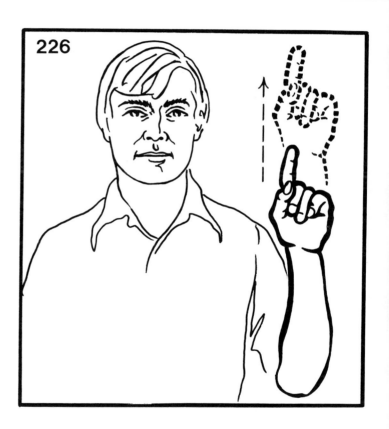

Left hand is elevated to shoulder height at left side of body. Palm faces forward with index pointing upward. Hand moves upward about one foot.

227. **WALK**
(kinetic)

go
hike
passage
path
promenade
road
run
saunter
sidewalk
stride
stroll
trail

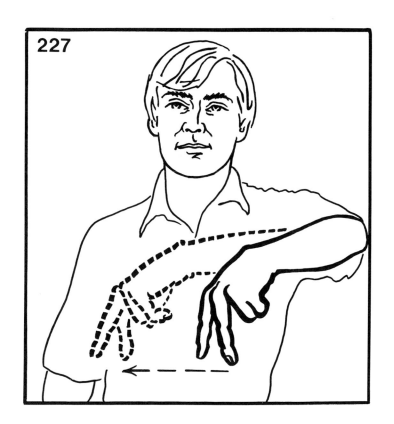

227

Left arm is extended in front of body with elbow at almost shoulder level. Hand's palm is down; index and middle finger are extended, pointing downward; others are folded. While the hand slowly advances toward right, the extended fingers alternately move forward (simulating action of legs in walking).

228. **WASH**

(kinetic)

bathe

clean

cleanse

launder

mop

rinse

scrub

shower

soak

soap

sponge

wet

wipe

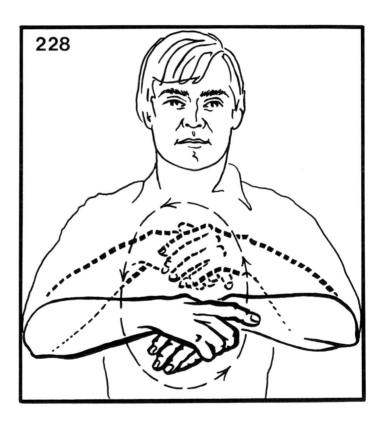

Both hands are placed in front of body, palms toward body. Right arm is resting on back of left hand. With a rotary motion, right hand slides forward and under left hand, which then slides forward and under right hand. Repeat three times.

229. **WATER**

(kinetic)

drink
flood
H$_2$O
lake
liquid
moisten
ocean
pond
pool
river
sea
sprinkle
stream
wet

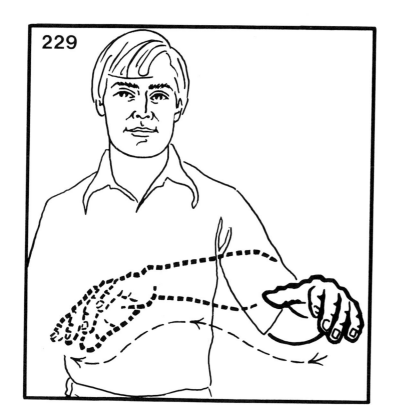

Left hand is extended forward at left side, palm down, fingers forward. Then it is moved across body three times in alternating upward and downward curves, tracing wave motion of water.

230. **WEST**

(static)

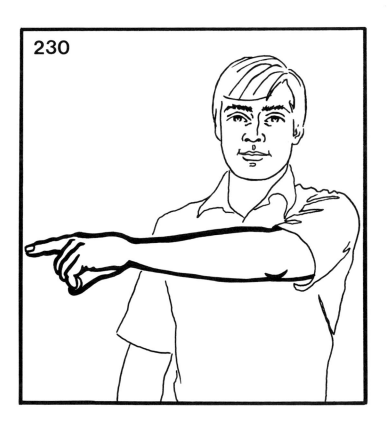

Left arm is extended across body, index finger pointing to the right; other fingers are folded, palm down. (Compare AFTERNOON.)

231. **WINDOW**
(kinetic)

clear	opening	transparent
obvious	see	window

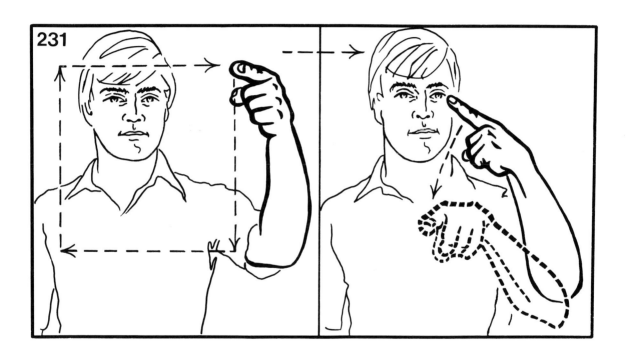

Left index (other fingers folded) traces large square before face. Left index then points to left corner of left eye, then points forward through window square.

232. **WOMAN**
(kinetic)

curved

female

feminine

form

girl

lady

maid

mistress

shape

shapely

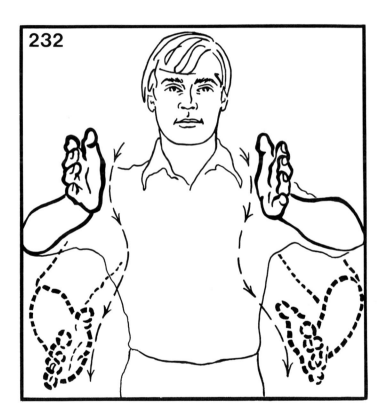

Hands are elevated to shoulder height, width of body apart. Palms are facing; fingers are extended and forward. Hands move in synchrony downward, tracing opposing curves: outward, inward, outward (female shape).

233. **WORK**

(kinetic)

chore	exertion	profession
do	job	task
effort	labor	toil
employment	make	trade [work]
energy	occupation	

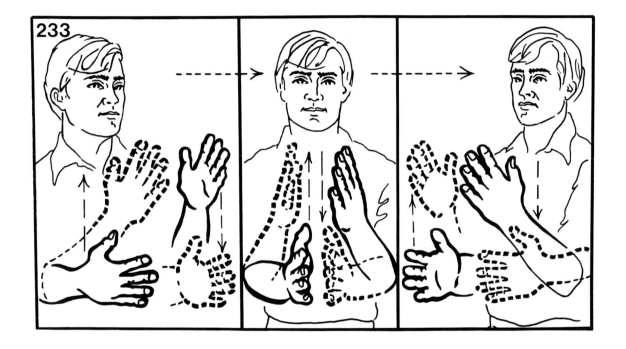

Hands are extended in front of body, palms facing, about six inches apart. Hands are alternately raised and lowered about six inches at left, at center, and at right. (Face should reflect effort. It clarifies signal if a forceful breath is exhaled after completion of sequence, emphasizing effort.)

234. **WRAP**

(kinetic)

bind
bundle
enclose
package
tie
wind [string]

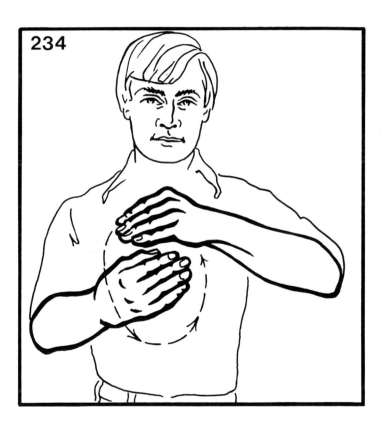

Right hand is placed at body center, chest high, palm toward body. Left hand, thumb tip touching bunched fingertips, circles right hand vertically, and then pulls down to left.

235. **WRITE**

(kinetic)

compose
copy
draft [written]
inscribe
letter
pen
pencil
signature
transcribe

Left hand is extended forward, palm down, index and thumb touching (as though holding a pencil). Hand moves from left to right on a slanted direction toward body in three jerky movements (as though writing).

236. **YOU**
(static)

yourself

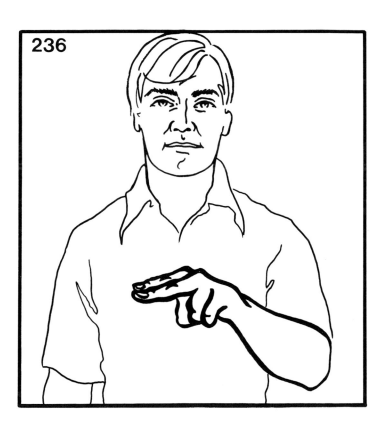

236

Left index and middle finger are extended forward, together; other fingers are folded. (Double fingers point at the person indicated. Single finger (index only) is generally used to indicate animals or things, not humans. Index alone can only be used for humans in the formal gesture for PERSON. Note: YOU + ALL = "you" (plural form); YOU + ME + ALL = "we."

Arithmetic Illustrations

148. **ZERO**

nothing

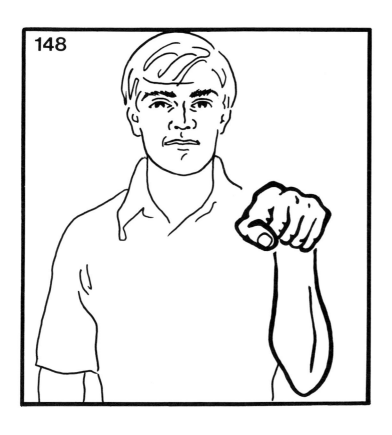

149. **NUMBERS**

[Arithmetic]

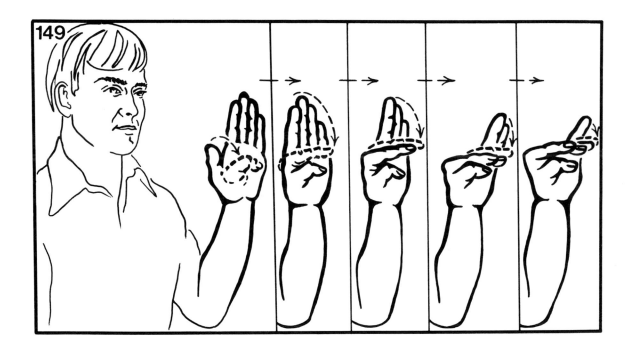

149-A. **ONE**

1

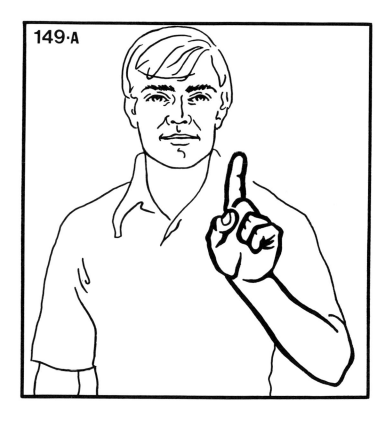

149-B. **TWO**

2

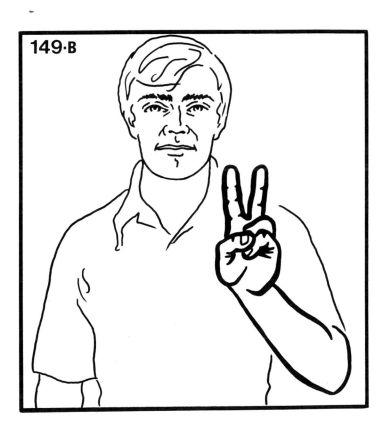

149-C. **THREE**

3

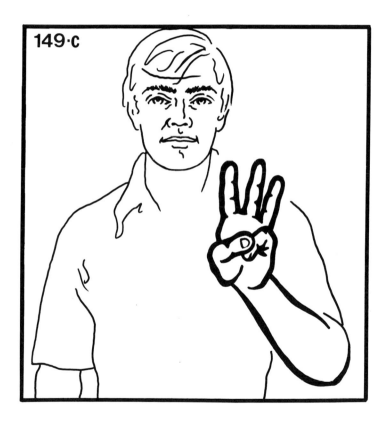

149-D. **FOUR**

4

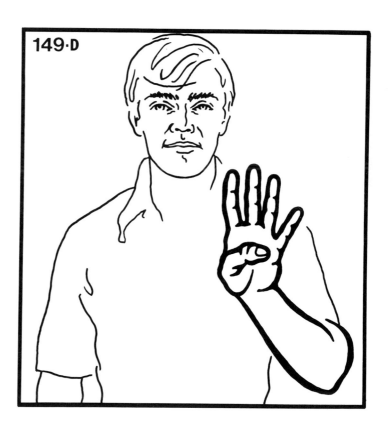

149-E. **FIVE**

5

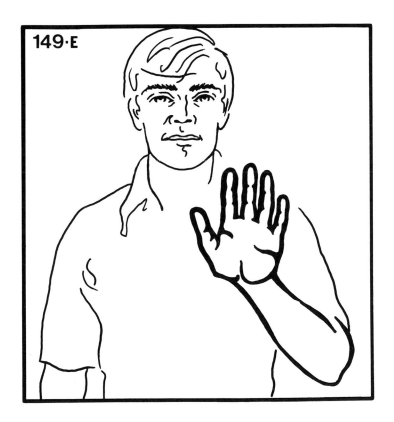

149-F. **SIX**

6

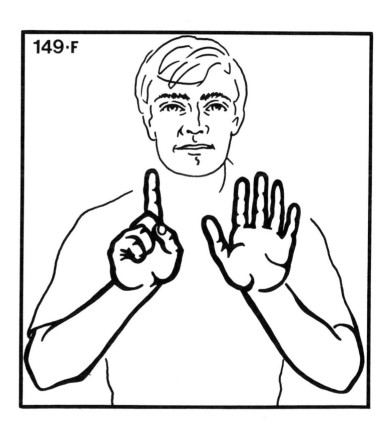

149-G. **SEVEN**

7

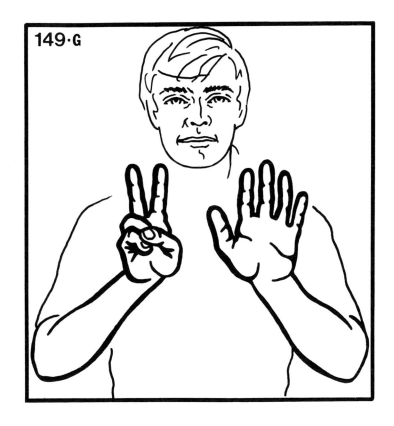

149-H. **EIGHT**

8

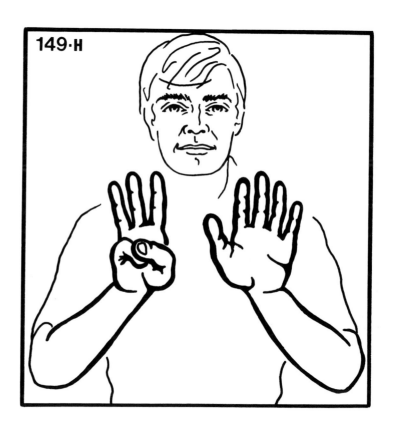

149-I. **NINE**

9

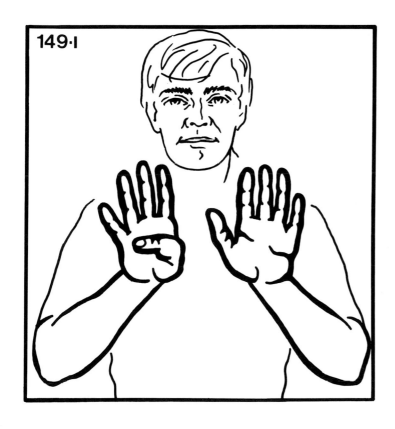

149·I

149-J. **TEN**

10

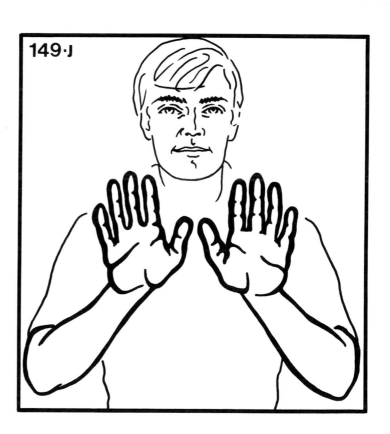

149-E + 238 + 149-E. **TEN**

(one-hand signal)

10

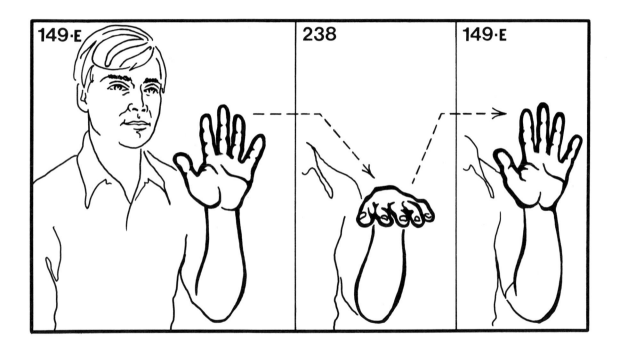

This panel, with the wrist flex, shows TEN performed with one hand only.

149-J + 238 + 149-A. **ELEVEN**

11

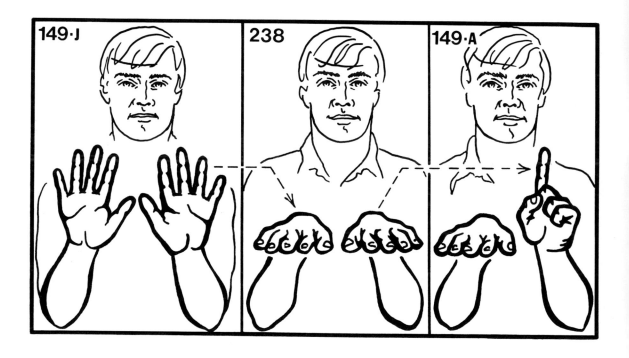

After an initial number has been executed, the wrist is flexed with hand dropped forward (238). Then a second number is executed. The wrist drop means the two numbers are to be added. Panel above shows the SUM ELEVEN (11) executed with two hands.

149-B + 139 + 149-J. **TWENTY**

20

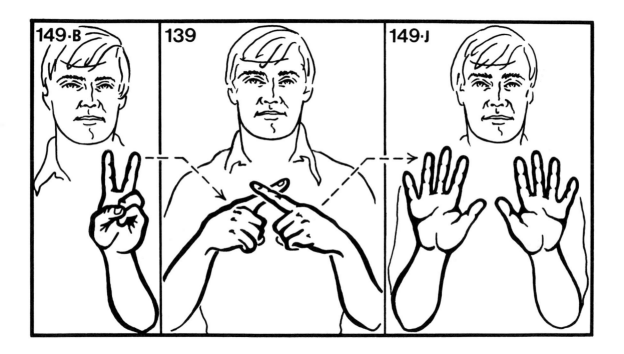

Panel shows TWENTY executed with two hands.

149-B + 237 + 148. **TWENTY**
(one-hand signal)

20

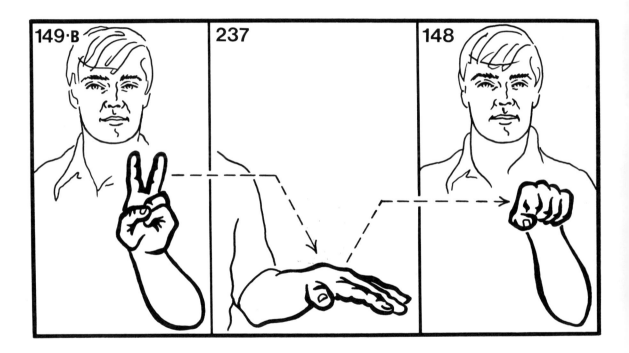

After an initial figure, if the elbow is flexed to drop the forearm, the signal (237) shifts the number to left column. The next executed number then occupies the right column. The panel shows TWENTY executed thus with only one hand. An additional (237) followed by ZERO would convey the number 200.

149-E + 237 + 149-E. **FIFTY-FIVE**

55

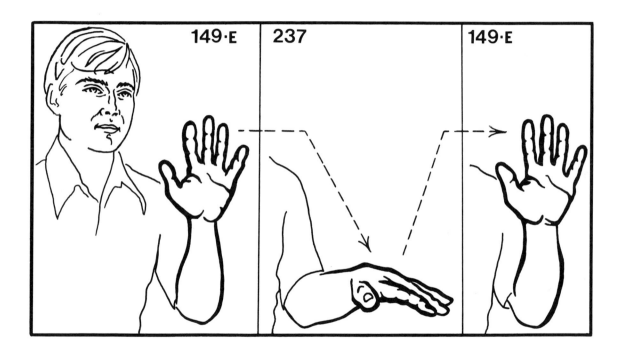

This panel, with the elbow flex, shows FIFTY-FIVE executed with one hand.

65 + 149 + 149.   **FRACTION**

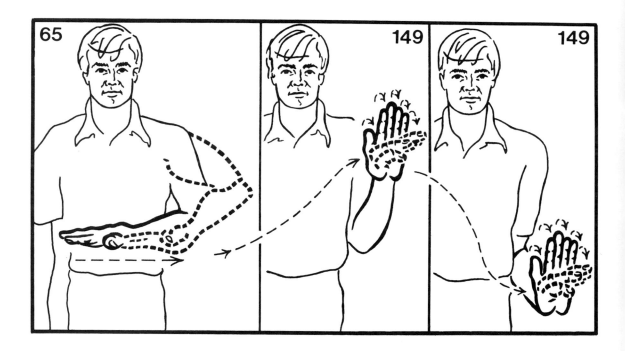

This panel shows the execution of concept FRACTION as a generalization, as opposed to a specific fraction. FRACTION is conveyed by using DIVIDE (65), then NUMBERS (149) held high, then NUMBERS (149) held lower.

65 + 149-A + 149-B. **ONE-HALF**

½

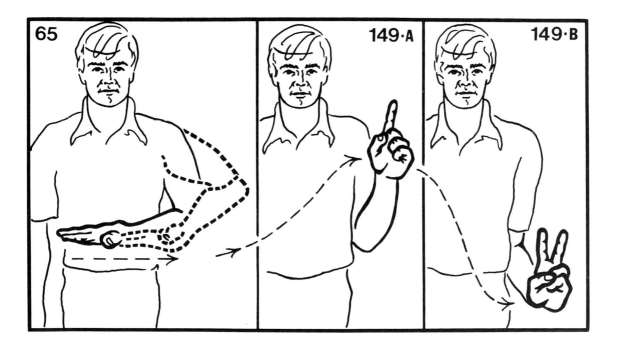

This panel shows the execution of concept ONE-HALF as a fraction, using DIVIDE (65), the ONE (149-A) held high, and TWO (149-B) held lower.

4. **ADD**

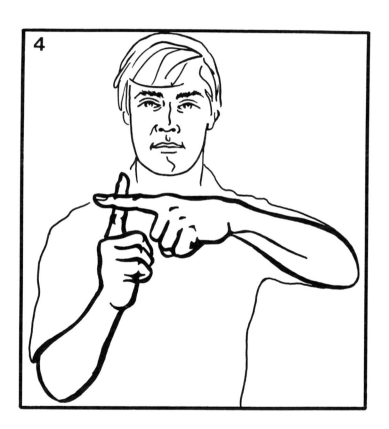

After an initial figure, if the elbow is flexed to drop the forearm, the signal (237) shifts the number to left column. The next executed number then occupies the right column. The panel shows TWENTY executed thus with only one hand. An additional (237) followed by ZERO would convey the number 200.

175. **REJECT**

subtract

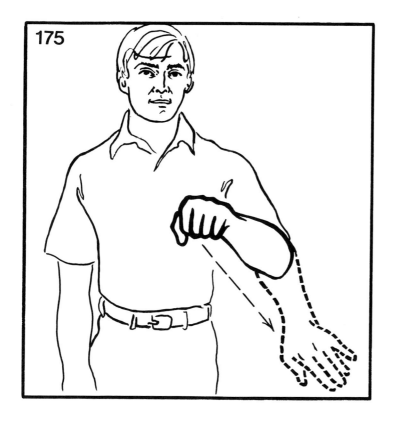

139. **MULTIPLY**

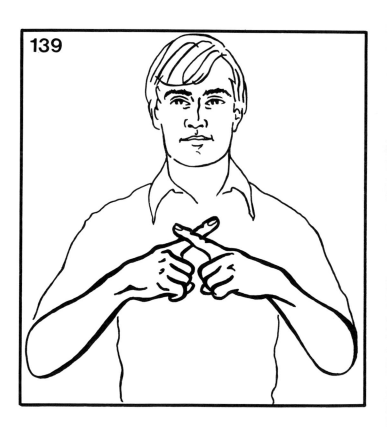

65. **DIVIDE**

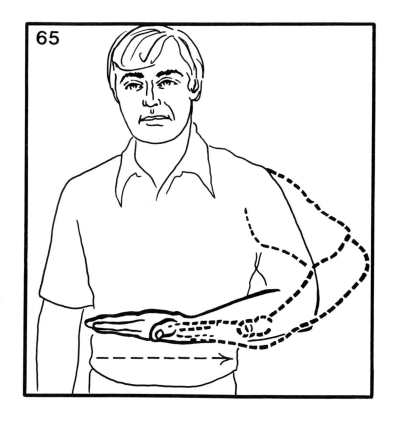

9. ALIKE

equal
same
sum

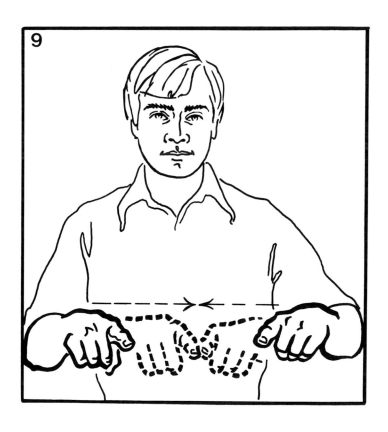

10. **ALL**

total

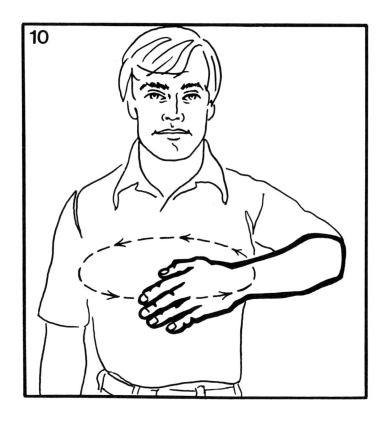

149-E + 238 + 149-E + 238 + 149-A. ELEVEN

11

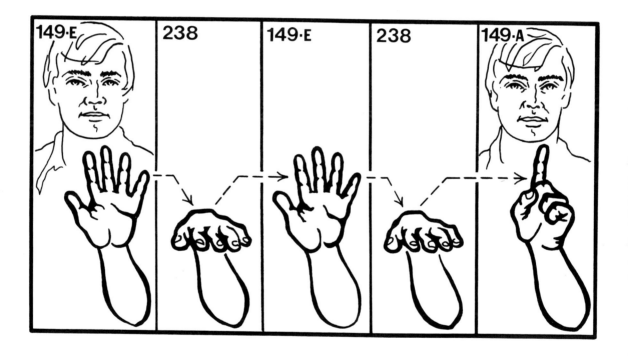

The panel shows ELEVEN with one hand, contrasting result (11) with wrist drop and result (551) with elbow drop.

Suggestions for Agglutinations

Ambulance	DRIVE + PAIN + SHELTER + FAST
Apology	BLAME + ME + ERASE + PLEASE
Bank	SHELTER + MONEY + LOCK
Bath	WASH + ME + ALL
Bitter	TASTE + REJECT
Blood	WATER + COLOR + POINT (lips)
Blue	COLOR + POINT (sky)
Bonfire	FIRE + BIG + ROUND
Bookmobile	SHELTER + READ + DRIVE + BIG
Boy	MAN + LITTLE
Bread	SPREAD + EAT
Breakfast	EAT + MORNING
Brief	TIME + LITTLE
Brown	COLOR + EARTH
Bus	DRIVE + BIG + MANY + MONEY
Buy	(1) EXCHANGE + MONEY
	(2) GIVE + MONEY + GET + OBJECT
Capable	MAN + WORK + OK
Cat	ANIMAL + MUSTACHE
Check	MONEY + WRITE
Church	SHELTER + PRAY
City	SHELTER + MANY
Closet	BOX + BIG + DOOR
Coffee	DRINK + HOT

Contact-lens	GLASSES + IN + LOOK (eye)
Cool	COLD + LITTLE
Cross	HEART + ANGRY
Cupboard	BOX + BIG + DOOR
Dentures	POINT (teeth) + OBJECT
Diet	EAT + FENCE
Dinner	EAT + AFTERNOON (evening)
	EAT + NOON + BIG
Earn	WORK + GET + MONEY
Egg	CHICKEN + GIVE + OBJECT
Everybody	ALL + PERSON
Everyplace	ALL + PLACE (here)
Everything	ALL + OBJECT
Father	(1) MAN + PROTECT + BABY
	(2) MAN + ADD + BABY
Fall	TIME + COLD + LITTLE
Feast	EAT + GOOD + BIG
Flash	FIRE + LITTLE + FAST
Flashlight	SUN + LITTLE + HOLD + HAND
Float	WALK + WATER
Flower	GRASS + UNFOLD + COLOR
Forget	ERASE + BRAIN
Forgive	BLAME + ME + ERASE + PLEASE
Garage	SHELTER + DRIVE
Generous	HEART + BIG
Girl	WOMAN + LITTLE
Green	COLOR + GRASS
Grocery	SHELTER + EAT + MONEY
Half	DIVIDE + ALIKE
Headache	PAIN + POINT (head)
Hi-Fi	MUSIC + ROUND
Hill	EARTH + HIGH
Home	SHELTER + ME
Hospital	SHELTER + PAIN
How	QUESTION + WORK
Hurry	(1) COME + FAST
	(2) WALK + FAST
	(3) DRIVE + FAST
Husband	MAN + RING
Ice	WATER + HARD + COLD
Impatient	HEART + ANGRY
Inherit	PERSON + DIE + GIVE
Insane	(1) BRAIN + REJECT
	(2) BRAIN + FLY + DISTANT
Interest	GET + MONEY + NO + WORK
Judge	PERSON + GIVE + JUSTICE
Kind	HEART + GOOD
Kleenex	NAPKIN + POINT (nose)
Lake	WATER + ROUND + BIG
Lamp	SUN + LITTLE + IN + SHELTER
Lawyer	PERSON + TALK + JUSTICE
Library	SHELTER + READ
Lunch	EAT + NOON

Mankind	(1) MAN + WOMAN + ALL
	(2) PERSON + ALL
Market	SHELTER + EAT + MONEY
Method	QUESTION + WORK
Microscope	GLASSES + WORK + BIG
Mother	WOMAN + BABY
Mouth Wash	WASH + POINT (mouth)
Neither	ONE + NO + TWO + NO
Never	TIME + NO + FUTURE
Newspaper	READ + BIG (wide)
Night	SLEEP + TIME
Now	HERE + TIME
Nurse	WOMAN + MEDICINE
Old	WALK + 3 + POINT (legs)
Orange	COLOR + SUN + POINT (lips)
Part	DIVIDE + NO + ALIKE
Party	ALL + PERSON + EAT + DANCE
Pasture	EARTH + GRASS + ANIMAL + EAT
Pepper(y)	EAT + HOT + ON + POINT (tongue)
Pillow	SLEEP + HEAD + OBJECT
Pink	COLOR + POINT (lips) + LITTLE
Power	(1) MAN + POINT (biceps)
	(2) MAN + POINT (biceps) + PUSH
Present (now)	HERE + TIME
Publisher	PERSON + WORK + READ + OBJECT
Purple	COLOR + POINT (lips) + POINT (sky)
Race (Auto)	(1) DRIVE + MANY + FAST
	(2) RIDE + MANY + FAST
Radio	MUSIC + TALK + HEAR
Record Player	MUSIC + ROUND
Red	COLOR + POINT (lips)
Refrigerator	BOX + COLD + EAT
Restaurant	SHELTER + EAT + MONEY + SIT
Road	OBJECT + DRIVE + ON
Room	SHELTER + DIVIDE (part)
Seek	LOOK + POINT (three places)
School	(1) SHELTER + READ + WRITE
	(2) SHELTER + LEARN
Shoe	OBJECT + POINT (foot) + IN
Shop	SHELTER + OBJECT + EXCHANGE + MONEY
Sing	MUSIC + TALK
Song	MUSIC + TALK + OBJECT
Sour	TASTE + NO
Spouse	PERSON + RING
Spring	TIME + HOT + LITTLE
Store	SHELTER + OBJECT + EXCHANGE + MONEY
Strong	MAN + POINT (biceps)
Stupid	BRAIN + WORK + LITTLE
Summer	TIME + HOT
Supper	EAT + AFTERNOON (evening) + LITTLE
Sweet	TASTE + OK
Taxi	DRIVE + MONEY
Teacher	PERSON + GIVES + KNOWLEDGE (know)

Telescope	GLASSES + LOOK + DISTANT
Television	BOX + LOOK + HEAR
Toilet	WATER + SIT (chair)
Tomorrow	DAY + FUTURE
Trouble	NOTHING + OK
Truck	DRIVE + BIG + OBJECT
Unhappy	CRY + HEART
Vegetable	GRASS + MAN + EAT
Warm	HOT + LITTLE
We	YOU + ME + ALL
Week	TIME + SEVEN + DAY
What	QUESTION + OBJECT
Wheel	ROUND (vertical) + WALK
When	QUESTION + TIME
Where	QUESTION + HERE (place)
Which	QUESTION + BETWEEN + 2
Who	QUESTION + PERSON
Why	QUESTION + THINK
Wife	WOMAN + RING
Winter	(1) TIME + COLD
	(2) TIME + SNOW
Year	ALL + MONTH
Yellow	COLOR + SUN
Yesterday	DAY + PAST

Clinical Signal Index

References

Brain W.R. (1964). *Clinical Neurology.* London: Oxford University Press.

Brown, J.W. (1968). A model for control of peripheral behavior in aphasia. Paper presented to the Academy of Aphasia, Rochester, MN.

Clark, W.P. (1885). *Indian Sign Languages.* Philadelphia: L.R. Hammersley & Co.

DeReuck, A.V.S., and O'Connor, M., eds. (1964). *Disorders of Language.* Boston: Little, Brown.

Donaldson, R.C., Skelly, M., and Paletta, F.X. (1968). Total glossectomy for cancer. *American Journal of Surgery* 116:585–590.

Duncan, J.L., and Silverman, F.H. (1977). Impacts of learning American Indian Sign on mentally retarded children. *Perceptual and Motor Skills* 4:1138.

Farb, P. (1968). *Man's Rise to Civilization as Shown by the Indians of North America.* New York: E.P. Dutton.

Goodglass, H., and Kaplan, E. (1972). *The Assessment of Aphasia and Related Disorders.* Philadelphia: Lea and Febiger.

Hadley, L.F. (1893). *Indian Sign Talk.* Chicago: Baker.

Hodge, F.W., ed. (1960). *Handbook of American Indians North of Mexico* (Part 2, Bulletin 30). Washington, DC: Bureau of Ethnology, Smithsonian Institution, pp. 567–568.

Keenan, J.S., and Brassell, E.G. (1975). *Aphasia Language Performance Scale.* Murfreesboro, Tenn.: VA Hospital.

Knapp, M.L. (1972). *Non-verbal Communication in Human Interaction.* New York: Holt, Rinehart and Winston.

Leiter, R.G. (1952). *International Performance Scale.* Los Angeles: Western Psychological Service.

Mallery, G. (1881). Sign language among North American Indians compared with that among other peoples and deaf mutes. In *First Annual Report of the Bureau of Ethnology to the Secretary of the Smithsonian Institution, 1879–1880.* Washington, DC Government Printing Office, pp. 263–552.

Nielson, J.M. (1962). *Agnosia, Apraxia, Aphasia.* New York: Hafner.

Perkins, W.H. (1971). *Speech Pathology.* St. Louis: C.V. Mosby.

Porch, B. (1971). *Porch Index of Communicative Ability.* Palo Alto: Consulting Psychologists.

Sanders, J.I., ed. (1968). *The ABC's of Sign Language.* Tulsa: Manca Press.

Sapir, E. (1929). *Selected Writings in Language, Culture and Personality.* Berkeley: University of California Press.

Silverman, F.H. (1977). *Research Design in Audiology and Speech Pathology.* Englewood Cliffs: Prentice-Hall.

Skelly, M., and Donaldson, R.C. (1972). Glossectomee speech rehabilitation procedures. In *Proceedings of XV International Congress of Logopedics and Phoniatrics.* Buenos Aires: Ares, pp. 249–256.

Skelly, M., and Donaldson, R.C. (1972). Glossectomee speech rehabilitation procedures. In *Proceedings of XV International Congress of Logopedics and Phoniatrics.* Buenas Aires: Ares, pp. 249–256.

Skelly, M., Donaldson, R.C., and Fust, R. (1972). Changes in phonatory aspects of glossectomee intelligibility through vocal parameter manipulation. *Journal of Speech and Hearing Disorders* 37:379–389.

Skelly, M., and Donaldson, R.C. (1972). Rehabilitation of speech after total glossectomy. In *Proceedings of World Congress of Rehabilitation.* Sydney, Australia.

Skelly, M., Donaldson, R.C. and Schinsky, L. (1972). Substitution consistency as a factor in glossectomee intelligibility. *Journal of the Missouri Speech and Hearing Association* 5:21–23.

Skelly, M., Schinsky, L., Donaldson, R.C., and Smith, R.W. (1972). Amer-Ind Sign: Gestural communication for the speechless. Paper and videotape exhibit presented at the Annual Convention of the American Speech and Hearing Association, San Francisco, 1972.

Skelly, M., Donaldson, R.C., and Fust, R. (1973). *Glossectomee Speech Rehabilitation.* Springfield, Ill.: Charles C. Thomas.

Skelly, M., Schinsky, L., Smith, R.W., and Fust, R.S. (1974). American Indian Sign (Amer-Ind) as a facilitator of verbalization for the oral verbal apraxic. *Journal of Speech and Hearing Disorders* 39:446–456.

Skelly, M. (1975) Aphasic patients talk back. *American Journal of Nursing* 75:1140–1142.

Skelly, M., Schinsky, L., Smith, R.W., Donaldson, R.C., and Griffin, J.M. (1975). American Indian Sign: A gestural communication system for the speechless. *Archives of Physical Medicine and Rehabilitation* 56:156–160.

Sklar, M. (1973). *Sklar Aphasia Scale.* Los Angeles: Western Psychological Service.

Tompkins, W. (1926, 1931). *Universal Sign Language.* San Diego: Published by the author.

Wechsler, I. (1958). *Clinical Neurology.* Philadelphia: W.B. Saunders.

Supplemental Bibliography

Asimov, I. (1963) *The Human Brain.* Boston: Houghton-Mifflin.

Cherry, C. (1957). *On Human Communication.* Cambridge, MA: MIT Press.

Darley, F.L., Aronson, A.F., and Brown, J.R. (1875). *Motor Disorders of Speech.* Philadelphia: W.B. Saunders.

Eisenson, J. (1973). *Adult Aphasia.* New York: Appleton-Century-Crofts.

Lesser, R. (1978). *Linguistic Investigations of Aphasia.* London: Edward Arnold.

Luria, A.R. (1963). *Restoration of Function After Brain Injury.* New York: Macmillan.

Schiefelbusch, R.L., and Lloyd, L.L., eds. (1974). *Language Perspectives—Acquisition, Retardation and Intervention.* Baltimore: University Park Press.

McLean, J.E., Yoder, D.E., and Schiefelbusch, R.L. (1972). *Language Intervention with the Retarded.* Baltimore: University Park Press.

Sagan, C. (1977). *The Dragons of Eden—Speculations on the Evolution of Human Intelligence.* New York: Random House.

Simeons, A.T.W. (1962). *Man's Presumptuous Brain.* New York: E.P. Dutton.

Smith, A.G., ed. (1966). *Communication and Culture.* New York: Holt, Rinehart and Winston.

Wooldridge, D.E. (1963). *The Machinery of the Brain.* New York: McGraw-Hill.

Williams, F. (1968). *Reasoning with Statistics.* New York: Holt, Rinehart and Winston.

Kaplan, A. (1964). *The Conduct of Inquiry.* San Francisco: Chandler.

Siegal, S. (1956). *Nonparametric Statistics for the Behavioral Sciences.* New York: McGraw-Hill.

Index

Madge Skelly, Ph.D., is Professor of Communication Disorders at St. Louis University, and Professor of Community Medicine at the St. Louis University School of Medicine. She also serves as Consultant in Communication to the Missouri State Department of Mental Health and to the Veterans Administration Medical Centers. She was formerly Chief of the Audiology and Speech Pathology Service at the St. Louis VA Hospital. Dr. Skelly is an ASHA fellow and a Missouri Licensee in Audiology and Speech Pathology. She is the author of *Glossectomee Speech Rehabilitation* (Springfield, IL: Charles C. Thomas, 1973). In 1974 she was awarded the Federal Medal for her contributions in the field of communication disorders. Part American Indian, Dr. Skelly was taught Hand Talk as a child by her Iroquois relatives.

Lorraine Schinsky, M.A., is a Speech Pathologist at the VA Hospital in St. Louis and the author of numerous journal articles in speech pathology.

John Dunivent, B.F.A., M.A., is a painter and designer whose work has been displayed at several museums. His designs have been used for a number of stage productions in both opera and theatre.